MODERN GREEN CHEMISTRY AND HETEROCYCLIC COMPOUNDS

Molecular Design, Synthesis, and Biological Evaluation

Innovations in Physical Chemistry: Monograph Series

MODERN GREEN CHEMISTRY AND HETEROCYCLIC COMPOUNDS

Molecular Design, Synthesis, and Biological Evaluation

Edited by
Ravindra S. Shinde, PhD
A. K. Haghi, PhD

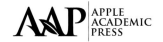

APPLE ACADEMIC PRESS

Apple Academic Press Inc.
4164 Lakeshore Road
Burlington ON L7L 1A4, Canada

Apple Academic Press, Inc.
1265 Goldenrod Circle NE
Palm Bay, Florida 32905, USA

© 2020 by Apple Academic Press, Inc.

First issued in paperback 2021

Exclusive worldwide distribution by CRC Press, a member of Taylor & Francis Group

No claim to original U.S. Government works

ISBN 13: 978-1-77463-520-9 (pbk)
ISBN 13: 978-1-77188-832-5 (hbk)

Library and Archives Canada Cataloguing in Publication

Title: Modern green chemistry and heterocyclic compounds : molecular design, synthesis, and
  biological evaluation / edited by Ravindra S. Shinde, PhD, A.K. Haghi, PhD.
Names: Shinde, Ravindra S., 1979- editor. | Haghi, A. K., editor.
Series: Innovations in physical chemistry.
Description: Series statement: Innovations in physical chemistry: monographic series | Includes
  bibliographical references and index.
Identifiers: Canadiana (print) 20200176994 | Canadiana (ebook) 2020017701X |
  ISBN 9781771888325 (hardcover) | ISBN 9780429328602 (ebook)
Subjects: LCSH: Heterocyclic compounds. | LCSH: Green chemistry.
Classification: LCC QD400 .M63 2020 | DDC 547/.59—dc23

CIP data on file with US Library of Congress

Apple Academic Press also publishes its books in a variety of electronic formats. Some content that appears in print may not be available in electronic format. For information about Apple Academic Press products, visit our website at **www.appleacademicpress.com** and the CRC Press website at **www.crcpress.com**

ABOUT THE EDITORS

Ravindra S. Shinde, PhD
Assistant Professor, Department of Chemistry and Industrial Chemistry,
Dayanand Science College, Latur, Maharashtra, India

Ravindra S. Shinde, PhD, is presently serving as Assistant Professor in the Department of Chemistry and Industrial Chemistry at Dayanand Science College, Latur, in Maharashtra, India. He is reviewer of many national and international of journals, including *Medicinal Chemistry Research,* the *United Journal of Chemistry,* and the *Journal of Emerging Technology and Innovation Research,* and is also an Advisory Board Member of the *European Journal of Biomedical and Pharmaceutical Sciences.* He has published many research papers in reputed national and international journals. He has completed his BSc, MSc, BEd, and PhD degrees from Swami Ramanand Teerth Marathwada University, Nanded, India.

A. K. Haghi, PhD
Professor Emeritus of Engineering Sciences, Editor-in-Chief,
International Journal of Chemoinformatics and Chemical Engineering &
Polymers Research Journal; Member, Canadian Research and
Development Center of Sciences and Cultures (CRDCSC), Canada

A. K. Haghi, PhD, is the author and editor of 165 books, as well as 1000 published papers in various journals and conference proceedings. Dr. Haghi has received several grants, consulted for a number of major corporations, and is a frequent speaker to national and international audiences. Since 1983, he served as professor at several universities. He is the former Editor-in-Chief of the *International Journal of Chemoinformatics and Chemical Engineering and Polymers Research Journal* and is on the editorial boards of many international journals. He is also a member of the Canadian Research and Development Center of Sciences and Cultures (CRDCSC), Montreal, Quebec, Canada. He holds a BSc in urban and environmental engineering from the University of North Carolina (USA), an MSc in mechanical engineering from North Carolina A&T State University (USA), a DEA in applied mechanics, acoustics and materials from the Université de Technologie de Compiègne (France), and a PhD in engineering sciences from Université de Franche-Comté (France).

INNOVATIONS IN PHYSICAL CHEMISTRY: MONOGRAPH SERIES

This book series offers a comprehensive collection of books on physical principles and mathematical techniques for majors, non-majors, and chemical engineers. Because there are many exciting new areas of research involving computational chemistry, nanomaterials, smart materials, high-performance materials, and applications of the recently discovered graphene, there can be no doubt that physical chemistry is a vitally important field. Physical chemistry is considered a daunting branch of chemistry—it is grounded in physics and mathematics and draws on quantum mechanics, thermodynamics, and statistical thermodynamics.

Editors-in-Chief

A. K. Haghi, PhD
Former Editor-in-Chief, *International Journal of Chemoinformatics* and *Chemical Engineering and Polymers Research Journal*; Member, Canadian Research and Development Center of Sciences and Cultures (CRDCSC), Montreal, Quebec, Canada
E-mail: AKHaghi@Yahoo.com

Lionello Pogliani, PhD
University of Valencia-Burjassot, Spain
E-mail: lionello.pogliani@uv.es

Ana Cristina Faria Ribeiro, PhD
Researcher, Department of Chemistry, University of Coimbra, Portugal
E-mail: anacfrib@ci.uc.pt

BOOKS IN THE SERIES

- **Applied Physical Chemistry with Multidisciplinary Approaches**
  Editors: A. K. Haghi, PhD, Devrim Balköse, PhD, and
  Sabu Thomas, PhD

- **Biochemistry, Biophysics, and Molecular Chemistry: Applied Research and Interactions**
  Editors: Francisco Torrens, PhD, Debarshi Kar Mahapatra, PhD, and
  A. K. Haghi, PhD

- **Chemistry and Industrial Techniques for Chemical Engineers**
  Editors: Lionello Pogliani, PhD, Suresh C. Ameta, PhD, and
  A. K. Haghi, PhD

- **Chemistry and Chemical Engineering for Sustainable Development: Best Practices and Research Directions**
  Editors: Miguel A. Esteso, PhD, Ana Cristina Faria Ribeiro, and
  A. K. Haghi, PhD

- **Chemical Technology and Informatics in Chemistry with Applications**
  Editors: Alexander V. Vakhrushev, DSc, Omari V. Mukbaniani, DSc,
  and Heru Susanto, PhD

- **Engineering Technologies for Renewable and Recyclable Materials: Physical-Chemical Properties and Functional Aspects**
  Editors: Jithin Joy, Maciej Jaroszewski, PhD, Praveen K. M.,
  and Sabu Thomas, PhD, and Reza Haghi, PhD

- **Engineering Technology and Industrial Chemistry with Applications**
  Editors: Reza Haghi, PhD, and Francisco Torrens, PhD

- **High-Performance Materials and Engineered Chemistry**
  Editors: Francisco Torrens, PhD, Devrim Balköse, PhD,
  and Sabu Thomas, PhD

- **Methodologies and Applications for Analytical and Physical Chemistry**
  Editors: A. K. Haghi, PhD, Sabu Thomas, PhD, Sukanchan Palit,
  and Priyanka Main

- **Modern Physical Chemistry: Engineering Models, Materials, and Methods with Applications**
  Editors: Reza Haghi, PhD, Emili Besalú, PhD,
  Maciej Jaroszewski, PhD, Sabu Thomas, PhD, and Praveen K. M.

- **Molecular Chemistry and Biomolecular Engineering: Integrating Theory and Research with Practice**

- Editors: Lionello Pogliani, PhD, Francisco Torrens, PhD, and
  A. K. Haghi, PhD

- **Modern Green Chemistry and Heterocyclic Compounds: Molecular Design, Synthesis, and Biological Evaluation**
  Editors: Ravindra S. Shinde, and A. K. Haghi, PhD

- **Physical Chemistry for Chemists and Chemical Engineers: Multidisciplinary Research Perspectives**
  Editors: Alexander V. Vakhrushev, DSc, Reza Haghi, PhD, and J. V. de Julián-Ortiz, PhD

- **Physical Chemistry for Engineering and Applied Sciences: Theoretical and Methodological Implication**
  Editors: A. K. Haghi, PhD, Cristóbal Noé Aguilar, PhD, Sabu Thomas, PhD, and Praveen K. M.

- **Practical Applications of Physical Chemistry in Food Science and Technology**
  Editors: Cristóbal Noé Aguilar, PhD, Jose Sandoval Cortes, PhD, Juan Alberto Ascacio Valdes, PhD, and A. K. Haghi, PhD

- **Research Methodologies and Practical Applications of Chemistry**
  Editors: Lionello Pogliani, PhD, A. K. Haghi, PhD, and Nazmul Islam, PhD

- **Theoretical Models and Experimental Approaches in Physical Chemistry: Research Methodology and Practical Methods**
  Editors: A. K. Haghi, PhD, Sabu Thomas, PhD, Praveen K. M., and Avinash R. Pai

- **Theoretical and Empirical Analysis in Physical Chemistry: A Framework for Research**
  Editors: Miguel A. Esteso, PhD, Ana Cristina Faria Ribeiro, PhD, and A. K. Haghi, PhD

CONTENTS

CONTRIBUTORS

Cristóbal N. Aguilar
Bioprocesses and Bioproducts Group, Department of Food Research, School of Chemistry, Autonomous University of Coahuila–25280, Saltillo, Coahuila, México, E-mail: cristobal.aguilar@uadec.edu.mx

Pedro Aguilar-Zárate
Bioprocesses and Bioproducts Group, Department of Food Research, School of Chemistry, Autonomous University of Coahuila–25280, Saltillo, Coahuila, México

Ajay N. Ambhore
Department of Chemistry, Padmabhushan Dr. Vasantraodada Patil College, Tasgaon, Sangli (MS) India, E-mail: ambhorevijay1@gmail.com, rss.333@rediffmail.com

Jaman A. Angulwar
Department of Chemistry, Dayanand Science College, Latur–413512, Maharashtra, India

Gloria Castellano
Department of Experimental Sciences and Mathematics, Faculty of Veterinary and Experimental Sciences, Valencia Catholic University Saint Vincent Martyr, Guillem de Castro-94, E-46001 Valencia, Spain

Juan C. Contreras-Esquivel
Bioprocesses and Bioproducts Group, Department of Food Research, School of Chemistry, Autonomous University of Coahuila–25280, Saltillo, Coahuila, México

Reynaldo De la Cruz-Quiroz
Bioprocesses and Bioproducts Research Group, Food Research Department, Autonomous University of Coahuila, 25280, Saltillo, México

Sylvain Guyot
INRA, UR1268 BIA, Team Polyphenol, Reactivity and Processing (PRP), BP–35327, 35653 Le Rheu, France

A. K. Haghi
Professor Emeritus of Engineering Sciences, Former Editor-in-Chief, *International Journal of Chemoinformatics and Chemical Engineering & Polymers Research Journal;* Member, Canadian Research and Development Center of Sciences and Cultures (CRDCSC), Canada E-mail: akhaghi@yahoo.com

Kishan Prabhu Haval
Department of Chemistry, Dr. Babasaheb Ambedkar Marathwada University, Sub-Campus, Osmanabad–413501, Maharashtra, India, E-mail: havallpp11@gmail.com, rss.333@rediffmail.com

Daniel Hernandez-Castillo
Agricultural Parasitology Department, Antonio Narro Agrarian Autonomous University, Buenavista, Saltillo, Coahuila, México

Shrikaant Kulkarni
Assistant Professor, Vishwakarma Institute of Technology, Department of Chemical Engineering, 666, Upper Indira Nagar, Bibwewadi, Pune–411037, India, Mobile: +91-9970663353, E-mail: shrikaant.kulkarni@vit.edu

Shreyas S. Mahurkar
Department of Chemistry, Dayanand Science College, Latur–413512, Maharashtra, India, E-mail: mahurkar.shrayas1@gmail.com, rss.333@rediffmail.com

Sangita S. Makone
School of Chemical Sciences, Swami Ramanand Teerth Marathwada University, Nanded–431606, Maharashtra, India

Sunil R. Mirgane
Department of Chemistry, J.E.S. College, Jalna–431203 Maharashtra, India

Palani Natarajan
Assistant Professor, Department of Chemistry and Center for Advanced Studies in Chemistry, Punjab University, Chandigarh–160014, U.T., India, E-mail: pnataraj@pu.ac.in

Ajay M. Patil
Department of Chemistry, Pratishthan Mahavidyalaya, Paithan–431107, Maharashtra, India, E-mail: patilan4@gmail.com, rss.333@redifffmail.com

Priya
Research Scholar, Department of Chemistry and Center for Advanced Studies in Chemistry, Punjab University, Chandigarh–160014, U.T., India

Raúl Rodríguez-Herrera
Bioprocesses and Bioproducts Research Group, Department of Food Research, School of Chemistry, Autonomous University of Coahuila–25280, Saltillo, Coahuila, México

Sevastianos Roussos
Mediterranean Institute of marine and terrestrial Biodiversity and Ecology, Marseille, France

Ravindra S. Shinde
Research Center in Chemistry, Dayanand Science College, Latur–413512, MS, India, E-mail: rshinde.33381@gmail.com

Francisco Torrens
Institute for Molecular Science, University of Valencia, PO Box 22085, E-46071 Valencia, Spain, E-mail: torrens@uv.es

Jorge E. Wong-Paz
Bioprocesses and Bioproducts Group, Department of Food Research, School of Chemistry, Autonomous University of Coahuila–25280, Saltillo, Coahuila, México

ABBREVIATIONS

^{13}C NMR	carbon nuclear magnetic resonance
^{1}H NMR	proton nuclear magnetic resonance
AA	ascorbic acid
AAE	aqueous acetone extract
AAs	amino acids
Ac	acetyl
AcOH	acetic acid
AEs	adverse effects
AIDS	acquired immunodeficiency syndrome
Aq	aqueous
Ar	aryl
ART	artemisinin
ARTDs	ART derivatives
BC	breast cancer
BCA	biological control agents
BEC	bleaching earth clay
But	butyl
Cat	catalyst
CC	corn cob
CC	cyanuric chloride
CDCl$_3$	deuterated chloroform
CDMT	2-chloro-4,6-dimethoxy-1,3,5-triazine
CF	coconut fiber
CLSI	Clinical and Laboratory Standards Institute
CONACYT	Coahuila and the National Council of Science and Technology
Conc.	concentrated
CVD	chemical vapor deposition
D	doublet
d	doublet
DBSA	dodecylbenzene sulfonic acid
Dd	doublet of doublet
DHP	dihydropyridines

DM	diabetes mellitus
DMF	N,N-dimethyl formamide
DMSO	dimethyl sulfoxide
DNA	deoxyribonucleic acid
DPPH	diphenylpicrylhyride
EBX	ethynylbenziodoxolone
EDA	electron donor acceptor
EDTA	ethylene diamine tetraacetic acid
ESI-MS	infusion in electrospray mass spectrometry
Et	ethyl
EtOAc	ethylacetoacetate
EtOH	ethanol
g	gram
GHE	greenhouse effect
HAT	hydrogen atom transfer
HCl	hydrochloric acid
hr	hours
HTMAB	hexadecyltrimethylammonium bromide
Hz	hertz
IR	infrared
K_2CO_3	potassium carbonate
KBr	potassium bromide
Kg	kilogram
M	molar/multiplet
m	multiplet
M.P.	melting point
MASS	mass-spectroscopy
MCRs	multicomponent reactions
MDR	multidrug resistance
Me	methyl
MeOH	methanol
mg	milligram
MHz	megahertz
MIC	minimum inhibitory concentration
Min	minute
ML	methylene-lactone
mL	milliliters
mm	millimeter

mmol	milimol
MPLC	medium pressure liquid chromatography
Mtb	mycobacterium tuberculosis
Na_2CO_3	sodium carbonate
NHS	N-hydroxysuccinimide
nM	nanometer
NMR	nuclear magnetic resonance
NSCLC	non-small cell lung cancer
OH	hydroxy
PDA	potato dextrose agar
PEG-400	poly ethylene glycol-400
Ph	phenyl
PKC	palm kernel cake
ppm	parts per million
PTE	periodic table of the elements
RCC	radiochemical conversion
ROS	reactive oxygen species
RT	room temperature
S	singlet
SAR	structure-activity relationship
SCB	sugarcane bagasse
$SO_4{}^{\cdot-}$	sulfate radical anions
SOR	superoxide anion radical
SSF	solid-state fermentation
STL	sesquiterpene lactone
T	triplet
t-But	tert-Butyl
TEA	triethylamine
TEAB	tetraethyl ammonium bicarbonate
TEBA	triethyl benzyl ammonium chloride
TEM	transmission electron microscope
THR	*Trichoderma harzianum*
TLC	thin-layer chromatography
TMS	tetramethylsilane
UAAAN	Universidad Autónoma Agraria Antonio Narro
ZOI	zone of inhibition

PREFACE

Green chemistry, or environmentally benign chemistry, is the design of chemical products and processes that reduce or eliminate the use and generation of hazardous substances.

Rather than focusing only on those undesirable substances that might be inadvertently produced in a process, green chemistry also includes all substances that are part of the process. Therefore, green chemistry is a tool not only for minimizing the negative impact of those procedures aimed at optimizing efficiency, although clearly both impact minimization and process optimization, which are legitimate and complementary objectives of green chemistry. Green chemistry applies to industrial prospects, organic chemistry, inorganic chemistry, biochemistry, analytical chemistry, and even physical chemistry.

The wide range of applications of green chemistry includes uses in the pharmaceutical industry as well as new approaches that reduce or eliminate the use of solvents or render them safer and more efficient. Green chemistry has also inspired a growing number of ways to synthesize traditionally petroleum-based chemicals from biological materials, such as using plant matter or waste.

Heterocyclic compounds are of very much interest in our daily life. They have a high significance in our living system. Heterocyclic compounds have a wide range of applications in agrochemicals, pharmaceuticals, veterinary products, etc. They are also used as a starting material in the synthesis of organic compounds. These compounds may be aromatic or anti-aromatic. Heterocyclic compounds widely found in nature, e.g., pyramiding and purine, are the parts of DNA, vitamins, and enzymes. This book focuses on the importance of heterocyclic compounds in our life in different ways.

On the other hand, heterocyclic rings are present in the majority of known natural products, contributing to enormous structural diversity. In addition, they often possess significant biological activity. Medicinal chemists have embraced this last property in designing most of the small molecule drugs in use today.

Heterocyclic chemistry comprises at least half of all organic chemistry research worldwide. This book covers the general properties of heterocyclic compounds and general methods for their preparation. It provides the basis for understanding the chemistry of individual ring systems that are described in different chapters.

Heterocyclic compounds are an important class of molecules in organic chemistry, due to their presence in natural products and their use in pharmaceuticals and new materials.

Meanwhile, heterocyclic compounds play a vital role in the metabolism of living cells. The range of known compounds is enormous, encompassing the whole spectrum of physical, chemical, and biological properties.

This research-oriented volume is ideal for readers who want to fully realize the almost limitless potential to discover new and effective pharmaceuticals among heterocyclic compounds, the largest and most varied family of organic compounds. The book features several case studies and step-by-step descriptions of synthetic methods and practical techniques. It also serves as a guide for chemists, offering them new insights and new paths to explore for effective drug discovery.

The book introduces a selection of important heterocyclic compounds and the vital role that they play in life.

This book provides a balanced, concise, and informative account of heterocyclic chemistry that will be suitable for graduate students and a convenient reference book for research workers, for both specialists in the field and those whose expertise lies in other areas but who nevertheless need information on green chemistry heterocyclic compounds.

This research-oriented book is illustrated throughout with clearly drawn chemical structures. The highly systematic coverage given to the subject makes this the most authoritative one-volume account of modern green chemistry and heterocyclic compounds available. It also provides a balanced, concise, and informative account of heterocyclic chemistry.

CHAPTER 1

AN OVERVIEW OF THE ORGANIC SYNTHESIS AND TRANSFORMATIONS INITIATED BY SULFATE RADICAL ANIONS (SO$_4$$^{\cdot-}$) PRODUCED FROM AQUEOUS PERSULFATE SOLUTIONS UNDER TRANSITION METAL-FREE CONDITIONS

PRIYA and PALANI NATARAJAN[*]

Department of Chemistry and Center for Advanced Studies in Chemistry, Punjab University, Chandigarh, India

[*]*Corresponding author. E-mail: pnataraj@pu.ac.in*

ABSTRACT

In recent times, the sulfate radical anions (SO$_4$$^{\cdot-}$) are largely being utilized for the functionalization of drugs (taxol, pregabalin, nicotine, etc.) and synthesis of various organic compounds including heterocyclic compounds, fertilizers, nanoparticles, and polymers. Moreover, they are also employed for the destruction of a variety of organic contaminants such as perfluoro carboxylic acids, chlorinated solvents, polycyclic aromatic hydrocarbons, textile dyes, pharmaceuticals, xylenes, and so on. SO$_4$$^{\cdot-}$ have a very strong one-electron oxidation potential, i.e., 2.43 V vs. NHE in aqueous solutions, and they are well generated through the scission of the peroxide bond of persulfates. To date, some important reviews are available that summarize the metal-catalyzed productions of $SO_4^{\bullet-}$ and their applications toward organic functional group transformations as well as the extinction of organic pollutants. To the best of our knowledge, however, there is still no article exclusively discourses about the transition metal-free formation of $SO_4^{\bullet-}$ in aqueous solutions and their applications for the organic synthesis and functional group transformations. Therefore, in this chapter, we provide an overview of the transition metal-free protocols deal with the generation of $SO_4^{\bullet-}$ from persulfates in aqueous media. Also, we highlight the utilization of *in situ* formed $SO_4^{\bullet-}$ toward syntheses and functionalization of various small organic molecules.

1.1 INTRODUCTION

In recent times, sulfate radical anion ($SO_4^{\bullet-}$) has largely been utilized by academicians and industrialists in a broad range of chemical processes such as polymerization, soil remediation, and chemical oxidation for groundwater treatment, organic transformations, and syntheses. The sulfate radical anion is a very strong one-electron oxidant with an estimated reduction potential of 2.43 V vs. NHE in aqueous media. Normally, such a redox-activity is found only in (heavy) metals. This parallelism of properties enables the replacement of traditional metal-based materials with sulfate radical anions ($SO_4^{\bullet-}$). In addition, the use of $SO_4^{\bullet-}$ as a reagent has many advantages, including mild reaction conditions, ease of use, environmental-friendly, high tolerance towards functional groups, astonishing solubility in water and other aqueous solvents like acetone, acetonitrile, and alcohols.

The chemistry of $SO_4^{\bullet-}$ has been reviewed from time to time. Recently, two review articles on transition metal-catalyzed productions of $SO_4^{\bullet-}$ and their applications toward organic functional group transformations, as well as destruct of organic pollutants, have been compiled. In this chapter, we provide an overview of the transition metal-free protocols deal with the generation of $SO_4^{\bullet-}$ from persulfates in aqueous media. Also, we highlight the utilization of *in situ* formed $SO_4^{\bullet-}$ toward syntheses and functionalization of various organic compounds. The (radical) reactions, especially free from transition metals and occur in aqueous solutions, have attracted great attention of chemists due to environmental friendliness. In addition, residual transition-metal contamination could adversely affect the biological properties of the final products.

Generally, the $SO_4^{\bullet-}$ initiate organic reactions through either of hydrogen abstraction, one-electron oxidation, oxidative-decarboxylation, and hydrogen abstraction followed by decarboxylation. Accordingly, this chapter has been divided into four sections:

1. Hydrogen abstraction by sulfate radical anion;
2. Hydrogen abstraction by sulfate radical anion followed by decarboxylation;
3. One-electron oxidation by sulfate radical anion; and
4. Indirect involvement of sulfate radical anion in organic synthesis.

1.2 GENERATION OF SULFATE RADICAL ANIONS ($SO_4^{\bullet-}$) FROM PERSULFATES

Persulfates ($S_2O_8^{2-}$) are low priced crystalline solids, stable, non-hygroscopic, soluble in aqueous solutions, and ecologically friendly oxidants with high reduction potential. Regardless of high reduction potential, persulfates in their native form are inactive and usually give no reaction. For enhanced reactivity, they are activated through cleavage of O-O bond either by the Fenton redox process (Eq. 1) or thermolysis (Eq. 2) or photolysis (Eq. 2). Notice that the homolytic cleavage (Eq. 2) of O-O bond of persulfates affords two $SO_4^{\bullet-}$ whereas heterolytic cleavage (Eq. 1) provides one sulfate radical anion and one sulfate ion. Normally, the persulfates in the form of $Na_2S_2O_8$, $K_2S_2O_8$, and $(NH_4)_2S_2O_8$ are highly used as a reagent due to their ready availability in markets.

1.3   HYDROGEN ATOM ABSTRACTION BY SULFATE RADICAL ANION

1.3.1   FUNCTIONALIZATION OF N-HETEROCYCLIC COMPOUNDS THROUGH HYDROGEN ATOM ABSTRACTION BY SULFATE RADICAL ANION

The heterocyclic center is the significant theme of the vast majority of commercial drugs because of their natural biological properties. It is widely used to fight against numerous neurotic and physiological infirmities. These days, C-C bond arrangement by means of C-H functionalization through cross dehydrogenative coupling is becoming quite an alluring tool for the syntheses of imperative organic compounds as it is atom and step economical. Understanding this approach, Shi et al. in 2013 (Scheme 1.1) [1] developed a transition metal-free, green approach for the synthesis of substituted pyridines (1^8). Shi protocol worked by the reaction of unprotonated pyridine derivatives (1) with 1,4-dioxane (8) by using $K_2S_2O_8$ as an oxidant in aqueous solution in the absence of any harmful acid or toxic metal [1].

A variety of substituted pyridine derivatives (1^8a) were combined with 1,4-dioxane; however, non-substituted one provided the trisubstituted product (1^8b). The electron-donating substituents (1^8c) on the pyridine ring gave lower yields when contrasted with the electron-withdrawing ones (1^8d). The pyridine ring with cyano- as a substituent indicated diverse reactivities under the same reaction conditions such that C-2 substituted cyano (1^8e) afforded mixture of mono substituents in 45% yield, C-4 (1^8f), and C-3 (1^8g) cyano pyridine gave di- and tri-substituted products in 65% and 61% yields, respectively [1].

Along with pyridines, the enormous literature is available on the C-H functionalization of other heteroarenes. Singh and collaborators in 2015 (Scheme 1.1) [2] built up an exceptionally productive green methodology for the coupling of alicyclic ethers (9), cyclic ethers and alkanes (8) with diverse electron-deficient heteroarenes like pyridine (1), quinoline (2), isoquinoline (3), pyrazine (4) and pyrimidine (7) in admirable yields. The reaction continued under transition metal-free conditions in an aqueous solution of acetone, avoiding the utilization of any acid that was earlier required for the protonation of N-heteroarenes [2].

The reaction protocol was further stretched out to naphthoquinones (**10**). Pyridines (**1⁸h**), Quinolines (**2⁸a**), isoquinolines (**3⁸a**), pyrazine (**4⁸a**) gave high yields up to 90% with cyclic ethers. In the case of pyrimidine (**7⁸a**), the mixture of mono and disubstituted products were obtained. With alkanes (**7⁸a**) or alicyclic ethers (**3⁹a**), the reaction yield was enhanced by the addition of TBAB in DCE: water mixture [2]. Several control experiments with radical scavenger like TEMPO confirmed the radical mechanism as reaction yield reduced to a great extent in its presence.

Later in 2016, Shah and Dewari (Scheme 1.1) [3] reported a similar convention for the C-H arylation of ethers using CFL light as irradiation sources. The reaction continued at room temperature by means of dual C(sp²)–H and C(sp³)–H functionalization through the HAT pathway leading to the synthesis of N-heterocycles [3]. In the prior works revealed by Minisci, the acidic catalyst was essentially utilized for the protonation of heteroarenes, but, in this reaction, the yield is 77% even without utilizing trifluoroacetic acid, along these lines, it was expected that protonation of amines was likely happened through *in situ* generations of H⁺ ions from water.

This convention was compliant to the assortment of electron-deficient N-heteroarenes, for example, pyridines (**1**), quinolines (**2**), isoquinolines (**3**), pyrazines (**4**), quinoxalines (**5**) and it was further extended to the preparation of functionalized benzothiazoles (**6**) and naphthoquinones (**10**) [3]. The variety of cyclic (**8**) and non-cyclic ethers (**9**) was explored, and the best outcomes were acquired with 1,4-dioxane. It was discovered that 1,2-dimethoxyethane with isoquinolines (**3⁸b**) yielded regiomers where arylation occurred at methylene C-H and methoxy C-H positions. Similarly, yield up to 61% was obtained with benzothiazole (**6⁸a**). Substituted pyridines (**1⁸i**) also reacted well with 1,4-dioxane.

In 2016, Zhang et al. (Scheme 1.1) [4] envisioned the cross dehydrogenative coupling reaction of benzothiazole (**6**) with ethers in the biphasic solvent mixture of water and ether at 29°C. The reaction proceeded in visible light by making use of household 26W CFL bulb as irradiation sources [4].

Similarly, in 2016, Barriault, and coworkers [5] detailed the oxidative C(sp²)H and C(sp³)H cross-coupling reaction amongst heteroarenes and unactivated ethers (Scheme 1.1) [5]. According to the substrate scope, best outcomes were obtained with ether substituted pyridine (**1⁸j**), quinoline (**2⁸c**), isoquinoline (**3⁸c, 3⁹b**), and pyrazine (**4⁸c**) [5].

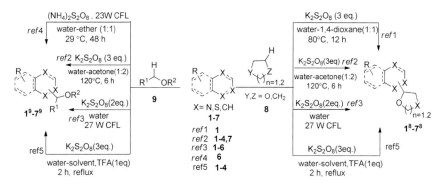

SCHEME 1.1   Transition metal-free persulfate mediated cross dehydrogenative coupling of ethers with N-heteroarenes in aqueous media.

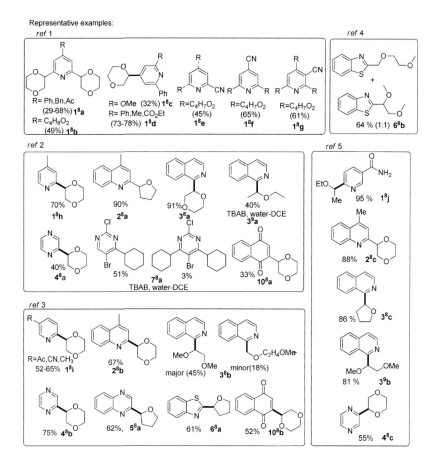

1.3.1.1 MECHANISM

Initially, $SO_4^{\bullet-}$ was formed by the homolytic cleavage of persulfate either in the presence of heat (Eq. 1) or through the formation of electron donor-acceptor (EDA) complex of heteroarenes and $S_2O_8^{2-}$ in the presence of visible light (eq2). Subsequently, hydrogen atom transfer (HAT) from the ether (**8/9**) to $SO_4^{\bullet-}$ resulted in nucleophilic α oxyalkyl radical (**8ª/9ª**), which at that point reacted with in situ generated protonated heteroarenes (**1ª–7ª**) leading to aminyl radical cation (**1ᵇ–7ᵇ**). This either through HAT or oxidative deprotonation formed substituted heteroarenes.

1.3.2 THE C–F FUNCTIONALIZATION THROUGH HYDROGEN ATOM ABSTRACTION BY SULFATE RADICAL ANION

The C–H functionalization of organic compounds through tandem cross-coupling reactions is a very significant and ever-demanding field in organic transformations due to minimal waste production and highly atom and step economic. This protocol has largely been utilized for the formation of C-F bond in organic molecules. Also, fluorinated chemistry is quite fascinating these days due to the application of fluorine-containing compounds in the dye and polymer industry, in research centers, pharmaceuticals, agrochemicals, and material science, etc. Chai and partners in 2015 (Scheme 1.2) [6] reported a direct, significantly competent strategy for mono (**14**) and di-fluorination (**15**) of essential arenes (**11**) through C(sp³)- H functionalization to C-F bond development utilizing $K_2S_2O_8$ as initiator and selectfluor (**12**) as fluorinating agent relying upon the measure of $K_2S_2O_8$

used as a part of aqueous acetonitrile solution. The reaction continued by means of one-pot two-stage fluorination processes where persulfate is utilized to activate the benzylic H atom specifically.

An array of functional groups on benzene (**14a**) together with fused cyclic compounds (**14b**) was amenable for mono-fluorination aside from anisole, benzyl bromides (**14c**), likewise in the case of difluorinated products (**15a**). Electronic factors influenced the yield of mono (**14d**) and di-fluorinated (**15c**) products to a great extent. Similarly, methyl quinines (**14b**) can also be difluorinated. Since persulfate can go about as a radical initiator and an oxidant, a competitive mechanism should happen amongst oxidation and fluorination such that oxidation product commands under-neath 60°C, whereas fluorinated products ruled over 80°C [6].

Taking forward this protocol of alkylfluorination, Tang et al. in 2015 (Scheme 1.2) [7] revealed the selective aliphatic C(sp^3)- H fluorination in an aqueous medium under metal-free conditions at 50°C utilizing selectfluor (**13**) as an effortlessly accessible fluorinating agent. Here, rela-tive radical stability of carbon chooses the position for fluorination. The methine or methylene position that was distant from electron-withdrawing groups (**14e**) and substrates with smaller chain lengths (**14f**) is more selec-tive for fluorination. The substrates with amino acid derivatives (**14g**) and cyclic ones (**14h**) were well tolerated. This convention was additionally reached out to the late-stage fluorination of complex biologically active compounds (sclareolide, diterpene, and taxol) in moderate to high yields. Deuterium kinetic isotope effect demonstrated that C-H bond cleavage is the rate-determining step towards fluorination [7].

By knowing the significance of ^{18}F in medical diagnosis as its use in PET imaging, a similar mechanism for the fluorination of benzylic C-H bond was proposed by Liang and co-workers in 2016 (Scheme 1.2) [8]. In this procedure, the authors revealed the transition metal-free radio fluori-nation of pseudo-p-benzyl halides (**16**) to (**11**) followed by activation of benzylic C-H bond of (**11**) to C-F for the synthesis of (18F) aryl-CF$_2$H (**14**) by using selectfluor (**12**) as fluorinating agent [8]. The optimized conditions demonstrated that better radiochemical conversion (RCC) 50±5% and high specific activity was acquired without silver salt. The reaction basically proceeded in two steps, where, initial step included the radio fluorination of pseudo benzyl halide (**16**) in which pseudo halide atom was replaced by ^{18}F in the presence of tetraethylammonium bicarbonate (TEAB) in aceto-nitrile within 10 minutes at 130°C with RCC of 98±2%. Once ^{18}F labeled arene (**11**) was obtained, it was then subjected to the fluorination of the benzylic C-H bond in the second step. The electron-deficient ketones with a variety of functional groups on the para position were fluorinated (**14i**). The convention was relevant on sterically hindered substrates (**14j**) as well as on N-heteroaromatic substituted substrates (**14k**) [8].

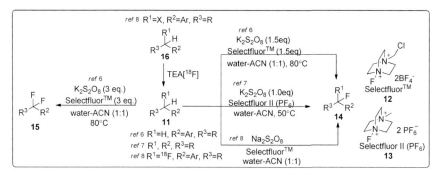

SCHEME 1.2 Transition metal-free persulfate mediated fluorination of C(sp³)-H bonds in aqueous media.

ref 6

ref 7

ref 8

1.3.2.1   MECHANISM

At first, the homolytic cleavage of persulfate produced $SO_4^{\bullet-}$ which on hydrogen abstraction from the substrate (11) gave carbon radical (11ª). At that point, the exchange of fluorine radicals from selectfluor (12/13) to intermediate (11ª) provided the required fluorinated product (14).

1.3.3   THE CF₃-FUNCTIONALIZED ORGANIC COMPOUNDS SYNTHESIS THROUGH HYDROGEN ATOM ABSTRACTION BY SULFATE RADICAL ANION

The CF_3 containing organic compounds are very essential in pharmaceuticals and engineered science, however, the past strategies for trifluoromethylation incorporated the transition metal-catalyzed coupling of aryl halides, aryl borons, anilines, and so forth with diverse trifluoromethylation agents, but this technique is extremely costly for the regular syntheses of fluorinated compounds, hence, Tian et al. in 2016 (Scheme 1.3) [9] endeavored to utilize the arene sulfonyl hydrazides as proficient trifluoromethyl source by means of C-S bond cleavage for vicinal halo trifluoromethylation of alkenes under environment friendly conditions. The authors detailed the trifluoromethylation of N-arylacrylamides (17) with stable and easily accessible trifluoromethane sulfonylhydrazides (TfNHNHBoc) (18) as a convincing trifluoromethylating reagent by methods for cascade trifluoromethylation took after by cyclization of 17 yielding trifluoromethylated oxindoles (19) with the high regio-selectivity.

The aryl alkenes with various functional groups at para (19a) and ortho (19b) positions of aniline moiety were well tolerated. Also, α substituted alkenes (**19c**) were acceptable in good yields along with the synthesis of tricyclic oxindoles (**19d**).

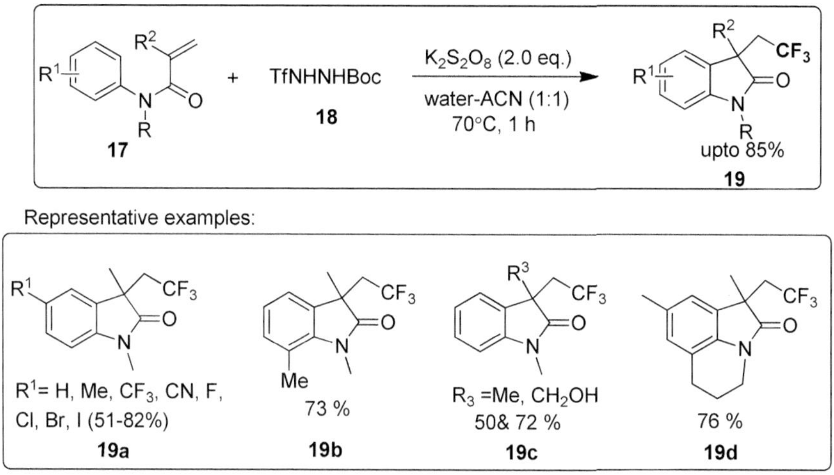

SCHEME 1.3 Transition metal-free persulfate mediated trifluoromethylation/cyclization of N-aryacrylamides leading to CF$_3$ containing oxindoles in an aqueous medium.

1.3.3.1 MECHANISM

Initially, diazene (**18ᵃ**) was formed from TfNHNHBoc (**18**) by oxidation and its decomposition to (**18ᵇ**) with the loss of N$_2$, and then SO$_2$ gave CF$_3$• radical (**18ᶜ**). The radical (**18ᶜ**) attacks on the double bond of N-arylacryl-amides (**17**) forming alkyl radical (**17ᵃ**), which on intramolecular radical cyclization produces intermediate (**17ᵇ**). In the end, oxidative deproton-ation leads to the desired product (**19**).

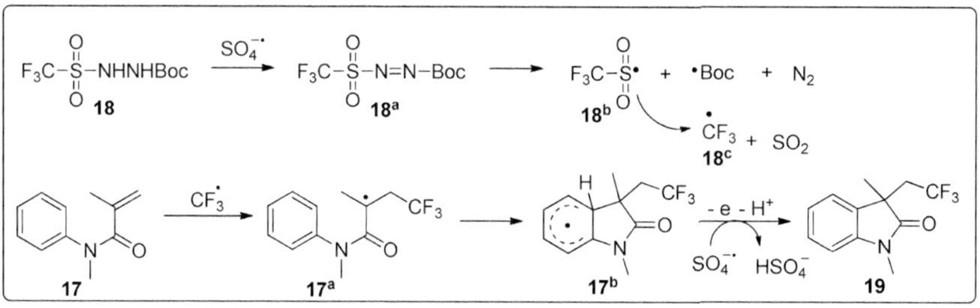

1.3.4   SYNTHESIS OF AZIDE-FUNCTIONALIZED ORGANIC COMPOUNDS THROUGH HYDROGEN ATOM ABSTRACTION BY SULFATE RADICAL ANION

With the revelation of organic azides by Peter Grieb around 140 years back, these have been broadly used in many organic transformations, so Tang and co-workers in their published research article in 2015 asserted that sulfonyl hydrazides had not been utilized as azide source till date. The authors reported the selective oxidation of unactivated C-H bonds (**11**) using sulfonyl azides (**20**) as azide source in aqueous acetonitrile solution under a nitrogen atmosphere for 4 hours (Scheme 1.4) [10].

The substrates with diverse functional groups on aryl ring (**21a**) have been azidated in moderate to good yields along with heteroaromatic rings (**21b**). Further, azidation of many biologically active compounds and natural products (diterpene, sclareolide, artemisinin (ART)) was carried out to make them more potent in drug discovery. Control experiments uncovered that reaction proceeded by means of a free radical pathway, not via carbocation formation. Deuterium isotope effect showed that C-H bond cleavage is not the rate-determining step in this particular transformation. The reaction of **21d** can also be scaled up to gram levels.

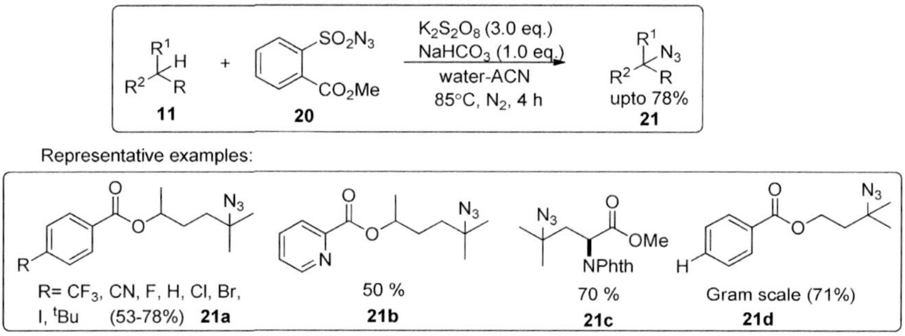

SCHEME 1.4   Transition metal-free persulfate mediated oxidative azidation of aliphatic C-H bonds in aqueous acetonitrile solution.

A similar type of methodology was reported in 2016 in which authors endeavored to couple carbon-based radicals with azide radical obtained from pyridine sulfonyl azide. Shi et al. in 2016 (Scheme 1.5) [11] reported the conversion of tertiary aliphatic C(sp^3) H bonds (**22**) into C-N$_3$ (**24**) using pyridine sulfonyl azide (**23**). The N-phthamines with different alkyl chains (**24a**) were recognized in significant yields. Varied functional groups on alkyl chain (**24b**), as well as cyclic substrates (**24c**), were tolerated in good yields. Being electron affluent, tertiary C-H bonds (**24a-c**) provided higher yields than secondary (**24d**) ones.

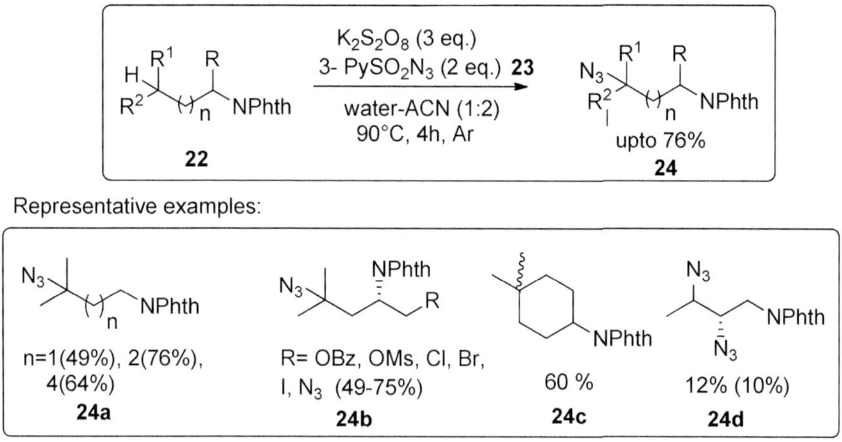

Representative examples:

n=1(49%), 2(76%), 4(64%)
24a

R= OBz, OMs, Cl, Br, I, N₃ (49-75%)
24b

60 %
24c

12% (10%)
24d

SCHEME 1.5 Transition metal-free persulfate mediated oxidation of tertiary aliphatic C(sp³)-H bonds in an aqueous medium.

1.3.4.1 MECHANISM

The $SO_4^{\bullet-}$ formed through thermolysis of persulfate salt abstracted the hydrogen atom from an aliphatic C-H bond of **11**, resulting in the formation of carbon radical intermediate (**11ᵃ**). The radical (**11ᵃ**) further reacted with the terminal nitrogen atom of sulfonyl azide (**20/23**) to form intermediate (**20ᵃ/23ᵃ**), which on the release of sulfonyl radical (**20ᵇ**) gave the azidation product (**21**). This sulfonyl radical on oxidation with $SO_4^{\bullet-}$ and then by nucleophilic attack of water formed sulfinic acid (**20ᶜ**).

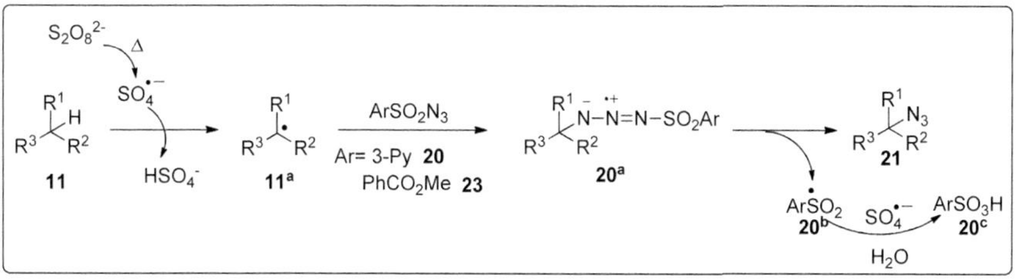

1.3.5 SYNTHESIS OF SPIRO-OXINDOLES THROUGH HYDROGEN ATOM ABSTRACTION BY SULFATE RADICAL ANION

Spiro-oxindoles are highly robust biological compounds and widely used as a part of pharmaceuticals were synthesized by Duan and co-workers in 2013 (Scheme 1.6) [12] using simple transition metal-free and exceedingly proficient protocol. The authors published the oxidative spirocyclization of hydroxymethyl acrylamide (17) with 1,3-dicarbonyl compounds (25) by means of cascade dual C-H functionalization followed by intramolecular dehydration which brings about the formation of spiro-oxindoles (26).

Aniline moiety of N-arylacrylamides with different substituents at para (26a) and ortho (26b) positions were well tolerated. In the case of dibenzoylmethane (26c), no bicyclized product obtained due to two phenyl groups. Apart from N-methyl, N-benzyl acrylamide (26d) was also acceptable in good yields.

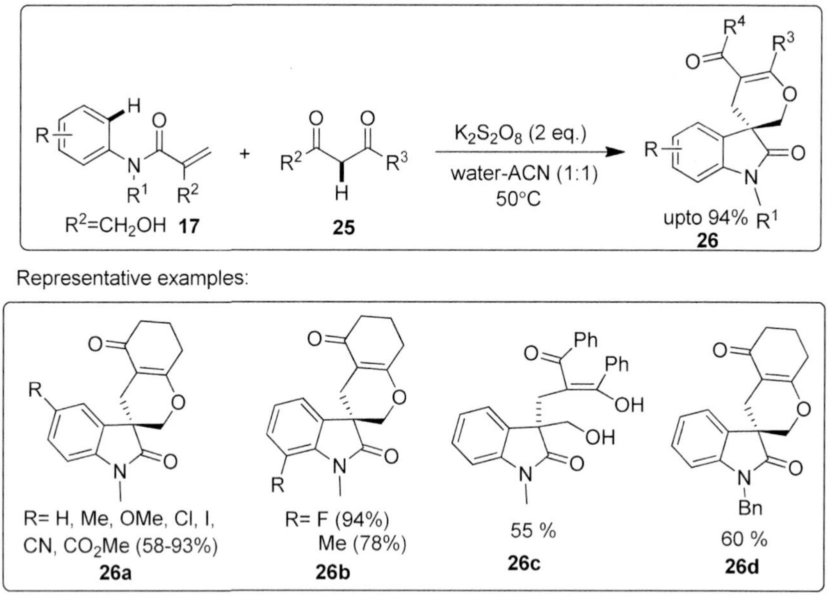

SCHEME 1.6 Transition metal-free persulfate mediated synthesis of spirooxindoles in aqueous acetonitrile solution.

1.3.5.1 MECHANISM

The $SO_4^{\bullet-}$ through HAT from dione (25) afforded the alkyl radical (25ᵃ), which on reaction with N-arylacrylamides (17) gave 17ᵃ followed by intramolecular radical cyclization and generated radical (17ᵇ). 17ᵇ on oxidative deprotonation or HAT produced the annulated oxindoles (17ᶜ); subsequently, the loss of water as a byproduct yielded the spirooxindole product (26).

1.3.6 SYNTHESIS OF BENZOCOUMARIN DERIVATIVES THROUGH HYDROGEN ATOM ABSTRACTION BY SULFATE RADICAL ANION

Gevorgyan in 2013 (Scheme 1.7) [13] demonstrated the oxidative intramolecular cyclization of electron-deficient aryl benzoic acids (27) promoted by $K_2S_2O_8$ at 50–60°C for the synthesis of benzocoumarin derivatives (28). The eco- friendly convention can also be scaled up to gram levels for the synthesis of 28a. This protocol was appropriate to a wide range of electron-deficient arenes at meta (28b) and para (28c) positions.

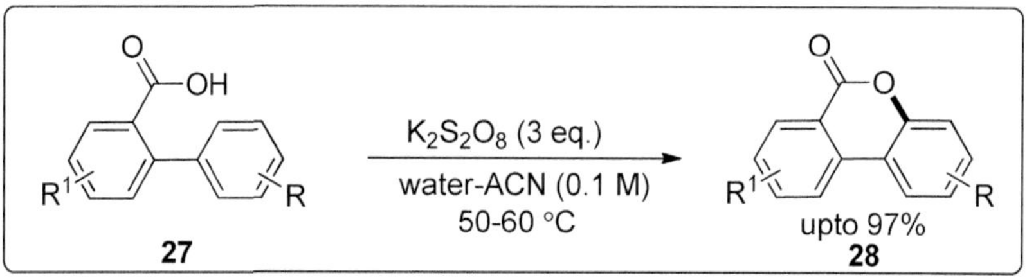

Representative examples:

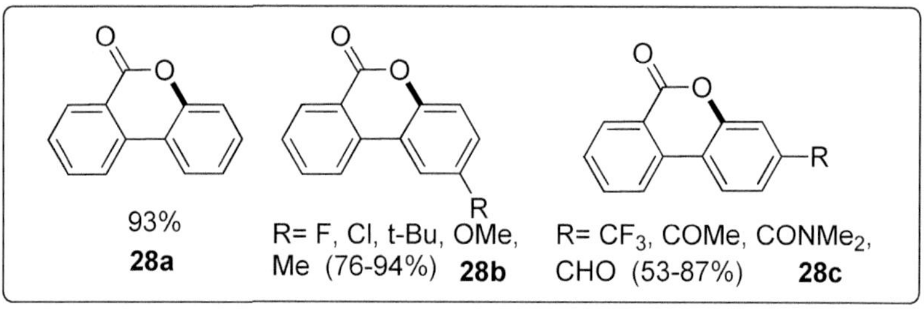

93%	
28a	R= F, Cl, t-Bu, OMe,
	Me (76-94%) **28b**

R= CF$_3$, COMe, CONMe$_2$,
CHO (53-87%) **28c**

SCHEME 1.7   Transition metal-free persulfate mediated C-H oxygenation of arenes in an aqueous acetonitrile solution.

1.3.6.1   MECHANISM

Upon thermolysis, persulfate decomposes to SO$_4$$^{•-}$ which on hydrogen abstraction from carboxylic acid (**27**) produce **27**^{a}. Then intramolecular cyclization gave aryl radical (**27**^{b}), which on oxidative deprotonation in the presence of SO$_4$$^{•-}$ gave the required product (**28**).

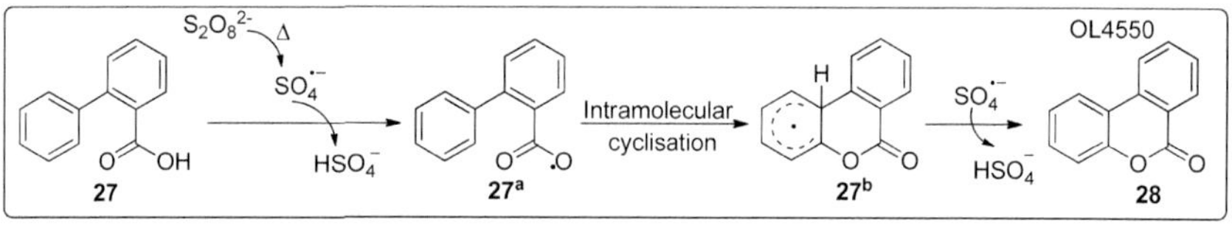

1.3.7   SYNTHESIS OF SULFONATED OXINDOLES THROUGH HYDROGEN ATOM ABSTRACTION BY SULFATE RADICAL ANION

Sulfonated oxindoles being potent biologically active molecules widely found in drug delivery and synthetic intermediates. Thus, in 2014, Wang et al. (Scheme 1.8) [14] reported the simple, transition metal-free, one-pot synthesis of sulfonated oxindoles (30) with the use of sulfonic acid (29) as a sulfonating agent and $K_2S_2O_8$ as an oxidant. The scope of N arylacrylamides with varied functional groups was compatible at para (30a) and sterically obstructed ortho positions (30b). However, meta-substituted (30c) gave a mixture of regiomers. Also, benzene sulfonic acids with different substrates (30d) were acceptable in good yields.

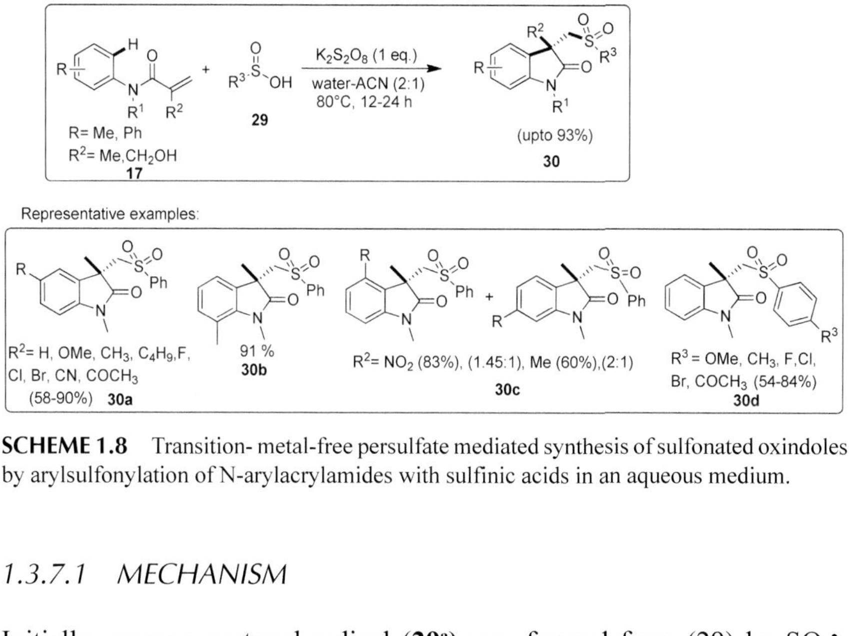

Representative examples:

SCHEME 1.8 Transition-metal-free persulfate mediated synthesis of sulfonated oxindoles by arylsulfonylation of N-arylacrylamides with sulfinic acids in an aqueous medium.

1.3.7.1 MECHANISM

Initially, oxygen centered radical (29^a) was formed from (29) by SO$_4$$^{•-}$ through SET followed by deprotonation in the presence of $S_2O_8^{2-}$. The radical (29^a) resonate with sulfonyl radical (29^b), which on an addition to the double bond of acrylamide (17), generated the alkyl radical (17^a). 17^a on intramolecular cyclization gave 17^b followed by oxidative deprotonation in the presence of SO$_4$$^{•-}$ providing the required product 30.

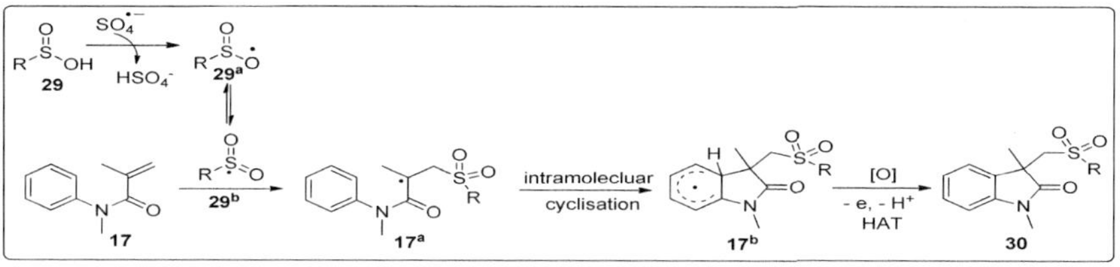

1.3.8 SYNTHESIS OF SUBSTITUTED DIHYDROFURANS THROUGH HYDROGEN ATOM ABSTRACTION BY SULFATE RADICAL ANION

After that, Guo in 2015 (Scheme 1.9) [15] revealed the synthesis of substituted dihydrofurans (**32**) through cascade radical addition of 1,3-dicarbonyl compounds (**25**) with styrenes (**31**) followed by cyclization resulting in the formation of the desired product in moderate to high yields. A variety of non-activated alkenes with substituents at the ortho (**32a**), meta (**32b**), and para (**32c**) positions of aryl ring were very much acknowledged. α-methyl styrenes (**32d**) with quaternary carbon center were acquired. The protocol was well amenable to cyclized product (**32e**) for 1-H indene.

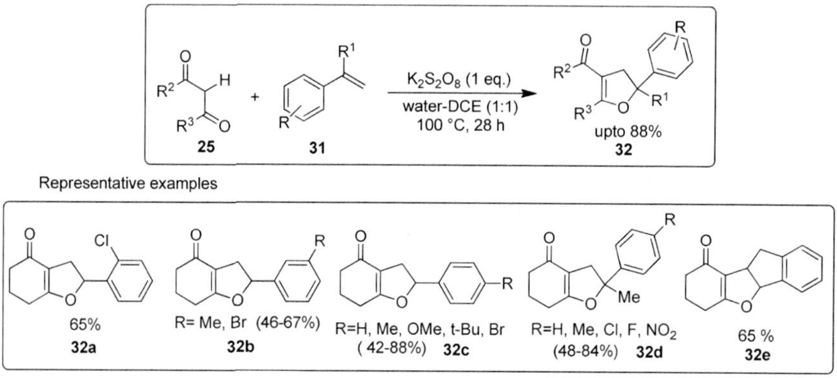

SCHEME 1.9   Transition metal-free synthesis of dihydrofurans by radical cyclization of 1,3-Dicarbonyl Compounds with Styrenes in aqueous media.

1.3.8.1 MECHANISM

$S_2O_8^{2-}$ on homolytic cleavage in the presence of heat generated the $SO_4^{\bullet-}$ that abstract hydrogen atom from dione (**25**) to form carbon radical (**25a**). **25a** attacked the double bond of styrene (**31**) to form radical (**31a**) that was converted to carbocation intermediate (**31b**) through oxidation by $SO_4^{\bullet-}$. The carbocation (**31b**) with loss of proton and intramolecular cyclization formed the desired product **32**.

1.3.9 SYNTHESIS OF β-ALKYNYLATED KETONES THROUGH HYDROGEN ATOM ABSTRACTION BY SULFATE RADICAL ANION

The combination of strained cycloalkanes with hypervalent alkylating agents was first announced by Duan et al. in 2015 (Scheme 1.10) [16]. The series of β, γ, δ alkynylated ketones (35^1–35^3) were synthesized by radical tandem ring-opening of tertiary cycloalkanols (33) followed by coupling with alkynyl hypervalent iodide reagent EBX (ethynyl-1,2-benziodoxol-3(1H- one) (34) through a succession of C-C bond cleavage and formation.

Cyclopropanols with different groups at the para position of benzene (35^1a) and benzyl ring (35^1b) were tolerated yielding β alkynylated ketones (35^1). Similarly, δ alkynylated ketones (35^2) were successfully synthesized using this green transition metal-free protocol by the reaction of series of cyclobutanols. The cyclopentanone that is somehow less strained yielded δ alkylated ketones (35^3) in the presence of silver salts.

A similar procedure of the ring-opening of cycloalkanes was then reported in 2016 by Li-Na Guo and group for the synthesis of oxindoles (Scheme 1.10) [17]. The authors reported the oxidative ring opening of strained cycloalkanols (33) followed by tandem radical cyclization of N arylacrylamides (17) in one pot procedure resulting in the formation of alkylated oxindoles (36) incorporating the remote carbonyl group via C-C bond cleavage and two new C-C bond formations. Cyclopropanols with varied electron-donating and withdrawing groups at the para position of benzene (36a) were very much acknowledged. After that, varied functional groups on the ortho (36b), as well as para (36c) position of the aniline moiety, were amiable to this transformation together with varied N-protecting groups (36d). Using this protocol, less strained cyclopentanol furnished no product.

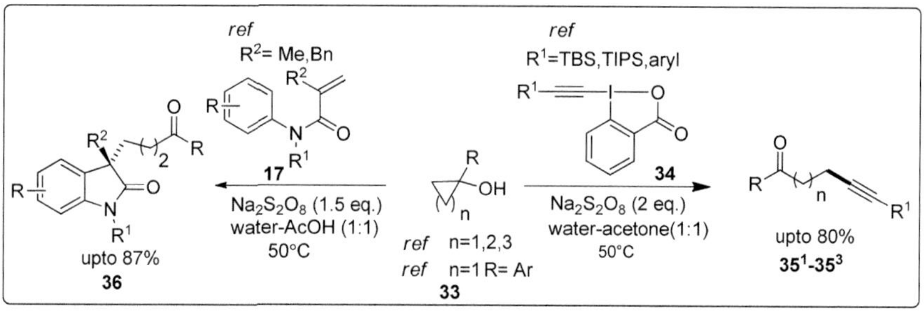

Representative examples:

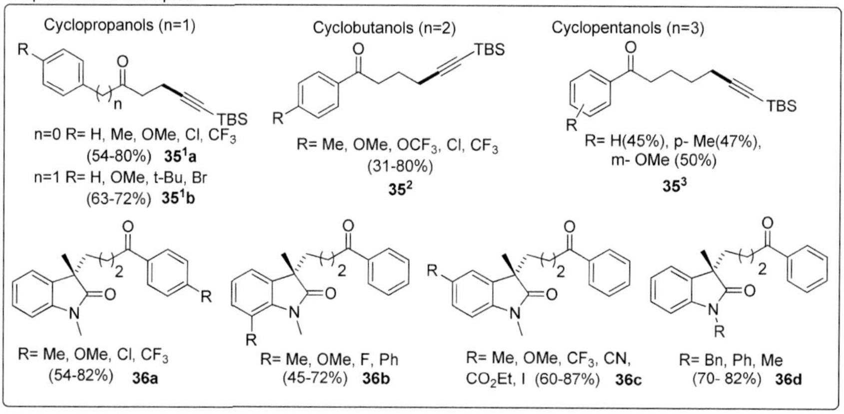

SCHEME 1.10 Transition metal-free persulfate mediated synthesis of alkylated oxindoles by the reaction of N-arylacrylamides with tertiary cycloalkanols in an aqueous medium.

1.3.9.1 MECHANISM

Upon thermolysis, persulfate salt decomposed to $SO_4^{\bullet-}$. The single-electron oxidation by $SO_4^{\bullet-}$ from cycloalkanol (**33**) produced oxygen centered radical (**33^a**), which on further arrangement gave keto radical (**33^b**). This radical attacked the double bond of acrylamide (**17**), providing the alkyl radical (**17^a**) and then aryl radical intermediate (**17^b**) by intramolecular cyclization. **17^b** on oxidative deprotonation gave alkylated oxindoles (**36**). Also, the attack of keto radical (**33^b**) on the triple bond of (**34**) gave alkyl radical (**34ª**). Then β elimination afforded the alkynylated product (**36**) and intermediate (**34ᵇ**), which on reductive protonation gave two iodobenzoic acids (**34ᶜ**).

1.3.10   ARYL RADICALS THROUGH HYDROGEN ATOM ABSTRACTION BY SULFATE RADICAL ANION

Aryl boronic acids (**38**) being stable, readily obtainable substrates have been employed by Ilangovan in 2015 (Scheme 1.11) [18] for the preparation of arylquinones (**39**) by direct C(sp²)–H functionalization of quinones (**37**) with boronic acids (**38**) in an aqueous medium using $K_2S_2O_8$.

Boronic acids with a variety of functional groups at para (**39a**) and ortho (**39b**) positions furnished products in good yields. As per the quinone derivatives, 2,6-dimethoxy (**39c**) and 2-methyl substituted (**39d**) were also acceptable. After that, this convention was applied to 1,4- naphthoquinone in the presence of a base and a good yield of 45% obtained with **39e**. The reaction was well applicable on the gram scale level with 61% yield using 3.1g of substrate permitting huge-scale use of this convention.

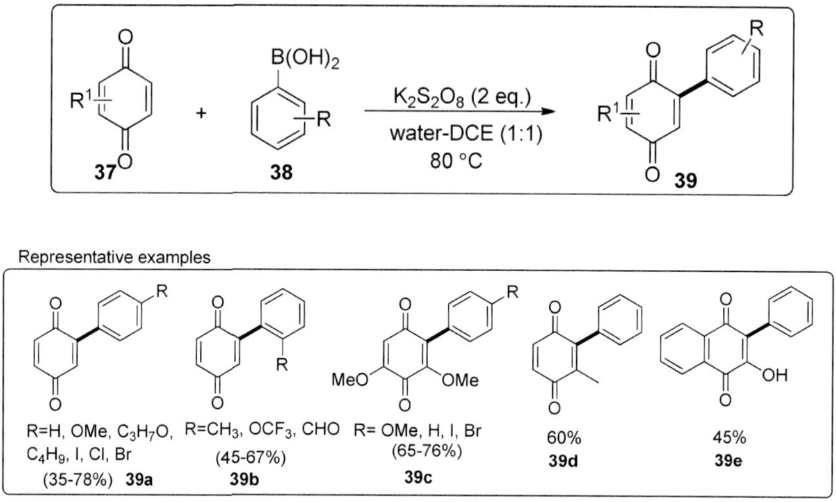

Representative examples

SCHEME 1.11   Transition metal-free persulfate mediated C-H functionalization of quinines with aryl boronic acids in an aqueous medium.

1.3.10.1   MECHANISM

Boronic acid (**38**) through HAT by $SO_4^{\bullet-}$ generated the aryl radical (**38ª**). This radical (**38ª**) on reaction with quinone (**37**) gave alkyl radical (**37ª**) following oxidative deprotonation by $SO_4^{\bullet-}$ gave product (**39**).

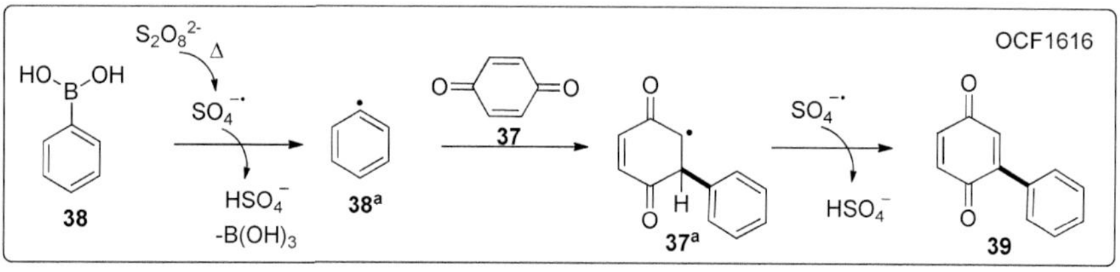

1.3.11   ALIPHATIC C-H BOND OXIDATION BY HYDROGEN ATOM ABSTRACTION BY SULFATE RADICAL ANION

In continuation of C-H functionalization protocols, Shi et al. in 2016 (Scheme 1.12) [19] demonstrated the transition metal-free oxidation of phthaloyl protected primary amines and amino acid derivatives (**22**) to corresponding carbonyl compounds (**40**) with high regioselectivity with the help of persulfate as initiator as well as an oxidizing agent.

The differing amino acids (AAs) (**40a**), including cyclic substrates (**40b**) were altogether continued with good functional group tolerance. Similar is the case with varied amines (**40c, d**). In the case of substrates with tertiary CH bonds (**40e**), hydroxyl derivatives were obtained instead of carbonyl compounds. With O^{18} labeling experiments, it was found that O of carbonyl comes from water. The reaction was also extended to gram scale levels.

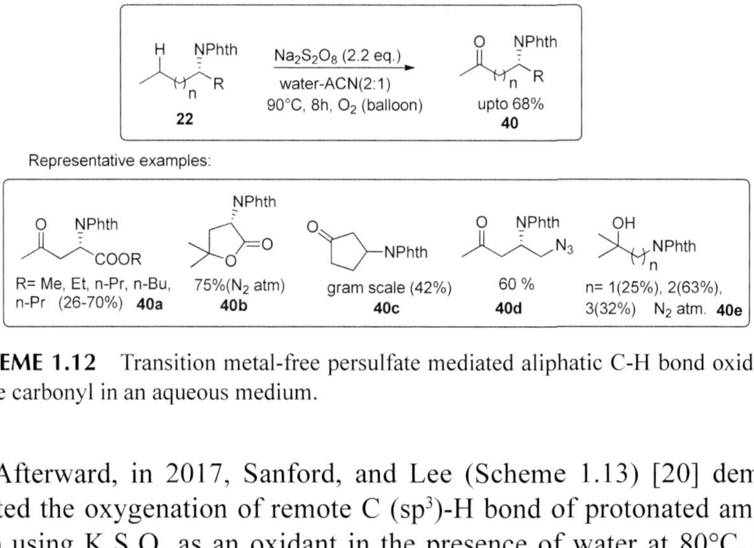

SCHEME 1.12   Transition metal-free persulfate mediated aliphatic C-H bond oxidation to the carbonyl in an aqueous medium.

Afterward, in 2017, Sanford, and Lee (Scheme 1.13) [20] demonstrated the oxygenation of remote C (sp³)-H bond of protonated amines (**41**) using $K_2S_2O_8$ as an oxidant in the presence of water at 80°C. The authors explored that protonation of amines (**41**) with the assistance of sulfuric acid was carried out so as to make N group strongly electron-withdrawing, thereby deactivating the C(sp³)-H bond. Primary (**42a**), secondary (**42b**), tertiary (**42c**) amine substrates with good functional group tolerance were hydroxylated. It was found that higher selectivity was acquired in the case of protonated amines with tertiary C-H bond at a separation of 2 or 3 carbon atoms from N (**42d**). The ecological protocol was relevant in the late-stage oxidation of pharmaceutical important drugs like memantine (Alzheimer's drug), pregabalin (epilepsy drug), and leucine (important amino acid).

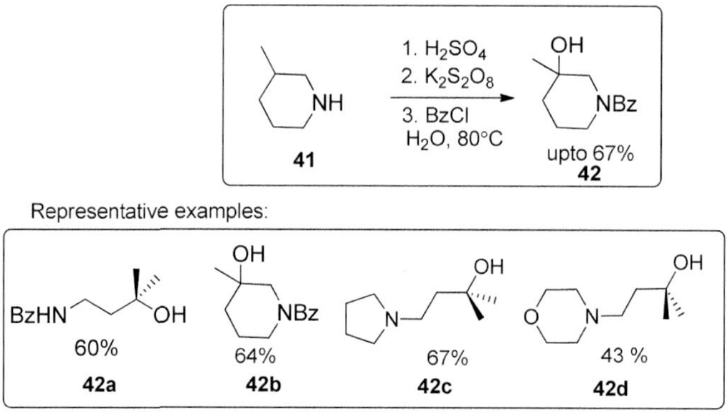

SCHEME 1.13   Transition metal-free persulfate mediated oxygenation of C(sp³)-H bond of protonated aliphatic amines in an aqueous medium.

1.3.11.1   MECHANISM

The $SO_4{}^{\bullet-}$ abstract the hydrogen atom from **22** to form alkyl radical (**22ª**), which again on oxidation by $SO_4{}^{\bullet-}$ gave carbocation (**22ᵇ**). Then alcohol (**22ᶜ**) was formed by the nucleophilic attack of water, which on further oxidation, provided the ketone (**40**) as the final product.

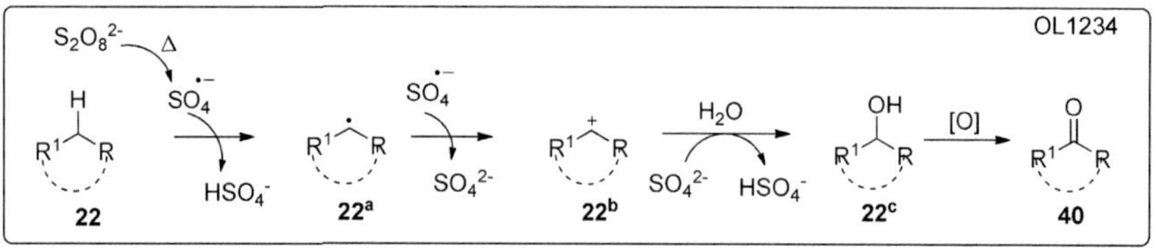

1.3.12   SYNTHESIS OF N-HETEROCYCLIC COMPOUNDS THROUGH HYDROGEN ATOM ABSTRACTION BY SULFATE RADICAL ANION

Wang group takes forward the eco-friendly protocol for the synthesis of N-heterocyclic compounds. In 2016, N-aryl-2-quinolinones (**44**) were synthesized via cascade intramolecular C(sp²)-H amidation of

Knoevenagel products (**43**) in a biphasic solvent mixture of n-butyl acetate and water (Scheme 1.14) [21].

The varied substituents on the phenyl ring of the benzylidene group of Knoevenagel products were investigated. Para substituted substrates (**44a**) were extremely compatible, but meta-substituted provided a mixture of regiomeric products (**44b**). Aniline ring with both electrons donating and withdrawing groups provided the corresponding product (**44c**) in good yields. Good reactivity was obtained in the case of sterically hindered substrates (**44d**) too. It was discovered that the cleavage of the C-H bond is not the rate deciding step, and it was investigated by the kinetic isotope effect.

Further effective aza analogs of phenanthridines were accounted for by the same group in 2017. Wang et al. (Scheme 1.15) [22] reported the synthesis of benzo[c][2,7]naphthyridine-6-ones (**47**) from 1,4-dihydropyridines (DHP) (**45**) by means of cascade C(sp^2)-H amidation process in 1.5 h only when refluxed at 80°C.

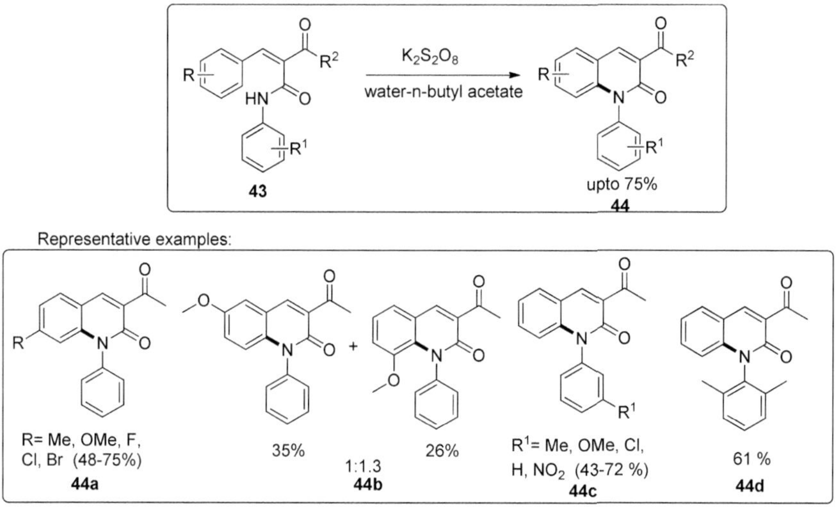

SCHEME 1.14   Transition metal-free persulfate mediated synthesis of N-Aryl 2-Quinolinones from Knoevenagel Products by Intramolecular C (sp^2)–H amidation in an aqueous medium.

Substituents at para (**47a**) and meta (**47b**) position of the phenyl ring of DHP were very much endured, yet sterically hindered ortho substituents provided no yield. The substituents at the aniline moiety of DHP (**47c**) were acceptable in good yields. Also, substituents with two amide groups (**47d**) functioned admirably.

Similarly, Wang et al. (Scheme 1.15) [23] reported the oxidative intramolecular cyclization of easily accessible Friedländer products, 4aryl-quinoline-3-carboxamides (**46**) to diverse functionalized dibenzo[2,7] naphthyridinones (**47**) under catalyst-free conditions in 32–78% yields. The authors researched the ortho-cyclization of quinoline derivatives providing corresponding products in good to moderate yields. The protocol worked well with the para-substituted quinoline derivatives (**47e**), m-substituted (**47f**) provided cyclization product in satisfactorily yield at less obstructed site whereas ortho-substituted (**47g**) failed to furnish any product. The diverse groups on the meta (**47h**) and para (**47i**) position of

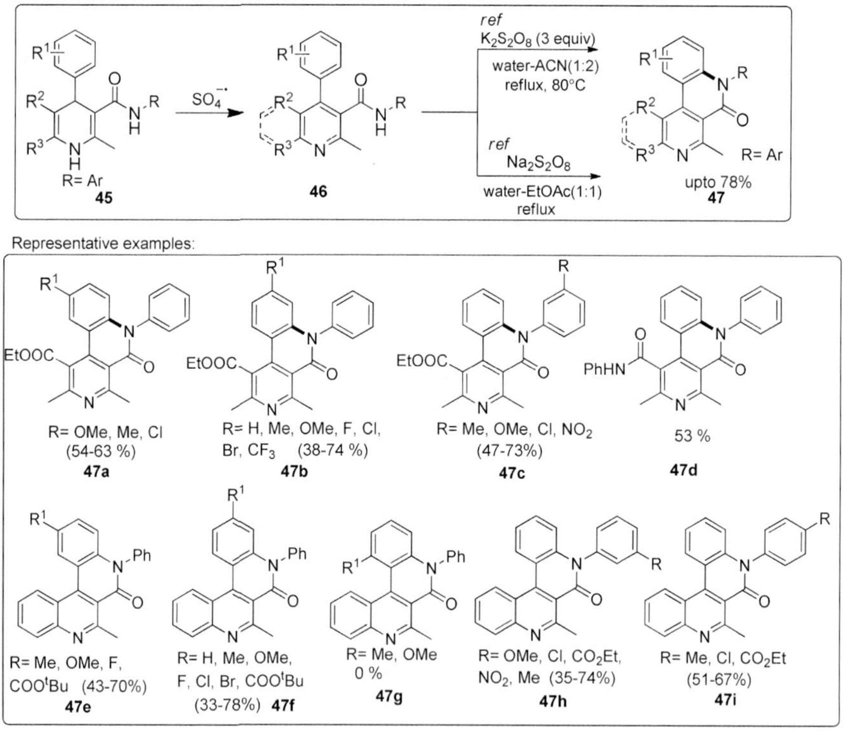

SCHEME 1.15 Transition metal-free persulfate mediated synthesis of benzo[*c*][2,7] naphthyridine-6-ones via C(sp^2)- H amidation of DHP derivatives in aqueous acetonitrile solution.

the aniline ring were also explored. The authors also investigated that the spiro product was obtained under the same optimizing conditions but by using silver salt $AgNO_3$. This silver salt mediated transformation brought about ipso-cyclization of quinoline derivatives instead of ortho-cyclization. Then O^{18} labeling experiments were conducted in the presence of H_2O^{18} to investigate that oxygen of carbonyl group originated from water, not from the persulfate salt.

1.3.12.1 MECHANISM

The thermal decomposition of persulfate salt produced the $SO_4^{\bullet-}$. Dihydropyridine (45) through oxidative deprotonation by $SO_4^{\bullet-}$ gave radical intermediate (45ᵃ), which further in the presence of $SO_4^{\bullet-}$ produces carboxamide (46). Then, hydrogen abstraction from the substrate (46) produced amidyl radical intermediate (46ᵃ). This radical (46ᵃ) on intramolecular ortho cyclization produce aryl radical (46ᵇ). Finally, hydrogen abstraction by $SO_4^{\bullet-}$ yielded the required product (47).

Carbazoles, a fused heterocyclic compound, have varied applications in the field of medical science as it possesses potent biological activities like antimalarial, antibiotic, psychotropic, and so forth, likewise having huge applications in the field of material science for the syntheses of organic electronics. In 2017, we (Scheme 1.16) [24] discovered the transition metal-free persulfate mediated approach for the synthesis of substituted carbazoles (49) in water by means of intramolecular radical cyclization of N substituted 2-aminobiaryls (48) through C(sp²)-H functionalization and C-N bond formation. The reaction advanced under a nitrogen atmosphere with the use of phase transfer catalyst TBAB, which on reaction with Na$_2$S$_2$O$_8$ provided TBAPS (tetrabutylammonium persulfate), which acted as an oxidant in all the transformations.

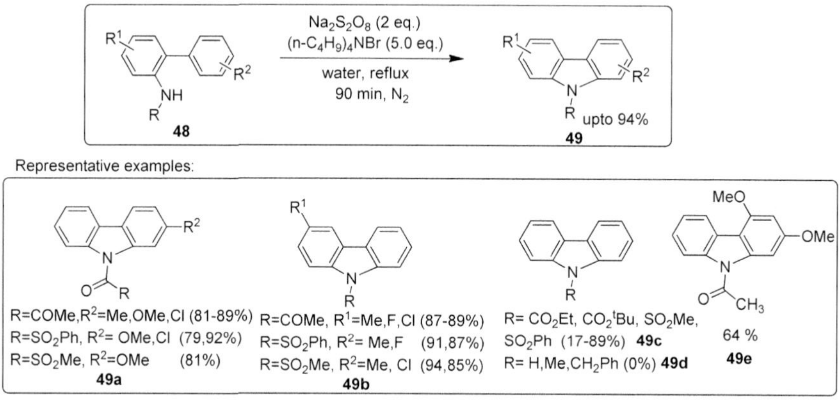

Representative examples:

SCHEME 1.16 Transition metal-free persulfate mediated synthesis of carbazoles by intramolecular oxidative cyclization of N-substituted 2-aminobiaryls in water as a solvent.

1.3.12.2   MECHANISM

The homolytic cleavage of persulfate salt produces SO$_4$•− which on hydrogen abstraction from **48** generated the aminyl radical (**48^a**). **48^a** on intramolecular cyclization produce aryl radical (**48^b**) followed by oxidative deprotonation in the presence of SO$_4$•− resulting in the formation of cyclized product (**49**).

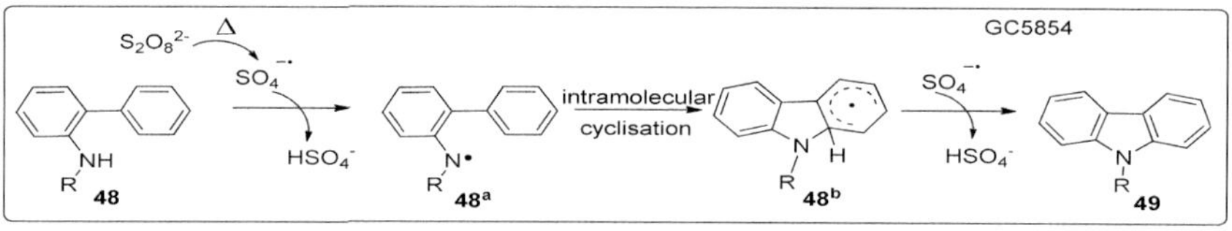

1.3.13   SYNTHESIS OF BIARYLS THROUGH HYDROGEN ATOM ABSTRACTION BY SULFATE RADICAL ANION

In 2017, Jegan Mohan, and associates (Scheme 1.17) [25] detailed the oxidative homocoupling of phenols and naphthols in the biphasic solvent system of ACN/water employing persulfate as potent oxidant and a radical initiator. The reaction brought about the formation of unsymmetrical quinone derivatives (**39**) and para-para coupling biphenols (**51**). However, if trifluoroacetic acid is used instead of this solvent mixture, biphenols, and binaphthols were the significant products.

Varied substituted phenols were screened in aqueous ACN solution in the presence of $K_2S_2O_8$. The authors explored that π-π coupling product was obtained from 2,6-dimethyl and 2,6-dimethoxy phenols; however, o-substituted phenols and naphthols provided quinoid coupling products, and meta-substituted gave quinoline derivatives. For 2-methyl phenol, the reaction was scaled up to gram levels with a yield of 55% (580 mg) from 1 g of the substrate.

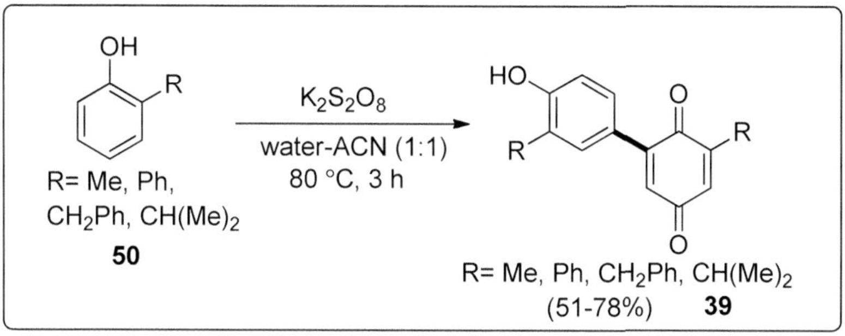

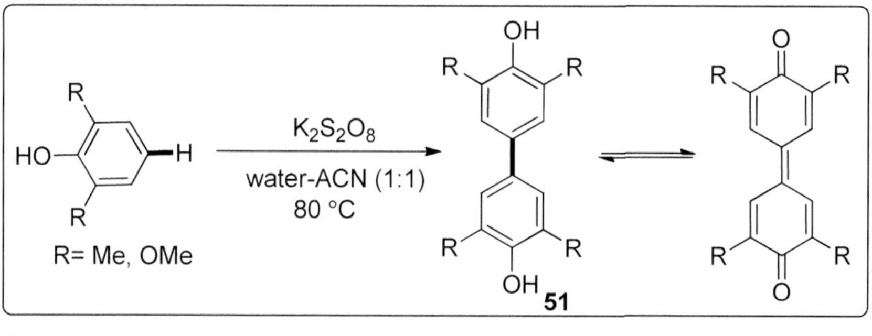

SCHEME 1.17 Transition metal-free persulfate mediated synthesis of biphenols and binaphthols by oxidative coupling reaction in an aqueous medium.

1.3.13.1 MECHANISM

Persulfate on activation with heat produces sulfate radical anion. This radical anion through proton abstraction from substrate generates phenoxyl radical intermediate which coupled with the similar radical to give symmetrical biphenols.

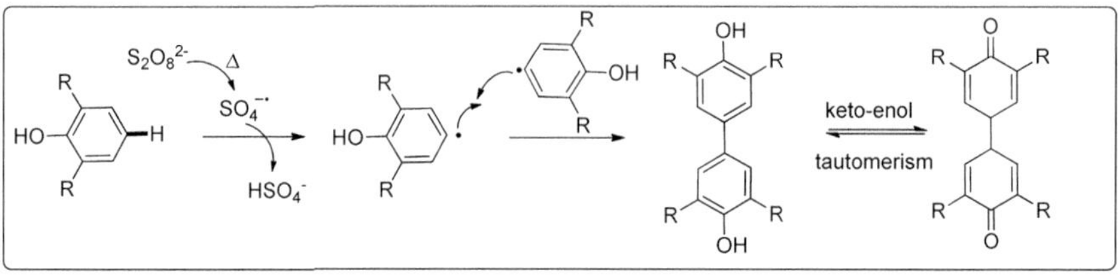

1.4 HYDROGEN ABSTRACTION BY SULFATE RADICAL ANION FOLLOWED BY DECARBOXYLATION

Carboxylic acids being steady, flexible, inexpensive, effectively available turned out to be the best choice for alkyl radical formation after the expulsion of non-toxic CO_2.

1.4.1 SYNTHESIS OF THIOESTERS THROUGH HYDROGEN ABSTRACTION BY SULFATE RADICAL ANION FOLLOWED BY DECARBOXYLATION

Organosulphur compounds are extremely important biological compounds vastly used in anti-toxin drugs, so the preparation of S containing moiety is of enormous interest for scientific experts. Wang and co-workers in 2015 (Scheme 1.18) [26] discovered the transition metal-free arylthiation of α-keto acids (52) with thiols (53) through one-pot oxidative radical decarboxylation

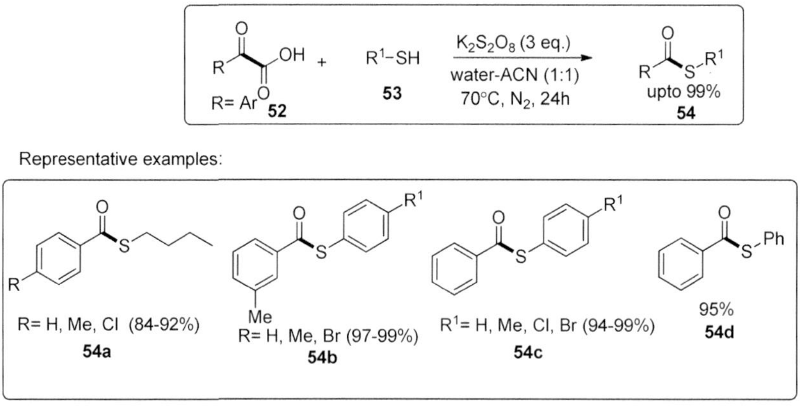

Representative examples:

SCHEME 1.18 Transition metal-free persulfate mediated decarboxylative coupling of α-keto acids with thiols in an aqueous medium.

leading to the formation of thioesters (**54**) with extrusion of CO_2 as the only by-product. Aromatic keto acids with varied groups at para (**54a**) and ortho (**54b**) position were acceptable. Similar is the case of aromatic (**54c**) and aliphatic (**54a**) thiols. Reaction with radical scavenger TEMPO demonstrated the radical mechanism, yet it was found that the reaction did not proceed via the condensation process. The reaction is also relevant for the gram-scale synthesis of thioesters (**54d**) in 96% yield with 1.03 g of the substrate taken.

1.4.1.1   MECHANISM

The $SO_4{}^{\bullet-}$ formed by thermal decomposition of $S_2O_8{}^{2-}$. The $SO_4{}^{\bullet-}$ through hydrogen atom abstraction generated thiyl radical (**53ª**) and acyl radical (**52ª**) on decarboxylation, which further on coupling provided the desired product (**54**).

1.4.2   SYNTHESIS OF ALKYNONES THROUGH HYDROGEN ABSTRACTION BY SULFATE RADICAL ANION FOLLOWED BY DECARBOXYLATION

In 2015, Duan, and co-workers (Scheme 1.19) reported the persulfate mediated decarboxylative alkynylation of α-keto acids (**52**) and oxamic acids (**52'**) with hypervalent ethynylbenziodoxolone (EBX) (**34**) as efficacious alkylating agents endowing ynones (**55**) and propiolamides (**55'**) in excellent yields.

The substrate scope revealed that stearic hindrance and electronic effect has little influence on the activity as good results were obtained with all ortho (**55a**), meta (**55b**), para (**55c**) substituted phenylglyoxylic acids. Substituted alkynyl reagents (**55d**) were all compatible however oxamic acids gave corresponding propiolamides (**55'c**) in lower yields, but yield somehow can be increased with the use of silver nitrate.

Later on, the effective synthesis of ynones (**55**) using stable starting materials in an aqueous medium with low-cost persulfate was demonstrated by Xu et al. in 2015. The authors envisioned the synthesis of ynones (**55**) through decarboxylative alkynylation of α keto acid (**52**) with EBX (**34**) as alkyne source (Scheme 1.19) [27].

α-keto acids with ortho (**55e**), meta (**55f**), and para (**55g**) substitution on benzene ring worked well. Also, alkyne bearing alkyl, aryl, and bulky silyl groups (**55h**) were all accepted.

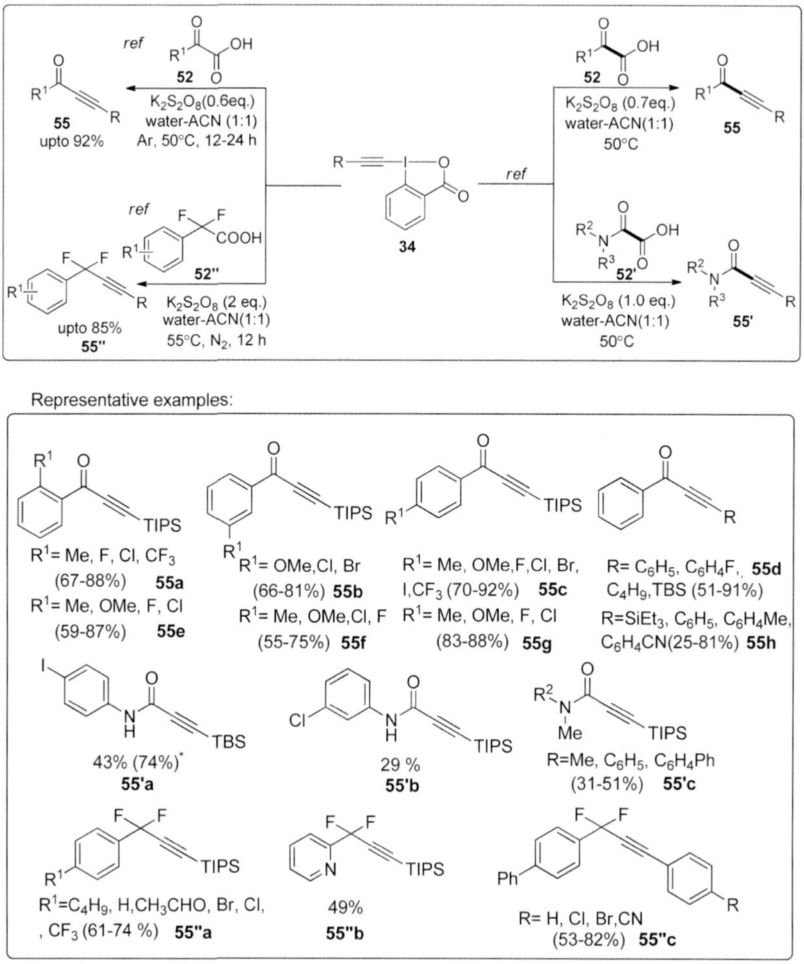

Representative examples:

SCHEME 1.19 Transition metal-free persulfate mediated syntheses of α,α-difluoro-methylated alkynes by direct decarboxylative alkynylation in aqueous media.

In 2016, Wua, and associates (Scheme 1.19) [28] envisioned greener system for the decarboxylative alkynylation of α,α difluoroarylacetic acids (52") with EBX (34) as hypervalent alkynylating agents furnishing α,α difluoromethylated alkynes (55") with varied functional group tolerance.

Difluoroarylacetic acids bearing varied groups on the aryl ring (55"a) functioned admirably, including N heteroaromatic ones (55"b). The various hypervalent alkynyl reagents like aryl (55"c) and alkyl (55"d) substituted EBX were tolerated in good yields. The radical mechanism was affirmed by control experiments with TEMPO/BHT.

1.4.2.1 MECHANISM

The thermolysis of persulfate salt produced $SO_4^{\cdot-}$. This was converted to HSO_4^- by abstraction of hydrogen atom from carboxylic acid (52). The carboxyl radical (52ª) so formed underwent decarboxylation to give radical (52ᵇ). This radical (52ᵇ) attacked the triple bond of alkynyl reagent (34) to give intermediate (34ª). This provided the desired alkynyl product (55) and radical (34ᵇ) through β elimination, afterwards reductive protonation of (34ᵇ) gave 2-iodobenzoic acid (34ᶜ).

1.4.3 SYNTHESIS OF AZAFLUORENONES AND FLUORENONES THROUGH HYDROGEN ABSTRACTION BY SULFATE RADICAL ANION FOLLOWED BY DECARBOXYLATION

Although intermolecular minisci reaction with improved reaction conditions has been accounted for by many research groups, at the same time, intramolecular minisci acylation reaction under transition metal-free environment is still under progress. The synthesis of azafluorenones (**57¹**) and fluorenones (**57²**) was exhibited by Laha et al. in 2017 through intra-molecular decarboxylative acylation of arenes or inactivated pyridines with α-oxocarboxylic acids (**56**) (Scheme 1.20) [29].

α-oxocarboxylic acids with diverse functional groups on arene (**57¹a**) and N-heteroarene (**57¹b**) yielded a mixture of 1-azafluorenone and 3-azafluorenone. However, methyl, and aldehyde groups provided 1-azafluorenone (**57¹c**) exclusively. Further, fluorenones (**57²**) have been synthesized using the same methodology with varied functional group tolerance. Screening tests showed that better yields were obtained with electron-rich α-oxycarboxylic acids (**57²a**) as compared to the electron-poor substrates (**57²b**).

Also, it was demonstrated by the cross experiments that intramolecular acylation reaction was preferred over intermolecular acylation. The reaction could also be scaled up to gram level with a yield of 78% from 1.36 grams of substrates.

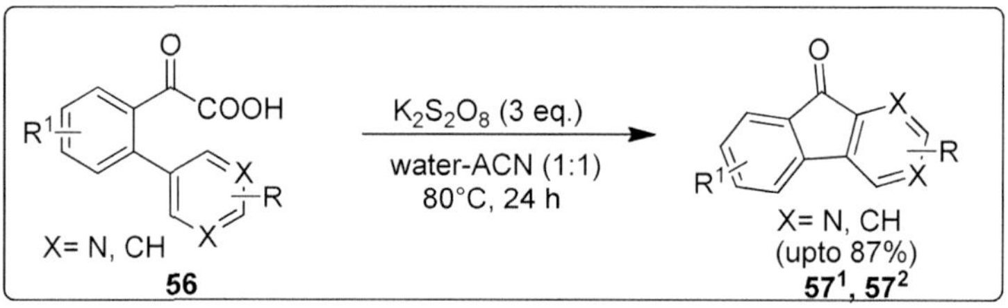

Representative examples:

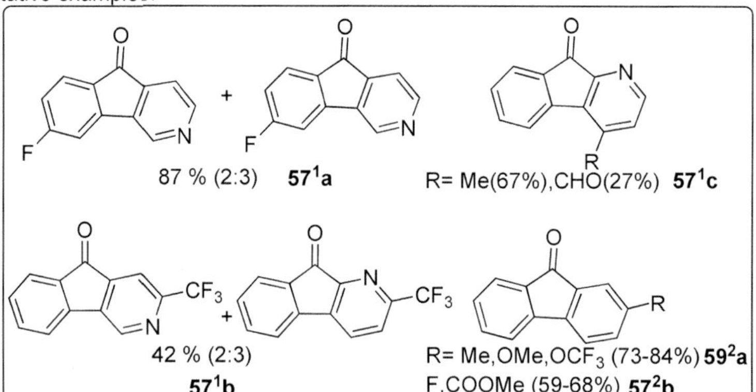

SCHEME 1.20 Transition metal-free persulfate mediated synthesis of azafluorenones and fluorenones through intramolecular decarbonylation in an aqueous medium.

1.4.3.1 MECHANISM

The hydrogen atom abstraction by $SO_4{}^{\bullet-}$ from **56** followed by decarboxylation produced the acyl radical **56^a**, which underwent intramolecular cyclization leading to aryl radical **56^b**, which on HAT to $SO_4{}^{\bullet-}$ gave desired product **57**.

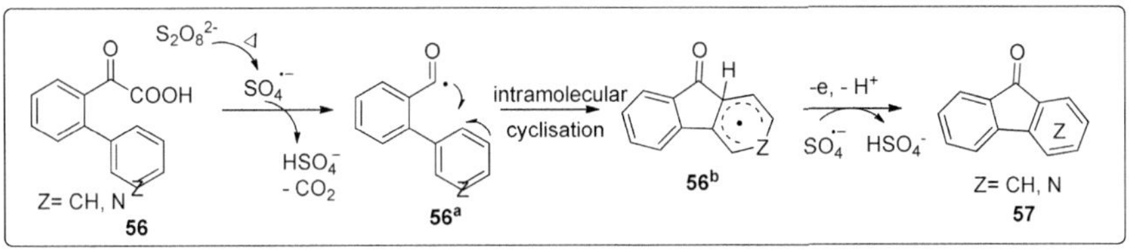

1.4.4 SYNTHESIS OF BENZOYLATED ISOQUINOLINES THROUGH HYDROGEN ABSTRACTION BY SULFATE RADICAL ANION FOLLOWED BY DECARBOXYLATION

The C (sp^2)H functionalization of isoquinolines (**3**) alongside some other N-heteroarenes with the help of α-keto acids (**52**) as acylating agents were accounted for by Singh and Chaubey in 2017 for the synthesis of C1 benzoylated isoquinolines (**3^{52}**) employing green solvent water at 100°C for 6 hours (Scheme 1.21) [30].

The protocol worked well with para-substituted arylglycoxylic acid (**3^{52}a**) as well as sterically congested mesityl glyoxylic acids (**3^{52}b**);

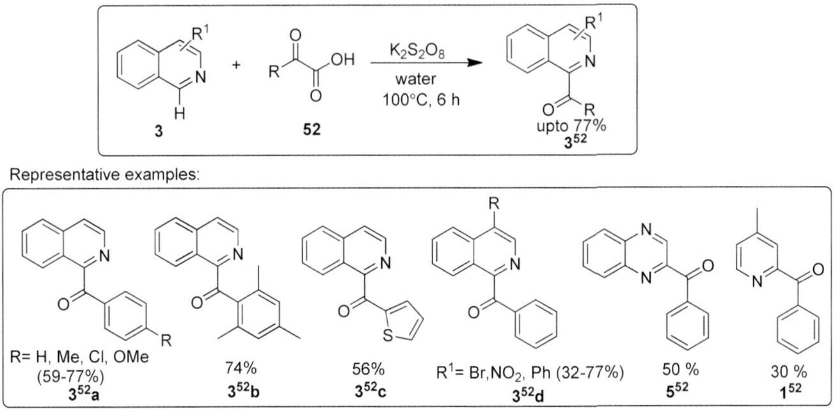

Representative examples:

SCHEME 1.21 Transition metal-free persulfate mediated decarboxylative acylation of isoquinolines in an aqueous medium.

however, lower product yield was obtained with heteroaromatic keto acid (3^{52}c). Also, isoquinolines with different substituents at C-4 position (3^{52}d) were compatible. Apart from it, acylation of quinoxaline (5^{52}) and pyridine derivatives (1^{52}) were also obtained.

1.4.4.1 MECHANISM

S$_2$O$_8^{2-}$ in the presence of heat gave SO$_4$$^{\bullet-}$. The hydrogen atom abstraction from keto acid (52) by SO$_4$$^{\bullet-}$ gave 52^a followed by decarboxylation yielded acyl radical (52^b). 52^b reacted with protonated heteroarenes (3) to give intermediate (3^a), which in the presence of base and SO$_4$$^{\bullet-}$ yielded required product (3^{52}).

1.4.5 SYNTHESIS OF KETONES THROUGH HYDROGEN ABSTRACTION BY SULFATE RADICAL ANION FOLLOWED BY DECARBOXYLATION

The synthesis of aldehydes and ketones (59) that are crucial substrates for divergent chemical transformations has been revealed by Bhat et al. in 2017 through transition metal-free, persulfate intervened oxidative decarboxylation of arylacetic acids (58) in water via direct decarboxylation of sp^3 hybridized carbon at 90°C for 12 h in open atmosphere (Scheme 1.22) [31]. Ibuprofen, a marketed medication has been converted to the corresponding ketones using this procedure.

Arylacetic acids with diverse groups (59a) were well endured, including naphthyl (59b) and heteroaromatic acids (59c). Apart from it, different phenylacetic acids (59d) were also acceptable. O^{18} labeled aldehydes/ketones can easily be prepared using this viable methodology without the need for any exchange experiments. The reaction was also applicable to the gram scale level.

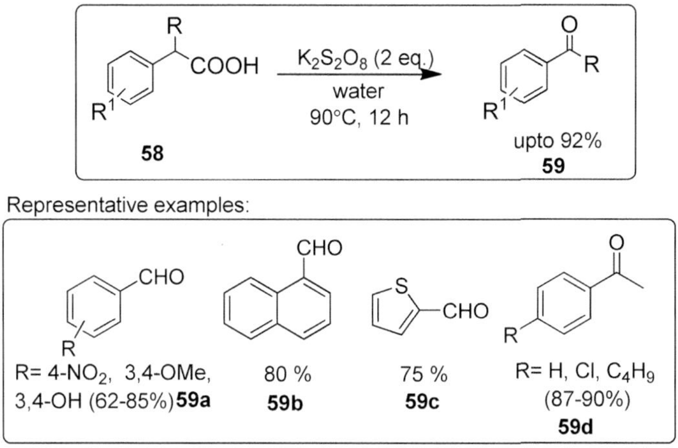

SCHEME 1.22 Transition metal-free persulfate mediated oxidative decarboxylation of aryl acetic acids in water.

1.4.5.1 MECHANISM

The homolytic cleavage of $K_2S_2O_8$ produces $SO_4^{\bullet-}$. This $SO_4^{\bullet-}$ through HAT and release of carbon dioxide from the substrate (**58**) gave **58ª**. This alkyl radical (**58ª**) in the presence of water and $SO_4^{\bullet-}$ gave (**58ᵇ**), which lead to the formation of carbocation (**58ᶜ**) and finally the required ketone (**59**) through oxidative deprotonation.

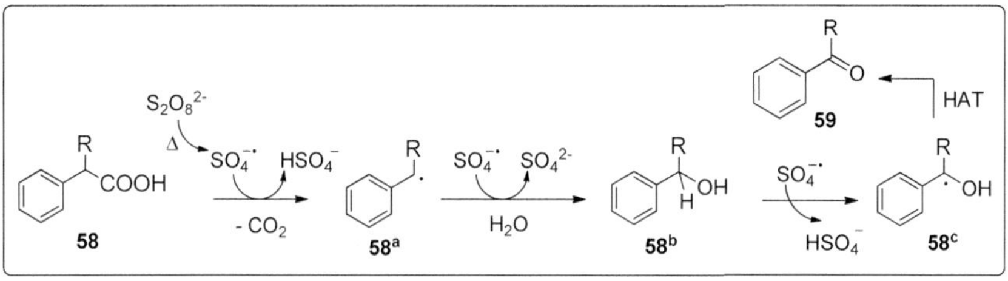

1.4.6 SYNTHESIS OF TRIFLUOROMETHYL ARENES THROUGH HYDROGEN ABSTRACTION BY SULFATE RADICAL ANION FOLLOWED BY DECARBOXYLATION

Taking forward the syntheses of trifluoromethylated arenes, Gong et al. in 2017 (Scheme 1.23) [32] revealed decarboxylative trifluoromethylation/ perfluoroalkylation of benzoic acid derivatives (**60**) utilizing modest and effortlessly accessible Langlois reagent (61) as CF_3 source in aqueous media at room temperature to such an extent that mixture of mono and di-substituted products (62) were obtained in all cases with great functional group tolerance. The reaction can be scaled up to gram level with a 68% yield.

The benzoic acids were trifluoromethylated/perfluoroalkylated in such a way that lower yields were obtained with sterically hindered aromatic acids (62b, 62d) than simple ones (62a, 62c). The reaction was highly selective in nature that asymmetric benzoic acids (62e) gave in situ generated products as major ones, and it was minor in the case of symmetric acids (62f).

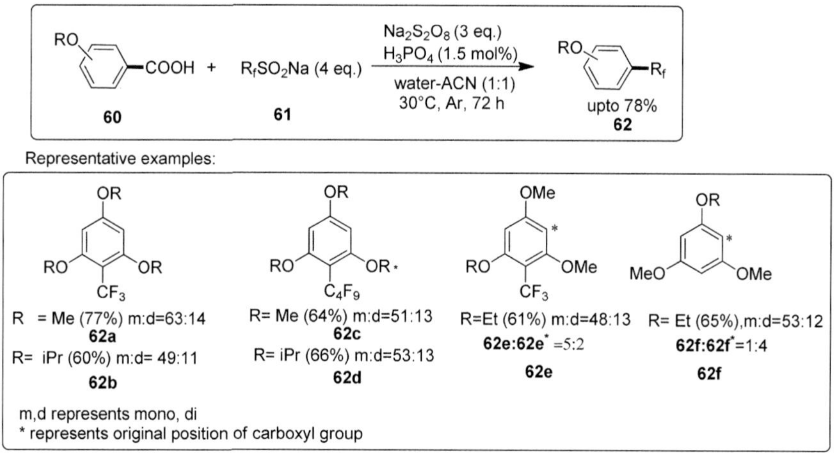

SCHEME 1.23   Transition metal-free persulfate mediated decarboxylative fluoroalkylation of benzoic acid derivatives in an aqueous medium.

1.4.6.1   MECHANISM

At first, $SO_4^{•-}$ was formed by the thermolysis of persulfate salt. In one step, $SO_4^{•-}$ through hydrogen atom abstraction from 60 followed by decarboxylation produced radical (60ᵃ). 60ᵃ in the presence of water formed 60ᵇ. Simultaneously, on the other hand, the CF_3 radical (61ᵃ) was formed by single elctron transfer from CF_3SO_2Na to $SO_4^{•-}$ with the release of SO_2. The CF_3 radical attacked on 60ᵇ resulting in the formation of intermediate (**60ᶜ**) that occurs in resonance with **60ᵈ**. The radical (**60ᶜ**) on hydrogen atom abstraction by $SO_4{}^{\bullet-}$ provided required product **62**.

1.5 ONE-ELECTRON OXIDATION BY SULFATE RADICAL ANION

1.5.1 OXYSULFONYLATION OF ALKENES VIA ONE-ELECTRON OXIDATION BY SULFATE RADICAL ANION

With the upsurge of radical chemistry in the field of organic synthesis, cheap, and green oxidants for the installation of O containing functionality is the need of the hour. In this shade, dioxygen is used as an effortlessly accessible, cost-effective oxidant, which in activated form can serve as the source of oxygen in organic compounds. However, with the purpose of making synthesis more reasonable, Ydav et al. in 2014 (Scheme 1.24) [33] reported the transition metal-free persulfate promoted oxysulfonylation reaction of inactivated olefins (**63**) with dioxygen and low-cost arenesulfinate salts (**64**) as sulfonylating agents in open flask at room temperature for the synthesis of β- ketosulfones (**65**).

Sulfinate salts with varied functional groups on the aryl ring (**65a**) were well tolerated. Similar is the case of alkenes with substitution on the aryl ring (**65b**) in spite of the position of the functional group (**65c**). Also, internal alkenes with substitution on both sides of the double bond (**65d**) were tolerated in good yields. From several test experiments, it was deduced that carbonyl oxygen of β- ketosulfone originated from dioxygen.

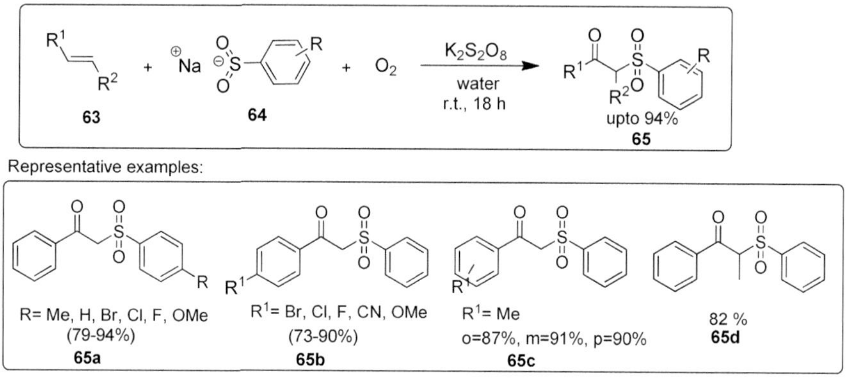

Representative examples:

R= Me, H, Br, Cl, F, OMe (79-94%) 65a	R^1= Br, Cl, F, CN, OMe (73-90%) 65b	R^1= Me o=87%, m=91%, p=90% 65c	82 % 65d

SCHEME 1.24 Transition metal-free persulfate mediated synthesis of β-ketosulfones through oxysulfonylation of alkenes in water.

1.5.1.1   MECHANISM

Initially, the sulfonate anion **64** in the presence of $SO_4^{•-}$ produced sulfonyl radical **64^a** through a one-electron oxidation process. **64^a** then attacked the double bond of alkene **63** to form alkyl radical intermediate **63^a**. Then in the presence of O_2 the oxygen centered intermediate **63^b** was formed, which lead to β hydroxyl sulfones **63^c** in the presence of $SO_4^{•-}$ and water. This **63^c** through Russel fragmentation with the loss of water and oxygen gave desired oxysulfonated compound **65**.

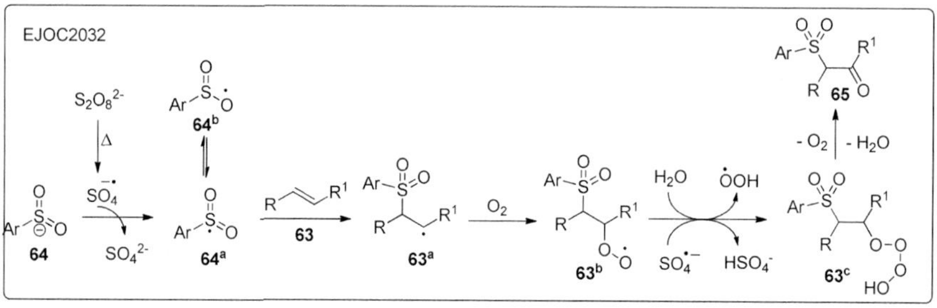

1.5.2   TRIFLUOROMETHYLATION OF N-ARYLACRYLAMIDES VIA ONE-ELECTRON OXIDATION BY SULFATE RADICAL ANION

At that point in 2014, Wang and collaborators (Scheme 1.25) [34] built up the technique for the development of trifluoromethylated oxindoles. The authors described the trifluoromethylation of N-arylacrylamides (17) for the syntheses of CF_3 containing oxindoles (19) utilizing easily accessible Langlois reagent (CF_3SO_2Na) (61) as steady solid CF_3 source in a heterogeneous reaction medium with water as co-solvent as it will expand the solubility of inorganic salts.

The moderate yields were obtained with substituents on para (19e) and ortho (19f) position of aniline moiety where, m-substituted (19g) provided a mixture of regiomers. Substrates bearing N aryl, alkyl (19h) protecting groups gave better yield than others (19i). The collection of α substituted alkenes (19j) was suitable with distinct functional groups.

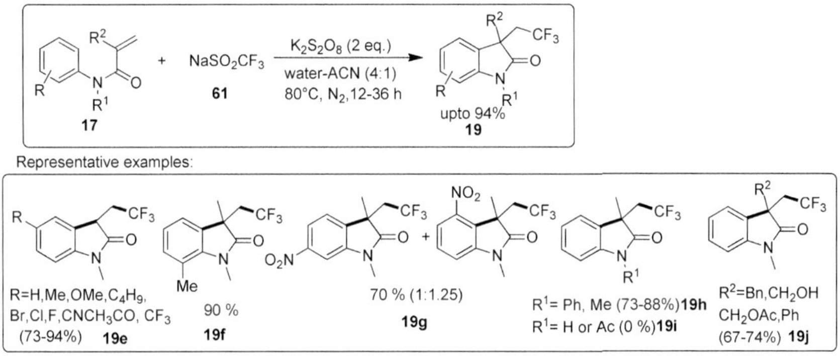

SCHEME 1.25 Transition metal-free persulfate mediated synthesis of CF_3 containing oxindoles in an aqueous medium.

Then in 2014, Zhan et al. (Scheme 1.26) [35] disclosed the synthesis of highly productive azide substituted oxindoles (67) via transition metal-free azidocarbocyclization of N-arylacrylamides (17) employing sodium azide (66) as azide source in a biphasic solution of water and acetone at 80°C for 8 h. In this paper, the authors detailed the electronic impact where higher yields were obtained for electron-donating substituents (67a) than electron-withdrawing (67b) at the para position while meta-substituted (67c) gave a mixture of regio-selective products. Stearic hindrance played its role as ortho-substituted (67d) gave comparatively lower yields. Variety of N-protecting groups (67e) were screened. Likewise, no yield was achieved on changing the heteroatom from N to O in the alkene framework. Higher yield of 94% was reported on changing the benzene ring to naphthalene (67f).

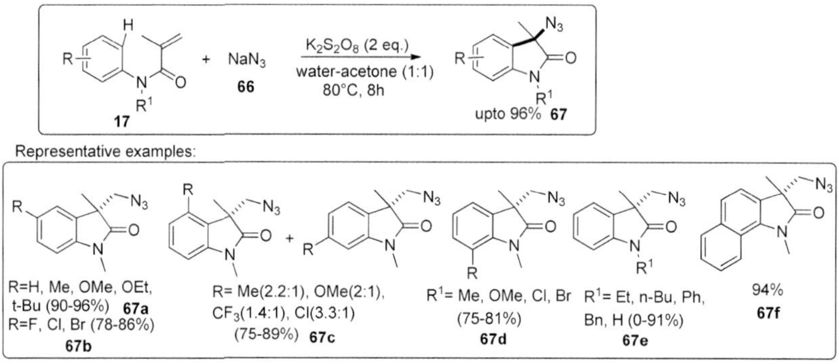

SCHEME 1.26 Transition metal-free persulfate mediated synthesis of azidooxindoles by carboazidation of acrylamides in an aqueous acetone solution.

1.5.2.1 MECHANISM

Initially, the $SO_4^{\bullet-}$ was formed through thermolytic cleavage of persulfate. The $SO_4^{\bullet-}$ through one-electron oxidation of sodium azide (66) and Langlois reagent (61) produced N_3 radical (66^a) and CF_3 radical (61^a) resp. These radicals then attacked the double bond of activated alkenes (17) to form alkyl radical intermediate (17^a), which on intramolecular cyclization afforded the aryl radical (17^b) and on oxidation and loss of H$^+$ in the presence of $SO_4^{\bullet-}$ gave functionalized oxindoles (19/67).

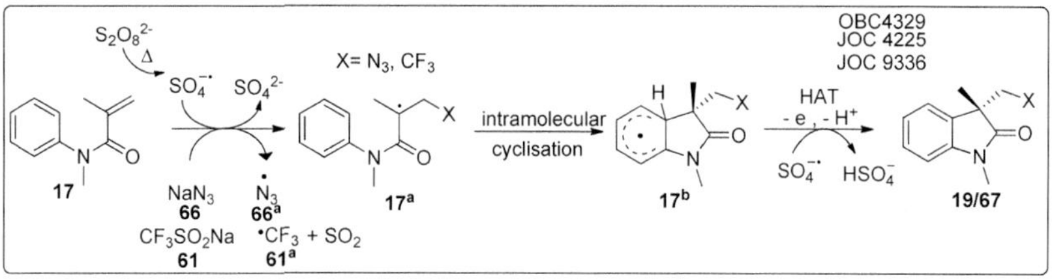

1.5.3 SYNTHESIS OF PHENANTHRIDINES VIA ONE-ELECTRON OXIDATION BY SULFATE RADICAL ANION

Substituted phenanthridines (70) because of their intense natural highlights like antiviral, antibiotic, antitumor, cytotoxic, etc. have been synthesized in the presence of Mn, Cu, Pd, and so forth. But its preparation by means of the productive green procedure is exceedingly required in the field of restorative science. Zhou et al. in 2015 (Scheme 1.27) [36] revealed the radical cascade decarboxylation followed by the cyclization of 2-cyanobiphenyls (**68**) with carboxylic acids (**69**) under transition metal-free conditions in aqueous media by utilizing $K_2S_2O_8$ as initiator and K_2CO_3 as a base. This convention is exceptionally robust and environment-friendly that brought about the arrangement of two C-C bonds and cleavage of C-COOH.

An assortment of aromatic carboxylic acids (**70a**) and aliphatic acids, including cyclic (**70b**), were acceptable in good yields. Additionally, 2-isocyanobiphenyls with diverse functional groups (**70c**) alongside heterocyclic ones (**70d**) were converted to phenanthridines.

After that, this protocol was extended to the synthesis of 6-trifluoromethylated phenanthridines (**70⁴**) by the reaction of 2-isocyanobiphenyls (**68**) with Langlois reagent (**61**).

Phenanthridines, in perspective of its flexible conformation and pharmacological activities, are very important in medicinal and synthetic chemistry. Li et al. in 2018 reported the synthesis of glycosylated phenanthridines (**70²**) by $K_2S_2O_8$ mediated oxidative radical decarboxylation of uronic acids with 2-isocyanobiphenyls (**68**) (Scheme 1.27) [37].

Then again, the synthesis of 6- substituted phenanthridines was accounted for by Xu et al. in 2017 (Scheme 1.27) [38], where unprotonated AAs were utilized as effective and easily available radical precursors. The reaction was performed in aqueous acetonitrile solution using $K_2S_2O_8$

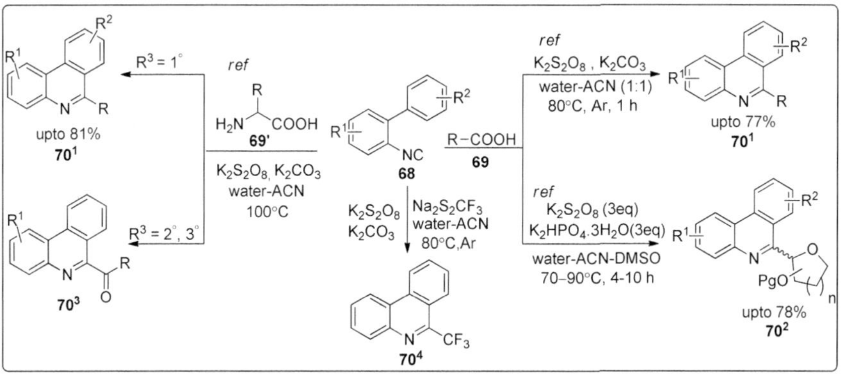

SCHEME 1.27 Transition metal-free persulfate mediated synthesis of 6- substituted phenanthridines by oxidative cyclization of isocyanobiphenyls with carboxylic acids in an aqueous medium.

as an oxidant under transition metal-free conditions. The authors investigated that alkyl-substituted phenanthridines (**70¹**) were the major product in the case of 1° alkylated AAs, whereas acyl substituted phenanthridines (**70³**) were obtained using 2° and 3° alkylated AAs. 2-isocyanobiphenyls (**68**) with substituents (**70¹e, 70¹f**) along with heterocyclic (**70¹g, 70¹h**) were obtained in respectable yields.

Representative examples:

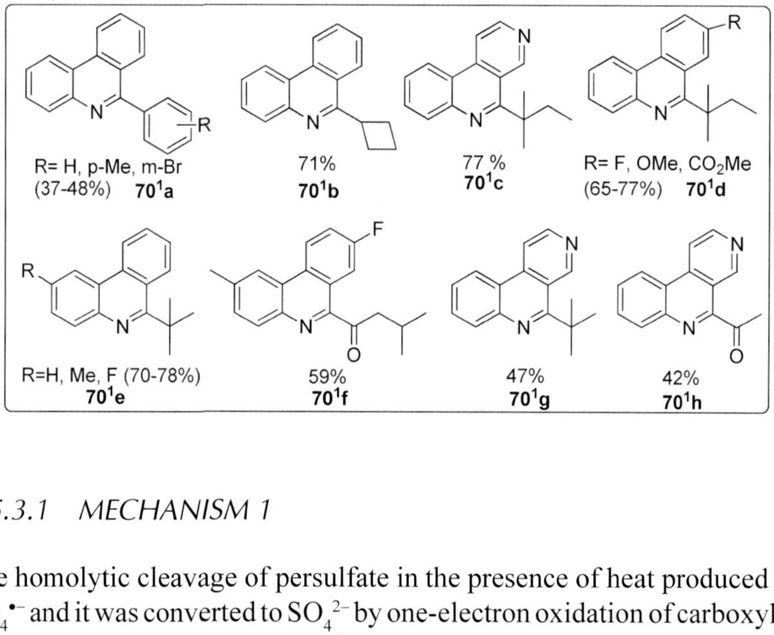

R= H, p-Me, m-Br
(37-48%) **70¹a**

71%
70¹b

77 %
70¹c

R= F, OMe, CO₂Me
(65-77%) **70¹d**

R=H, Me, F (70-78%)
70¹e

59%
70¹f

47%
70¹g

42%
70¹h

1.5.3.1   MECHANISM 1

The homolytic cleavage of persulfate in the presence of heat produced the $SO_4^{\cdot-}$ and it was converted to SO_4^{2-} by one-electron oxidation of carboxylate (**69**) to acyloxy radical intermediate (**69ᵃ**). This (**69ᵃ**) on decarboxylation produced the alkyl radical (**69ᵇ**), which then added to isocyanobiphenyl (**68**) to form imidoyl radical (**68ᵃ**) and then on intramolecular radical cyclization form aryl radical (**68ᵇ**). This on oxidative deprotonation under basic conditions and $SO_4^{\cdot-}$ produced (**70**).

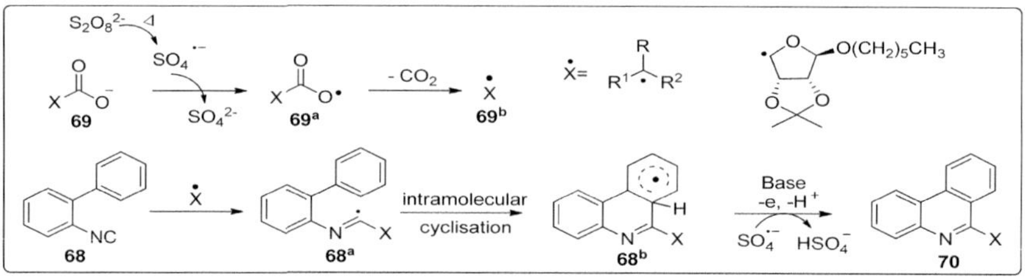

1.5.3.2 MECHANISM 2

The $SO_4^{\bullet-}$ formed through thermolysis of persulfate converted the amino acid anion (**69'**) to an alkyl radical (**69'ª**) through one-electron oxidation followed by decarboxylation. The alkyl radical (**69'ª**) in the presence of $SO_4^{\bullet-}$ oxidized to iminium cation (**69'ᵇ**) and then to aldehydes (**69'c**) in the presence of water with the loss of ammonia. Thus aldehydes through HAT formed acyl radical (**69'ᵈ**) or an alkyl radical (**69'e**) by further loss of CO. The acyl radical or alkyl radical attacked the isocyanides (**68**) to form imidoyl radical (**68ª**), which on intramolecular cyclization produced aryl radical (**68ᵇ**) and finally the desired product (**70**) through oxidation and loss of proton in the presence of a base.

1.5.4 SYNTHESIS OF TRIFLUOROMETHYLARENES VIA ONE-ELECTRON OXIDATION BY SULFATE RADICAL ANION

In 2014, Gong et al. showed the persulfate interceded transition metal-free syntheses of trifluoromethylated arenes (**72**) utilizing affordable, easily accessible Langlois reagent (**61**) as CF_3 source by means of C(sp^2)- H functionalization ensuing C(sp^2)- C(sp^3) bond development in aqueous ACN under Ar atmosphere (Scheme 1.28) [39].

It was discovered that all substrates incorporating active hydrogen (**72a**) functioned admirably with this convention, including heterocyclic substrates (**72b**); however, sterically congested ones gave lower yields (**72c**). The reaction can also be scaled to gram levels for the synthesis of **72d**.

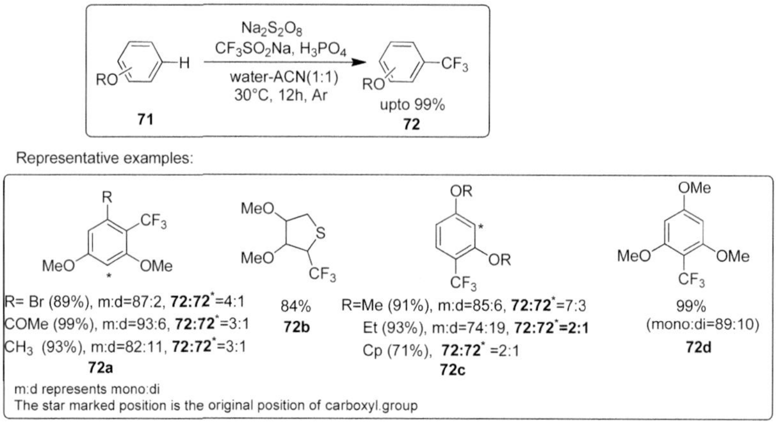

Representative examples:

R= Br (89%), m:d=87:2, **72:72***=4:1
COMe (99%), m:d=93:6, **72:72***=3:1
CH$_3$ (93%), m:d=82:11, **72:72***=3:1
72a

84%
72b

R=Me (91%), m:d=85:6, **72:72***=7:3
Et (93%), m:d=74:19, **72:72***=2:1
Cp (71%), **72:72*** =2:1
72c

99%
(mono:di=89:10)
72d

m:d represents mono:di
The star marked position is the original position of carboxyl group

SCHEME 1.28   Transition metal-free persulfate mediated trifluoromethylation of C(sp^2)-H arenes in aqueous acetonitrile solution.

1.5.4.1   MECHANISM

The CF$_3$ radical (**61ª**) was formed by single-electron oxidation in the presence of SO$_4$$^{•-}$ with the release of SO$_2$. This radical **61ª** attacked the alkoxide (**71**) to form radical intermediate (**71ª**), which occurs in resonance with (**71^b**). The radical on HAT to SO$_4$$^{•-}$ produced the required product (**72**).

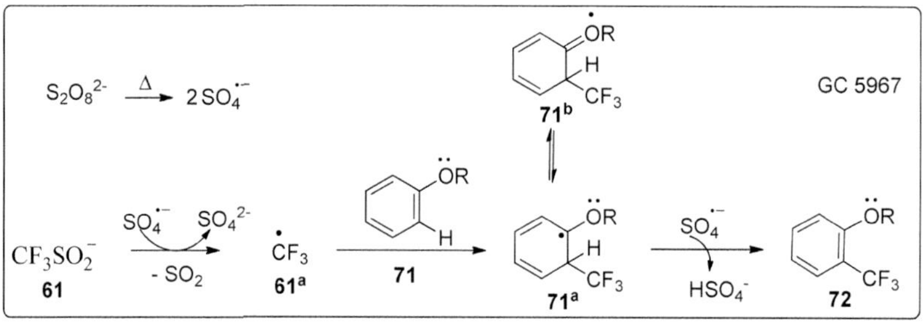

1.5.5   THIOLATION OF ALLENYL PHOSPHINE OXIDES VIA ONE-ELECTRON OXIDATION BY SULFATE RADICAL ANION

Thioethers, the sulfur analogs of ethers, are significant organosulfur compounds in the field of the agrochemical industry, heteroarene syntheses, pharmaceutical science, polymer chemistry, etc. Disulfides being easily available, less harmful, and stable substrates are extensively used as the source of thioethers. So taking forward the work in this direction, recently in 2018, Wu and co-workers (Scheme 1.29) [40] revealed the thiolation of allenyl phosphine oxide (**73**) with diaryl sulfides (**74**) in an aqueous medium. The reaction continued through the homolysis of disulfide to produce aryl thiyl radical followed by C-O bond cleavage of allenyl phosphine oxide furnishing potent S, P functionalized butadienes (**75**) in excellent yields.

The diaryl sulfides with various groups on the aryl ring (**75a**) were compatible along with heterocyclic (**75b**). Allenyl phosphine oxide with substrates at terminal C atom (**75c**) and cyclic substrates (**75d**) were also appropriate in good yields. Also, electron-rich allenes furnished a mixture of isomers with greater selectivity towards E isomer (**75e**) yet exclusive E isomer attained in case of electron-deficient ones (**75f**). Control experiments envisioned the radical mechanism by the trapping of thiyl radical species instead of α-alkenyl radical by the cleavage of the α allenyl C-O bond.

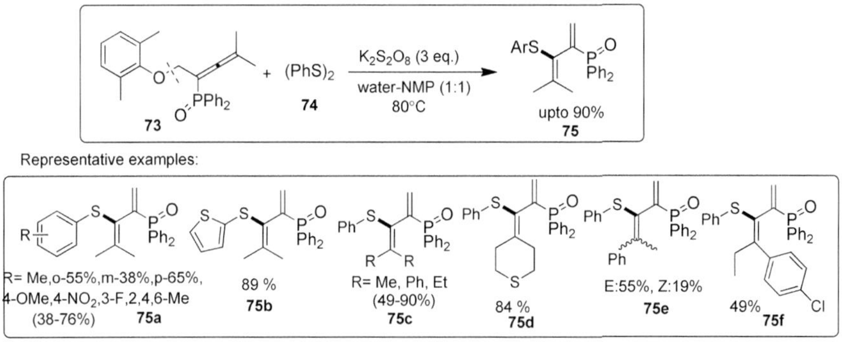

SCHEME 1.29   Transition metal-free persulfate mediated thiolation of allenyl phosphine oxides via cleavage of α-allenylic C-O bonds in an aqueous medium.

1.5.5.1   MECHANISM

The decomposition of persulfate in the presence of heat produced $SO_4^{\cdot-}$. The disulfides (**74**) through one-electron oxidation in the presence of $SO_4^{\cdot-}$ produced the thiyl radical (**74^a**), which then attacked the double bond of allenyl phosphine oxide (**73**) to form alkenyl radical intermediate (**73^a**). This again on β elimination and oxidation gave the required product (**75**).

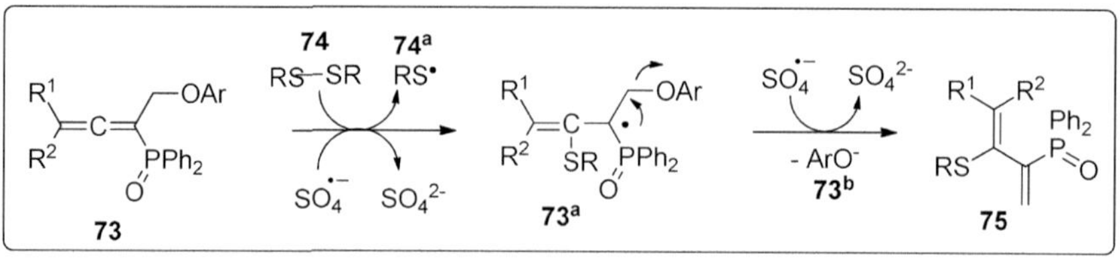

1.6 INDIRECT INVOLVEMENT OF SULFATE RADICAL ANION IN ORGANIC SYNTHESIS

The scientific community is attempting to synthesize the phosphorylated N-heterocycles as these are highly potent biological compounds with green and sustainable approaches. Wang et al. in 2015 (Scheme 1.30) [41] evinced the first example of oxidative cross-coupling reaction between ketene dithioacetals (76) with diaryl phosphine oxide (77) through direct C-H phosphorylation under transition metal-free conditions in an aqueous medium resulting in highly efficient tetra-substituted alkenes (78) with expansive substrate scope.

The alkenes with varied functional groups, including alkyl (78a) and aryl (78b) were tolerated in good yields. This convention was well applicable even on changing the dithioacetals to cyclic (78d) and acyclic (78c) alkyl thiols. This approach was further applied to the late-stage synthesis of phosphorylated N-heterocycles. Deuterium labeling experiments demonstrated that the C-H bond of alkene is not the rate-determining step.

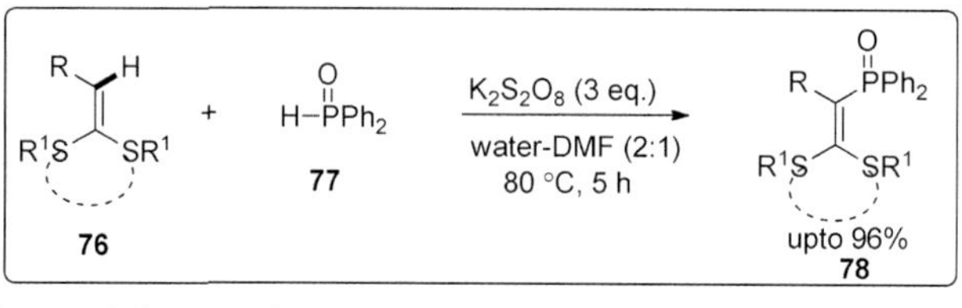

Representative examples:

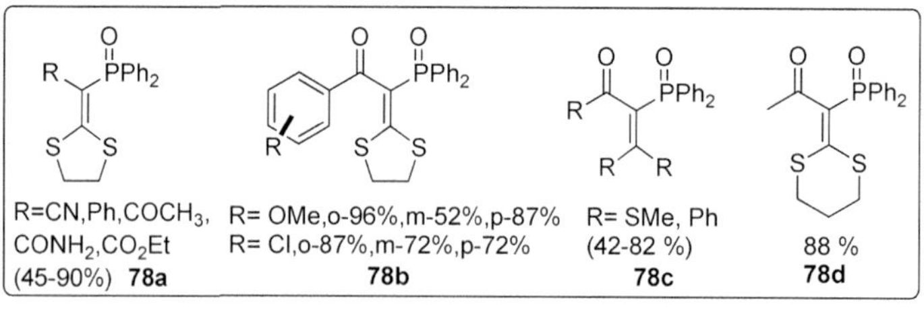

SCHEME 1.30 Transition metal-free persulfate mediated phosphorylation of ketene dithioacetals in aqueous DMF solution.

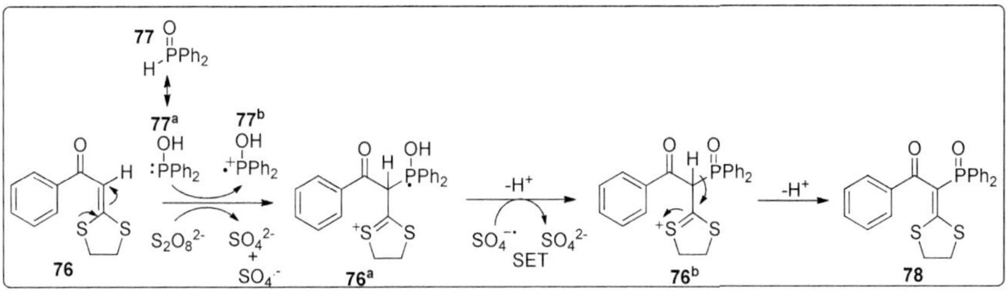

Gomez et al. in 2015 (Scheme 1.31) [42] revealed the photoredox synthesis of benzo-3,4-coumarin via lactonization of 2-aryl benzoic acids employing ammonium persulfate as radical initiator and oxidant in the presence of visible light at room temperature. The authors made use of 9-mesityl-10-methyl acridinium perchlorate [MesAcr] ClO_4 as organo photocatalysts having a very short lifetime of microseconds, which is an exceptionally strong oxidizing agent. 2-aryl benzoic acids with diverse functional groups were all around acknowledged. Kinetic isotope experiments revealed that C-H bond cleavage is not the rate-determining step, and the reaction proceeded by means of a radical pathway.

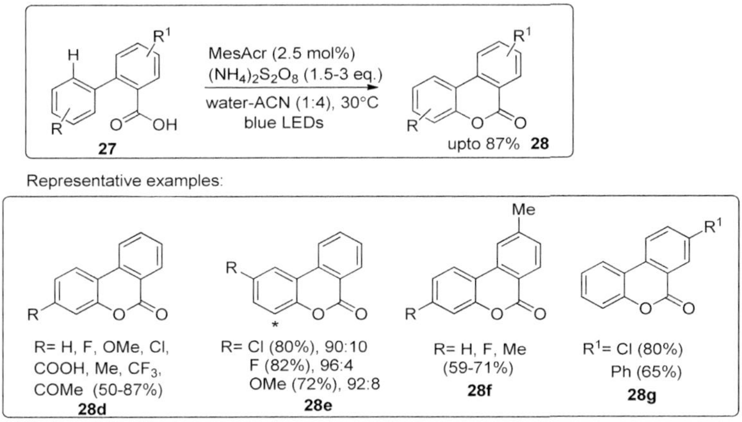

SCHEME 1.31 Transition metal-free lactonization of 2-arylbenzoic acids using MesAcr as a photocatalyst in an aqueous medium.

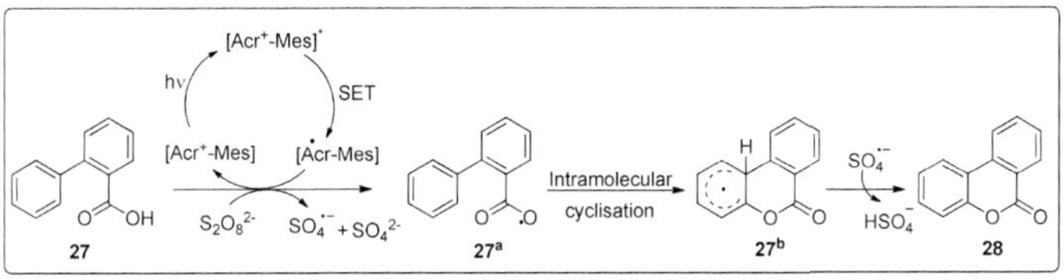

Xu and colleagues in 2016 (Scheme 1.32)[44] explored the α-oxyacylation of carbonyl compounds through the reaction of acetone (**79**) with carboxylic acids (**69**) prompting the syntheses of biologically active α acyloxy carbonyl compounds (**80**) in a highly efficient and operationally simpler manner. The reaction continued for 12 hours in the presence of $K_2S_2O_8$ as the oxidant, potassium iodide as a catalyst and K_2HPO_4 as a base at 80°C using the green solvent water. The practical relevance of this convention is that this can be effectively scaled up to gram levels with a good yield of 89% (1.6 g) from 1.22 g of benzoic acid. The kinetic isotope effect showed that C-H bond cleavage might be the rate-determining step.

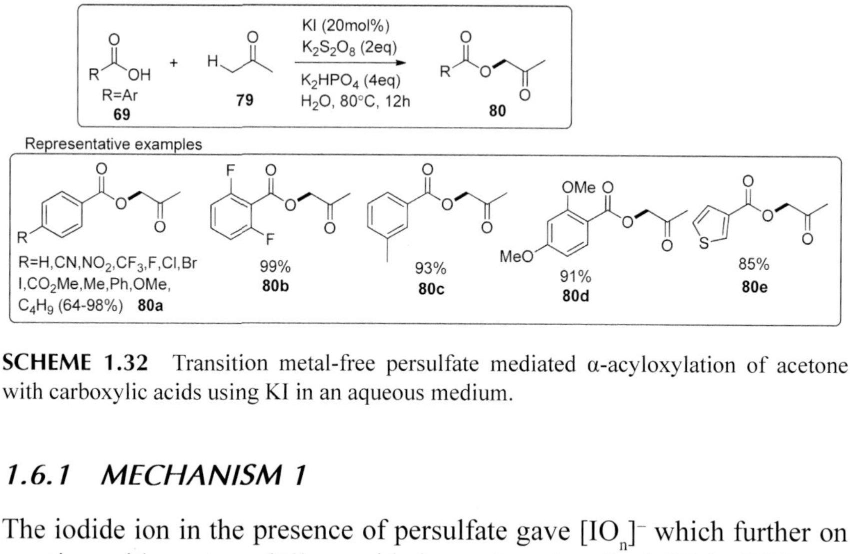

SCHEME 1.32   Transition metal-free persulfate mediated α-acyloxylation of acetone with carboxylic acids using KI in an aqueous medium.

1.6.1   MECHANISM 1

The iodide ion in the presence of persulfate gave $[IO_n]^-$ which further on reaction with acetone (**79**) provided α carbonyl radical (**79ᵃ**). (**79ᵃ**) was converted to carbocation (**79b**) by the loss of electron in the presence of $SO_4^{•-}$. (**79b**) on reaction with carboxylic anion (**69ᵃ**) generated from carboxylic acid (**69**) in the presence of base gave desired product (**80**).

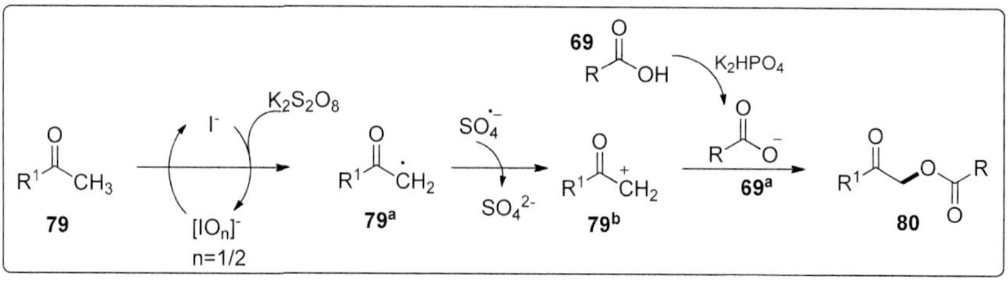

Molander and collaborators in 2017 (Scheme 1.33) [44] announced the synthesis of hetero-arylated chromanones (1^{81}–6^{81}) from the coupling of 2-trifluoroborate-4- chromanone (**81**) as radical precursors with different heteroarenes (**1–6**) in aqueous acetonitrile solution at room temperature in the presence of largely available visible light. Also, trifluoroacetic acid was used in order to activate the nitrogen of N-heteroarenes. Mesitylene acridinium perchlorate was used as photocatalyst, and $K_2S_2O_8$ was employed as a modest oxidant with great solubility in water.

The same group (Molander et al.) (Scheme 1.33) [45] extended the similar environment benign menisci type reaction utilizing the highly efficient organo-photocatalyst (MesAcr) under the same reaction conditions. Here, the authors reported the radical primary, secondary, tertiary alkylation of N-heteroarenes (**1–6**) with alkyltrifluoroborates (**82**) in the presence of persulfate as a radical initiator in aqueous acetonitrile solution. This protocol was adequate with alkyltrifluoroborates with a very good yield of 72%, however other organoboranes were not satisfactory.

A variety of laboratory and industrially important heteroarenes, including pyridines (**1**), quinolines (**2**), isoquinolines (**3**), quinoxalines

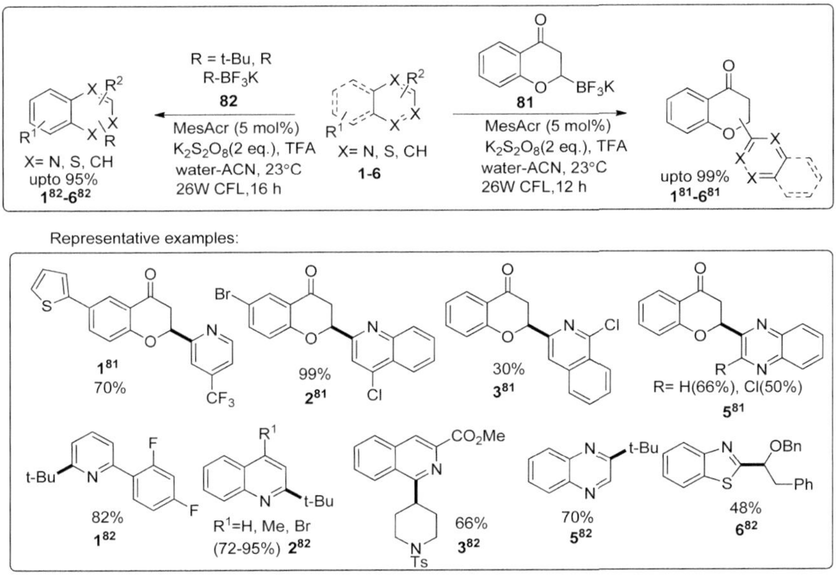

SCHEME 1.33 Transition metal-free persulfate mediated heteroarenes functionalization with alkyl trifluoroborates and 2-trifluoroboratochromanones in an aqueous medium.

(5), benzothiazoles (6), etc. with broad functional group tolerance were alkylated in moderate to excellent yields. It was further utilized for the late-stage C-H alkylation to induce biologically active alkyl moieties onto heteroarenes.

1.6.2 MECHANISM 2

Initially, the photocatalyst MesAcr was excited to higher energy state in the presence of visible light. This exciting complex is highly oxidizing and generated the alkyl radical (82ª) through a single electron transfer from the substrate (82). This radical (82ª) then attacked the protonated heteroarenes (1ª) to form radical cation intermediate (1ᵇ), which through HAT by $SO_4^{\bullet-}$ yielded substituted heteroarenes (1⁸²).

Wang et al. in 2017 (Scheme 1.34)[47] described the mild, metal free, NHS intervened cross dehydrogenative coupling reaction of N-hetero-arenes (1–3) with cyclic ethers (8) for the synthesis of ether substrates in the presence of ammonium persulfate in green solvent water at 40°C. This is essentially a Minisci type reaction involving C(sp³)-H heteroarylation of ethers by cross dehydrogenative coupling. In this transformation, N-hydroxysuccinimide (NHS) was used as an effective catalyst and mediator instead of the visible light that undergoes hydrogen atom transfer prompting N-centered radical cation. As contrasted to the conventional Minisci reaction, no acid is required in this transformation. Kinetic studies revealed that hydrogen atom transfer from C α position of tetrahydrofuran is fundamentally the rate deciding step.

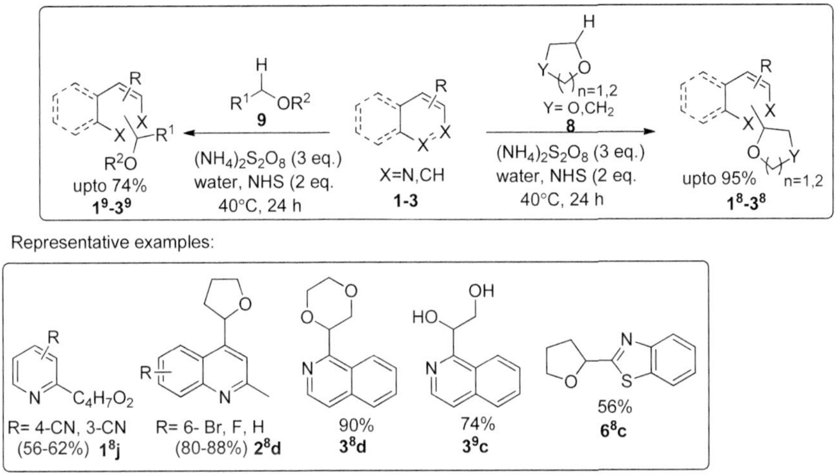

Representative examples:

SCHEME 1.34   Transition metal-free persulfate and NHS mediated Cα heteroarylation of ethers in water.

1.6.3   MECHANISM 3

Henceforth, Molander et al. in 2017 (Scheme 1.35) [47] revealed the ecofriendly transition metal-free convention for C-H alkylation of non-functionalized heteroarenes like pyridine (1), quinoline (2), isoquinoline (3), benzothiazole (6), pyrimidine (7) and 1,4-quinones (37) in aqueous medium with the help of 1,4-dihydropyridines (45) as coupling partner and C(sp^3) radical source.

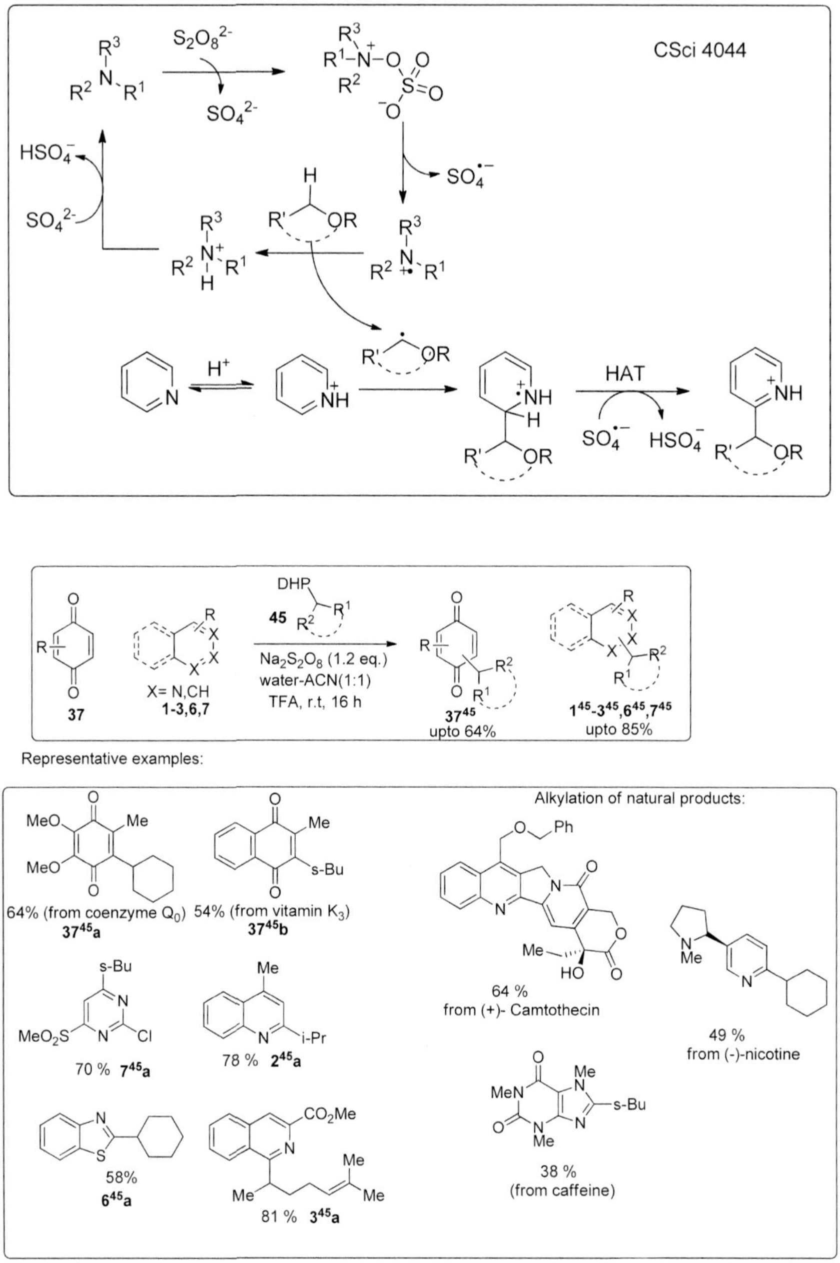

SCHEME 1.35 Transition metal-free persulfate mediated C-H alkylation of N-hetero-arenes and 1,4- quinines with DHP in aqueous acetonitrile solution.

This effective environment amiable protocol was further applied to the late-stage C-H alkylation of natural products and pharmaceutical important drugs. Numerous imperative medications like nicotine, caffeine, cinchonine, quinine, camptothecin were enhanced to comparing more strong natural subsidiaries. Deuterium labeling studies demonstrated that N-deuterated DHP experienced slow homolytic cleavage as contrasted with N-H DHP.

1.7   CONCLUSION

This chapter provides an overview of the transition metal-free protocols deal with the generation of $SO_4^{\bullet-}$ from persulfates in aqueous media. Also, it highlights the utilization of *in situ* formed $SO_4^{\bullet-}$ toward syntheses and functionalization of various small organic molecules, including heterocyclic compounds, acyclic compounds, and (hetero) aromatic compounds. It is worthy of mentioning that the (radical) reactions, especially free from transition metals and occur in aqueous solutions, have attracted great attention of chemists due to environmental friendliness. Therefore, (i) a skillful utilization of $SO_4^{\bullet-}$ produced under metal-free conditions may replace conventional methods used for the synthesis of pharmaceuticals with facile routes; and (ii) the present chapter may act as an accelerator in boosting the applications of $SO_4^{\bullet-}$ in organic syntheses as well as in the environmental remediation process.

KEYWORDS

- electron donor acceptor
- ethynylbenziodoxolone
- hydrogen atom transfer
- radiochemical conversion
- sulfate radical anions
- tetraethylammonium bicarbonate

REFERENCES

1. Li, X., Wang, H. Y., & Shi, Z. J., (2013). Transition metal-free cross-dehydrogenative alkylation of pyridines under neutral conditions. *New J. Chem., 37*(6), 1704–1706.
2. Ambala, S., Thatikonda, T., Sharma, S., Munagala, G., Yempalla, K. R., Vishwakarma, R. A., & Singh, P. P., (2015). Cross-dehydrogenative coupling of α-C(Sp₃)-H of ethers/alkanes with C(Sp₂)-H of heteroarenes under metal-free conditions. *Org. Biomol. Chem., 13*(46), 11341–11350.
3. Devari, S., & Shah, B. A., (2016). Visible light-promoted C-H functionalization of ethers and electron-deficient arenes. *Chem. Commun., 52*(7), 1490–1493.
4. Zhang, Y., Teuscher, K. B., & Ji, H., (2016). Direct α-heteroarylation of amides (α to nitrogen) and ethers through a benzaldehyde-mediated photoredox reaction. *Chem. Sci., 7*(3), 2111–2118.
5. McCallum, T., Jouanno, L. A., Cannillo, A., & Barriault, L., (2016). Persulfate-enabled direct C-H alkylation of heteroarenes with unactivated ethers. *Synlett, 27*(8), 1282–1286.
6. Ma, J. J., Yi, W., Bin, L. G. P., & Cai, C., (2015). Transition metal-free C-H oxidative activation: Persulfate-promoted selective benzylic mono- and difluorination. *Org. Biomol. Chem., 13*(10), 2890–2894.
7. Zhang, X., Guo, S., & Tang, P., (2015). Transition metal free oxidative aliphatic C-H fluorination. *Org. Chem. Front., 2*(7), 806–810.
8. Yuan, G., Wang, F., Stephenson, N. A., Wang, L., Rotstein, B. H., Vasdev, N., Tang, P., & Liang, S. H., (2017). Metal-free 18f-labeling of Aryl-CF2H via nucleophilic radiofluorination and oxidative C-H activation. *Chem. Commun., 53*(1), 126–129.
9. Guo, J. Y., Wu, R. X., Jin, J. K., & Tian, S. K., (2016). TfNHNHBoc as a trifluoromethylating agent for vicinal difunctionalization of terminal alkenes. *Org. Lett., 18*(15), 3850–3853.
10. Zhang, X., Yang, H., & Tang, P., (2015). Transition metal-free oxidative aliphatic C-H azidation. *Org. Lett., 17*(23), 5828–5831.
11. Li, X., & Shi, Z. J., (2016). Aliphatic C-H azidation through a peroxydisulfate induced radical pathway. *Org. Chem. Front., 3*(10), 1326–1330.
12. Wang, H., Guo, L. N., & Duan, X. H., (2013). Metal-free oxidative spirocyclization of hydroxymethylacrylamide with 1,3-dicarbonyl compounds: A new route to spirooxindoles. *Org. Lett., 15*(20), 5254–5257.
13. Wang, Y., Gulevich, A. V., & Gevorgyan, V., (2013). General and practical carboxyl-group-directed remote C-H oxygenation reactions of arenes. *Chem. – A Eur. J., 19*(47), 15836–15840.
14. Wei, W., Wen, J., Yang, D., Du, J., You, J., & Wang, H., (2014). Catalyst-free direct arylsulfonylation of N-arylacrylamides with sulfinic acids: A convenient and efficient route to sulfonated oxindoles. *Green Chem., 16*(6), 2988–2991.
15. Wang, S., He, L. Y., & Guo, L. N., (2015). Potassium persulfate mediated oxidative radical cyclization of 1,3-dicarbonyl compounds with styrenes for the synthesis of dihydrofurans. *Synth., 47*(20), 3191–3197.
16. Wang, S., Guo, L. N., Wang, H., & Duan, X. H., (2015). Alkynylation of tertiary cycloalkanols via radical C-C bond cleavage: A route to distal alkynylated ketones. *Org. Lett., 17*(19), 4798–4801.

17. Wang, H., Liu, Y., Li, M., Huang, H., Xu, H. M., Hong, R. J., & Shen, H., (2010). Multifunctional TiO_2 nanowires-modified nanoparticles bilayer film for 3D dye-sensitized solar cells. *Optoelectron. Adv. Mater. Rapid Commun., 4*(8), 1166–1169.

18. Ilangovan, A., Polu, A., & Satish, G., (2015). $K_2S_2O_8$-mediated metal-free direct C-H functionalization of quinones using arylboronic acids. *Org. Chem. Front., 2*(12), 1616–1620.

19. Li, X., Che, X., Chen, G. H., Zhang, J., Yan, J. L., Zhang, Y. F., Zhang, L. S., Hsu, C. P., Gao, Y. Q., & Shi, Z. J., (2016). Direct oxidation of aliphatic C-H bonds in amino-containing molecules under transition-metal-free conditions. *Org. Lett., 18*(6), 1234–1237.

20. Lee, M., & Sanford, M. S., (2017). Remote C(Sp3)-H oxygenation of protonated aliphatic amines with potassium persulfate. *Org. Lett., 19*(3), 572–575.

21. Luo, L., Tao, K., Peng, X., Hu, C., Lu, Y., & Wang, H., (2016). Synthesis of: N -aryl 2-quinolinones via intramolecular C(Sp2)-H amidation of knoevenagel products. *RSC Adv., 6*(106), 104463–104466.

22. Luo, L., Wang, Q., Peng, X., Hu, C., & Wang, H., (2017). Synthesis of Benzo[c] [2,7]naphthyridine-6-ones via cascade aromatization/C(Sp$_2$)–H amidation of 1,4-dihydropyridines. *Tetrahedron Lett., 58*(28), 2792–2795.

23. Dunham, J., Peacock, M., Tracy, C. R., Nielsen, J., & Vinyard, G., (1999). Assessing extinction risk: Integrating genetic information. *Ecol. Soc., 3*(1), NP.

24. Natarajan, P., Priya, & Chuskit, D., (2017). Transition metal-free and organic solvent-free conversion of N-substituted 2-aminobiaryls into corresponding carbazoles via intramolecular oxidative radical cyclization induced by peroxodisulfate. *Green Chem., 19*(24), 5854–5861.

25. More, N. Y., & Jeganmohan, M., (2017). Solvent-controlled selective synthesis of biphenols and quinones: Via oxidative coupling of phenols. *Chem. Commun., 53*(69), 9616–9619.

26. Yan, K., Yang, D., Wei, W., Zhao, J., Shuai, Y., Tian, L., & Wang, H., (2015). Catalyst-free direct decarboxylative coupling of α-keto acids with thiols: A facile access to thioesters. *Org. Biomol. Chem.,* 7323–7330.

27. Wang, P. F., Feng, Y. S., Cheng, Z. F., Wu, Q. M., Wang, G. Y., Liu, L. L., Dai, J. J., Xu, J., & Xu, H. J., (2015). Transition metal-free synthesis of ynones via decarboxylative alkynylation of α-keto acids under mild conditions. *J. Org. Chem., 80*(18), 9314–9320.

28. Li, X., Li, S., Sun, S., Yang, F., Zhu, W., Zhu, Y., Wu, Y., & Wu, Y., (2016). Direct decarboxylative alkynylation of α,α-difluoroarylacetic acids under transition metal-free conditions. *Adv. Synth. Catal., 358*(10), 1699–1704.

29. Laha, J. K., Patel, K. V., Dubey, G., & Jethava, K. P., (2017). Intramolecular minisci acylation under silver-free neutral conditions for the synthesis of azafluorenones and fluorenones. *Org. Biomol. Chem., 15*(10), 2199–2210.

30. Chaubey, N. R., & Singh, K. N., (2017). Metal-free decarboxylative acylation of isoquinolines using α-keto acids in water. *Tetrahedron Lett., 58*(24), 2347–2350.

31. Mete, T. B., Khopade, T. M., & Bhat, R. G., (2017). Oxidative decarboxylation of arylacetic acids in water: One-pot transition-metal-free synthesis of aldehydes and ketones. *Tetrahedron Lett., 58*(29), 2822–2825.

32. Wang, D., Fang, J., Deng, G. J., & Gong, H., (2017). Catalyst-free decarboxylative trifluoromethylation/perfluoroalkylation of benzoic acid derivatives in water-acetonitrile. *ACS Sustain. Chem. Eng., 5*(8), 6398–6403.

33. Chawla, R., Singh, A. K., & Yadav, L. D. S., (2014). $K_2S_2O_8$-mediated aerobic oxysulfonylation of olefins into β-keto sulfones in aqueous media. *European J. Org. Chem., 10*, 2032–2036.

34. Wei, W., Wen, J., Yang, D., Liu, X., Guo, M., Dong, R., & Wang, H., (2014). Metal-free direct trifluoromethylation of activated alkenes with Langlois' reagent leading to CF3-containing oxindoles. *J. Org. Chem., 79*(9), 4225–4230.

35. Qiu, J., & Zhang, R., (2014). Transition metal-free oxidative carboazidation of acrylamides via cascade C-N and C-C bond-forming reactions. *Org. Biomol. Chem., 12*(25), 4329–4334.

36. Lu, S., Gong, Y., & Zhou, D., (2015). Transition metal-free oxidative radical decarboxylation/cyclization for the construction of 6-alkyl/aryl phenanthridines. *J. Org. Chem., 80*(18), 9336–9341.

37. Zhou, X., Wang, P., Zhang, L., Chen, P., Ma, M., Song, N., Ren, S., & Li, M., (2018). Transition metal-free synthesis of c-glycosylated phenanthridines via $K_2S_2O_8$-mediated oxidative radical decarboxylation of uronic acids. *J. Org. Chem., 83*(2), 588–603.

38. Lu, S. C., Li, H. S., Gong, Y. L., Wang, X. L., Li, F. R., Li, F., Duan, G. Y., & Xu, S., (2017). Use of unprotected amino acids in metal-free tandem radical cyclization reactions: Divergent synthesis of 6-alkyl/acyl phenanthridines. *RSC Adv., 7*(88), 55891–55896.

39. Wang, D., Deng, G. J., Chen, S., & Gong, H., (2016). Catalyst-free direct C-H trifluoromethylation of arenes in water-acetonitrile. *Green Chem., 18*(22), 5967–5970.

40. Luo, K., (2018). *Syn Thesis Latent Radical Cleavage of α -Allenylic C-O Bonds : Potassium Persulfate Mediated Thiolation of Allenylphosphine Oxides Syn Thesis.*

41. Zhu, L., Yu, H., Guo, Q., Chen, Q., Xu, Z., & Wang, R., (2015). C-H bonds phosphorylation of ketene dithioacetals. *Org. Lett., 17*(8), 1978–1981.

42. Ramirez, N. P., Bosque, I., & Gonzalez-Gomez, J. C., (2015). Photocatalytic dehydrogenative lactonization of 2-arylbenzoic acids. *Org. Lett., 17*(18), 4550–4553.

43. Wu, Y. D., Huang, B., Zhang, Y. X., Wang, X. X., Dai, J. J., Xu, J., & Xu, H. J., (2016). KI-catalyzed α-acyloxylation of acetone with carboxylic acids. *Org. Biomol. Chem., 14*(25), 5936–5939.

44. Matsui, J. K., & Molander, G. A., (2017). Organocatalyzed, photoredox heteroarylation of 2-trifluoroboratochromanones via C-H functionalization. *Org. Lett., 19*(4), 950–953.

45. Matsui, J. K., Primer, D. N., & Molander, G. A., (2017). Metal-free C-H alkylation of heteroarenes with alkyltrifluoroborates: A general protocol for 1°, 2° and 3° alkylation. *Chem. Sci., 8*(5), 3512–3522.

46. Liu, S., Liu, A., Zhang, Y., & Wang, W., (2017). Direct Cα-heteroarylation of structurally diverse ethers: Via a mild N -hydroxysuccinimide mediated cross-dehydrogenative coupling reaction. *Chem. Sci., 8*(5), 4044–4050.

47. Gutiérrez-Bonet, Á., Remeur, C., Matsui, J. K., & Molander, G. A., (2017). Late-stage C-H alkylation of heterocycles and 1,4-quinones via oxidative homolysis of 1,4-dihydropyridines. *J. Am. Chem. Soc., 139*(35), 12251–12258.

CHAPTER 2

DESIGN AND SYNTHESIS OF TRIAZINE AMINE DERIVATIVES AS ANTIBACTERIAL AND ANTIFUNGAL AGENTS

RAVINDRA S. SHINDE* and SHREYAS S. MAHURKAR

Research Center in Chemistry, Dayanand Science College, Latur, Maharashtra, India

Corresponding author. E-mail: rshinde.33381@gmail.com

ABSTRACT

An efficient and convenient synthesis of 2-chloro-4,6-dimethoxy-1,3,5-triazine (CDMT) from cyanuric chloride in short reaction time followed by synthesis of novel substituted 4,6-dimethoxy-N-phenyl-1,3,5-triazin-2-amine(2a-x) using substituted anilines and heterocyclic amines, anhydrous K_2CO_3 in dry THF as a solvent. The advantages of this methodology are short reaction time, an excellent yield of products, easy work-up procedure. The synthesized compounds were confirmed by FT-IR, ¹HNMR, Mass spectral data. All the synthesized derivatives (2a-x) were biologically screened for their antibacterial and antifungal activities. Compounds **2c, 2e, 2f, 2g, 2i, 2l, 2o, 2q, 2s, 2t, 2u, 2x** are found antibacterial against human pathogenic microorganisms. Also compounds **2c, 2e, 2f, 2g, 2i, 2l, 2o, 2q, 2r, 2s, 2t, 2u** and **2x** are found potential anti-fungal against *Candida albicans* MTCC 227, *Candida glabrata* NCIM 3236, *Candida tropicalis* NCIM 3110, and *Aspergillus niger* NCIM 545 fungi were used for the study.

2.1   INTRODUCTION

The triazines are the well known and important nitrogen-containing hetero-cyclic. 1,3,5-triazine is the symmetric organic compound, which is also called s-triazine. The 1,3,5-triazine derivatives containing different amino groups on positions 2, 4, or 6 show with various biological activities. The merging of substituted heterocyclic amines in s-triazine would give a large range of structure which can be projected for attractive antibacterial and antifungal activity [1, 2].

Generally, the nucleophilic displacement reaction of chlorine from cyanuric chloride is the very common synthetic route for the synthesis of substituted 1,3,5-triazine derivatives was investigated by Bhat et al. [3]. The successive replacement of three chlorine atoms depends on the reaction condition, the addition of reagents, and the temperature of the reaction. This makes cyanuric chloride very expensive in the synthesis of various substituted 1,3,5-triazine hybrids [4]. Thurston et al. [5] revealed that this reaction consequently offers a suitable way for the synthesis of substituted amino, oxy-1,3,5-triazine hybrids.

Where, R_1, R_2, R_3 = Alkyl, Aryl   X = O, N, S

Microwave-assisted synthesis of various substituted triazine amine derivatives with different symmetrical and unsymmetrical amino substitu-ents has been carried out using microwave irradiation under solvent-free condition by Jose et al. [6]. This synthetic route offers excellent product yield and the high-speed reaction rate.

The triazine derivatives have been synthesized using solution and solid phases [7]. In solid-phase synthesis, the chlorine atoms in cyanuric chloride are replaced by coupling chlorotriazine to a support bound amino acid. By these methods, generally, 10,000 hybrid compounds are prepared using 45–50 amino acids (AAs). A solution-phase technique is well developed for the synthesis of triazine derivatives by coupling of cyanuric chloride with a various set of amines was performed by De Hoog et al. [8].

The trisubstituted derivatives of triazine were synthesized by a palladium-catalyzed cross-coupling methodology. The Suzuki coupling nucleophilic reaction of 6-chloro-2,4-diaminotriazine and aryl boronic acid. Unluckily authors Bork and Moon et al. [9] does not report the yield of the reaction.

In recent times, cyanuric chloride has attracted the attention of many researchers as its symmetrical structure facilitates to synthesize various sets of analogs and provides the basis for designing biological active molecules with a wide range of applications as therapeutics. The 1,3,5-triazine core has many applications such as medicinal chemistry, [10] herbicides, [11] catalysis, [12] polymer chemistry, [13] and supramolecular chemistry [14].

Some derivatives of cyanuric chloride, especially dimethoxy analog, is the middle first compound used for the synthesis of substituted 4,6-dimethoxy-N-phenyl-1,3,5-triazin-2-amine derivatives. In view of the above work on cyanuric chloride, with this, we account for the synthesis of 2-chloro-4,6-dimethoxy-1,3,5-triazine from cyanuric chloride in a little reaction time followed by synthesis of bioactive substituted 4,6-dimethoxy-N-phenyl-1,3,5-triazin-2-amine derivatives using substituted anilines/heterocyclic amines and anhydrous K_2CO_3 in dry THF. Many triazine derivatives have been prepared using this route.

2.2 PRESENT WORK

In the present chapter, we have developed novel strategies for an efficient and convenient method of synthesis of 2-chloro-4,6-dimethoxy-1,3,5-triazine

(2B) (CDMT) by using cyanuric chloride (2A), methanol, and catalytic amount of sodium bicarbonate (Scheme 2.1) followed by synthesis of substituted 4, 6-dimethoxy-N-phenyl-1,3,5-triazin-2-amines (2a-l) by using CDMT, substituted anilines/heterocyclic amines (2C) and anhydrous K_2CO_3 in dry THF as solvent (Scheme 2.2). The yield and melting points of substituted 4, 6-dimethoxy-N-phenyl-1,3,5-triazin-2-amine derivatives have shown in Table 2.1. All the synthesized compounds were screened against antimicrobial activity shown in Tables 2.4 and 2.5.

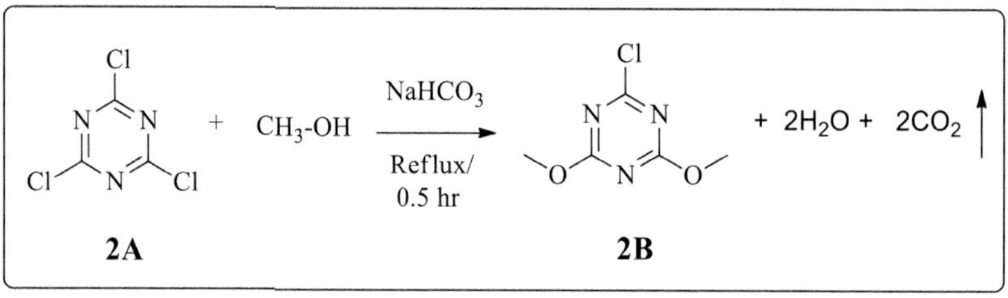

SCHEME 2.1   Synthesis of 2-chloro-4,6-dimethoxy-1,3,5-triazine.

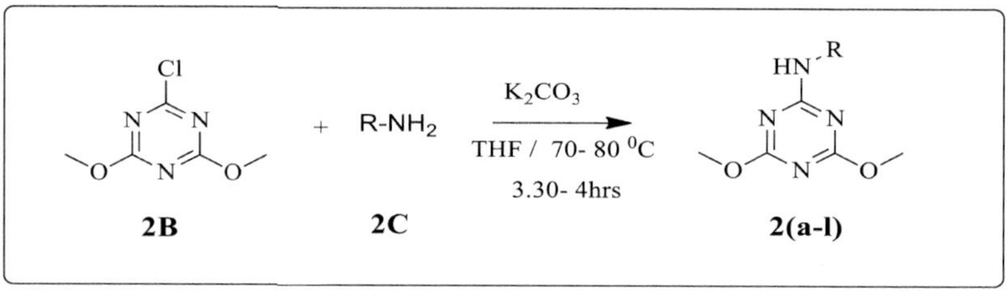

SCHEME 2.2   Synthesis of substituted 4,6-dimethoxy-N-phenyl-1,3,5-triazin-2-amine derivatives.

[R-NH$_2$ = 3,5-dimethoxybenzenamine, 3,4-dimethoxybenzenamine, 2-fluoropyridin-4-amine, 3-methoxybenzenamine, 3-(trifluoromethoxy) benzenamine, 3,4-difluorobenzenamine, 4-fluorobenzenamine, tetrahydro-2H-pyran-2-amine, 3-fluorobenzenamine, 6-methoxypyridin-3-amine, (pyridin-2-yl)methanamine, 1H-benzo[d]imidazol-5-amine].

2.3 EXPERIMENTAL

The aromatic amines, cyanuric chloride, methanol, and other chemicals were obtained from commercial sources and purified by distillation or recrystallization before use. Melting points were taken by the open capillary method and are uncorrected. The IR spectra are recorded on FT-IR Bruker with KBr disc, ^{1}H NMR spectra are recorded in DMSO-d$_6$ on a Bruker DRX-400 MHz, and mass spectra were obtained on Jeol-SX-102(FAB) spectrometer at S.A.I.F. Division, Punjab University, Chandigarh.

The preparation of substituted 4,6-dimethoxy-N-phenyl-1,3,5-triazin-2-amine derivatives (2a-l) was done in two steps: Step 1 and Step 2.

2.3.1 STEP-I

2.3.1.1 SYNTHESIS OF 2-CHLORO-4, 6-DIMETHOXY-1,3,5-TRIAZINE (2B)

Cyanuric chloride (**2A**)(18.5 g, 0.1 mol) was dissolved in 100 ml methanol, and 10 ml water in a 250 ml round bottom flask and sodium bicarbonate (16.8 g, 0.2 mol) was added slowly in the reaction mixture at room temperature. Then, the reaction mixture was refluxed for 30 minutes until the evolution of CO_2 was stopped. Then contents were poured into ice-cold water and filtered. The crude solid obtained was recrystallized from dichloromethane, which affords the pure white solid product (**2B**) and dried it in a desiccator.

Yield: 74%; M.P: 74–76°C; M. wt. = 175.01.
^{1}H NMR (400 MHz, DMSO-*d$_6$*): δ 4.05 (s, 6H, 2×OCH$_3$).
MS (*ESI*) *m/z*: 175.67 [M$^+$], 177.67 [M+2]$^+$.
Anal. Calcd for C$_5$H$_6$ClN$_3$O$_2$: C, 34.20; H, 3.44; N, 23.93%. Found: C, 33.98; H, 3.34; N, 23.70%.

2.3.2 STEP-II

2.3.2.1 GENERAL PROCEDURE FOR THE SYNTHESIS OF SUBSTITUTED 4,6-DIMETHOXY-N-PHENYL-1,3,5-TRIAZIN-2-AMINE DERIVATIVES (2A-L)

A mixture of CDMT (**2B**) (1 mmol), substituted aromatic amines (1 mmol) [3,5-dimethoxybenzenamine, 3,4-dimethoxybenzenamine, 2-fluoropyridin -4-amine, 3-methoxybenzenamine, 3-(trifluoromethoxy)benzenamine, 3,4-difluorobenzenamine, 4-fluorobenzenamine, tetrahydro-2H-pyran-2-amine,

3-fluorobenzenamine, 6-methoxypyridin-3-amine, (pyridin-2-yl)methena-mine, 1H-benzo[d]imidazol-5-amine] (**2C**) and anhydrous K_2CO_3 (2 mmol) were added in dry THF (10 ml) taken in a round-bottom flask. The reaction mixture was refluxed at 70°C for 4 hrs. The progress of the reaction was monitored by TLC. After completion of the reaction, crushed ice was added in the reaction mixture and extracted with ethyl acetate (20 ml X 3 times). The organic layer was separated and dried over anhydrous Na_2SO_4. The solvent was evaporated under vacuum, and the crude material was purified by using column chromatography (ethyl acetate and petroleum ether) to furnish the corresponding compounds (**2a-l**) with 70–75% yields.

2.4   RESULTS AND DISCUSSION

Herein, we have explored the synthetic utility of CDMT for the synthesis of substituted 4,6-dimethoxy-*N*-phenyl-1,3,5-triazin-2-amine derivatives. In accordance with our aim, we have performed the reaction of cyanuric chloride (**2A**) ((0.1 mol) with sodium bicarbonate (0.2 mol) in methanol and water to form 2-chloro-4, 6-dimethoxy-1,3,5-triazine (CDMT) (**2B**) Scheme 2.3. When we used an excess amount of sodium bicarbonate (0.3 mol), it furnished 2, 4, 6-trimethoxy-1,3,5-triazine.

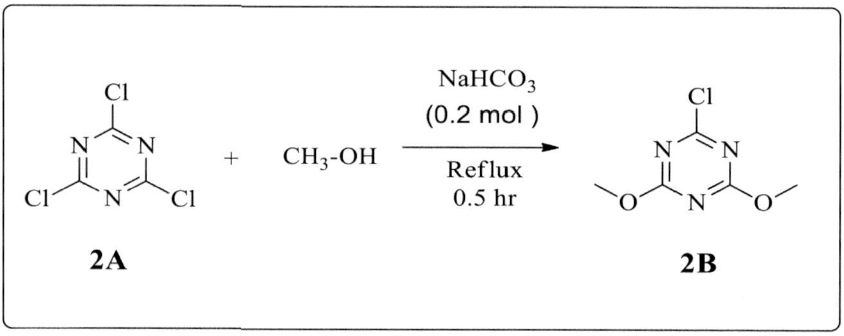

SCHEME 2.3   Synthesis of 2-chloro-4,6-dimethoxy-1,3,5-triazine (**2B**) (CDMT).

The possible mechanism of CDMT (**2B**) is as follows: Methanol (2 mol) acts as a nucleophile. Then two chlorine atoms of cyanuric chloride are substituted by methoxy anion with the formation of CDMT (**2B**).

Also, when we performed a reaction at a higher temperature and longer time resulted in 2, 4, 6-trimethoxy-1,3,5-triazine. Thus, by controlling the temperature, time, and mole of methanol, we achieved a suitable reaction condition for the synthesis of CDMT (**2B**).

The obtained CDMT is characterized by various analytical data. In ^{1}H NMR spectrum, chemical shift obtained at δ 4.04 (s, 6H) indicates the presence of two methoxy groups in CDMT and in mass spectrum peak at 175.5 confirms its molecular weight. The melting point is matching with literature. Then, CDMT (**2B**) was treated with various substituted aromatic/heterocyclic amines (**2C**) in the presence of anhydrous potassium carbonate in dry THF under reflux condition. Initially, we were using 1 equivalent K_2CO_3, but the reaction did not proceed to completion even after keeping for a longer time.

Hence, we increased the amount of K_2CO_3 to 2 equivalents and thus obtained the corresponding compounds (**2a-l**) with 70–75% yields (Scheme 2.2). All the reactions were completed within 4 hrs. The progress of the reaction was monitored by TLC. The structures of substituted 4,6-dimethoxy-*N*-phenyl-1,3,5-triazin-2-amine derivatives (**2a-l**) were confirmed by IR, ^{1}H NMR data, and mass spectrum analysis.

The IR spectra of compounds (**2a-l**) exhibit the characteristic absorption bands at 3225–3330 cm^{-1} (N-H stretching in secondary amine),

3000–2950 cm^{-1} (-C-H stretching in aliphatic), 1450–1650 cm^{-1},(-C=C, -C-H, aromatic stretching), 802–821 cm^{-1} (C$_3$N$_3$ in s-triazine ring).

The analytical, IR, and ^{1}H NMR data for compounds (**2a-l**) are given in Tables 2.1–2.3.

2.5 BIOLOGICAL EVALUATION

2.5.1 INTRODUCTION

The amazing progress represented by the appearance of antibiotics has changed the medical diagnosis of major and minor infections [15]. The bacterial resistance continues to expand and create a significant threat both in hospitals and more recently in the community [16]. The important information on the resistant antibacterial agent for human medicine is provided by World Health Organization and decided that the list of a critically imperative antibacterial agent should be restructured regularly as latest information become available, together with data on resistance pattern, new-fangled, and rising diseases and the growth of new drugs.[1] From the previous few years, the potential of s-triazine derivatives in medicinal and agrochemical properties have been subjected to investigation. Literature review indicates that amino-substituted triazine derivatives are connected with the numeral of significant antibacterial activities against gram-positive (*B. subtilius, B. sphaericus, S. aureus*, etc.) and gram-negative bacteria [17, 18] (*E. Coli, K. aerogenes, P. aeruginosa*, etc.). Since fluorine-containing compounds show potential bioactivity and promising metabolic stability and lipophilicity. The biological activities are physico-chemical properties of targeted molecules, and this consideration is made of a sort of chemical that fits into the active site.

2.5.2 ANTIBACTERIAL AND ANTIFUNGAL ASSAY

The compounds were diluted in dimethyl sulfoxide (DMSO) with 1 mg/mL concentrations for bioassay. The Antimicrobial activity was evaluated by

---

[1] Critically important antibacterial agents for human medicine for risk management strategies of non-human use. *Report of WHO Working Group Consultation*, Canberra, Australia, 15–18 Feb., 2005.

TABLE 2.1 Analytical and Mass Spectral Data of Triazine Amine Derivatives (2a-I)

Sr.No.	Mol. Formula	M.W.	Elemental Analysis Found (Calculated)			Mass (m/z)	M.P. (°C)	Yield%
			% C	% H	% N			
2a	$C_{13}H_{16}N_4O_4$	292.40	53.38 (53.42)	5.48 (5.52)	19.13 (19.17)	293[M+1]$^+$	126–128	75%
2b	$C_{13}H_{16}N_4O_4$	292.40	53.39 (53.42)	5.49 (5.52)	19.14 (19.17)	293[M+1]$^+$	120–122	73%
2c	$C_{10}H_{10}N_5O_2F$	251.22	47.78 (47.81)	4.58 (4.61)	27.85 (27.88)	252[M+1]$^+$	182–184	72%
2d	$C_{12}H_{14}N_4O_3$	262.11	54.90 (54.96)	5.35 (5.38)	21.35 (21.36)	263[M+1]$^+$	108–110	73%
2e	$C_{12}H_{11}N_4O_3F_3$	316.08	45.55 (45.58)	3.48 (3.51)	17.70 (17.72)	317[M+1]$^+$	125–126	70%
2f	$C_{11}H_{10}N_4O_2F_2$	268.08	49.25 (49.26)	3.74 (3.76)	20.85 (20.89)	269[M+1]$^+$	168–170	70%
2g	$C_{11}H_{11}FN_4O_2$	250.09	52.75 (52.80)	4.40 (4.43)	22.35 (22.39)	251[M+1]$^+$	142–144	72%
2h	$C_{10}H_{16}N_4O_3$	240.09	49.95 (49.99)	6.68 (6.71)	23.30 (23.32)	241[M+1]$^+$	110–111	73%
2i	$C_{11}H_{11}FN_4O_2$	250	52.02 (52.08)	4.40 (4.43)	22.35 (22.39)	251[M+1]$^+$	193–194	72%

TABLE 2.1 *(Continued)*

Sr.No.	Mol. Formula	M.W.	Elemental Analysis Found (Calculated)			Mass (m/z)	M.P. (°C)	Yield%
			% C	% H	% N			
2j	$C_{11}H_{13}N_5O_3$	263	50.15 (50.19)	4.95 (4.98)	26.31 (26.60)	$264[M+1]^+$	210–212	72%
2k	$C_{11}H_{13}N_5O_2$	247	53.40 (53.43)	5.25 (5.30)	28.29 (28.32)	$248[M+1]^+$	88–90	73%
2l	$C_{12}H_{12}N_6O_2$	272	52.90 (52.94)	4.40 (4.44)	30.83 (30.87)	$273[M+1]^{+\cdot}$	150–152	72%

R = different aromatic and heterocyclic amines.

TABLE 2.2 IR Spectral Data of Triazine Amine Derivatives (2a-l)

Sr. No.	Substituent R	IR Band Position (Wave Number cm−1)				
		-NH str. in 2° Amine	-C-H str. in (-OCH$_3$) Alkane	Ar-C=C- str. aromatic	C-O-C str. Aromatic Ether	-C-N- str. in Triazine
2a		3338	2980	1629	1207	809
2b		3339	2988	1614	1226	805
2c		3281	2984	1628	1202	809
2d		3280	2983	1618	1199	813
2e		3297	2988	1618	1225	804
2f		3250	2987	1637	1214	810

TABLE 2.2 *(Continued)*

Sr. No.	Substituent R	IR Band Position (Wave Number cm−1)				
		-NH str. in 2° Amine	-C-H str. in (-OCH₃) Alkane	Ar-C=C- str. aromatic	C-O-C str. Aromatic Ether	-C-N- str. in Triazine
2g	(structure)	3281	2982	1629	1198	807
2h	(structure)	3330	2979	1629	1222	809
2i	(structure)	3275	2950	1630	1210	809
2j	(structure)	3280	2960	1625	1207	812
2k	(structure)	3330	2975	1630	1200	815
2l	(structure)	3398	2985	1616	1231	801

TABLE 2.3 ¹H NMR Spectral Data of Triazine Amine Derivatives (2a-I)

Sr. No.	R	Assignments, Number of Proton, Multiplicity, and Chemical Shift in ppm				
		-OCH₃ in Triazine	Ar-OCH₃	Ar-H	Ar-H	-NH
2a		6H, s (3.72)	6H, s (3.77)	1H, s (6.21)	2H, s (7.05)	1H, s (10.06)
2b		6H, s (3.91)	6H, s (3.71–3.74)	1H, d (6.90)	1H, dd (7.14), 1H, d (7.52)	1H, s (9.95)
2c		6H, s (3.91)	—	1H, dd (7.19)	1H, m (8.27), 1H, dd (8.50)	1H, s (10.34)
2d		6H, s (3.91)	3H, s (3.74)	1H, m (6.62), 2H, m (7.24)	1H, m (7.51)	1H, s (10.12)
2e		6H, s (3.93)	—	1H, m (6.97), 1H, t (7.41)	1H, m (7.63), 1H,s (7.96)	1H, s (10.36)

TABLE 2.3 (Continued)

Sr. No.	R	Assignments, Number of Proton, Multiplicity, and Chemical Shift in ppm				
		-OCH$_3$ in Triazine	Ar-OCH$_3$	Ar-H	Ar-H	-NH
2f		6H, s (3.93)	—	1H, m (7.27–7.34), 1H, m (7.43–7.47)	1H, s (7.89)	1H, s (10.25)
2g		6H, s (3.91)		2H, m (7.09)	2H, m (7.71)	1H, s (10.07)
2h		-CH$_2$- 4H, m (1.49–1.89) 2H, q (1.90–1.93)	6H, s (3.83–3.88)	-CH$_2$- 2H, t (3.92–3.99)	-CH- 1H, t (4.01)	1H, s (8.22)
2i		6H, s (3.91)	—	1H, m (6.56) 2H, m (7.21)	1H, m (7.71)	1H, s (10.20)
2j		6H, s (3.90)	3H, s (3.71)	1H, m (7.15)	1H, m (8.23) 1H, m (8.45)	1H, s (10.31)

antimicrobial assay of the compounds by standard method [19], i.e., agar cup plate method against a panel of human pathogenic microorganisms: Gram-positive, *Staphylococcus aureus* NCIM 2178, *B. subtilis* NCIM 2250, Gram-negative, *Escherichia coli* NCIM 2137 and *Pseudomonas aeruginosa* NCIM 2036 while for the antifungal assay studies, *Candida albicans* MTCC 227, *Candida glabrata* NCIM 3236, *Candida tropicalis* NCIM 3110, and *Aspergillus niger* NCIM 545 fungi were used. The NA (Nutrient agar) was used as the culture media for antibacterial activity, and PDA (Potato Dextrose Agar) and YPD (Yeast Peptone Dextrose) agar were used as the culture media for antifungal activity. The commercial available Chloramphenicol and Griseofulvin in DMSO served as reference drugs for antibacterial and antifungal activity, respectively, to compare inhibition of growth. Both the plate containing the bacterial organisms and fungal organisms were incubated at 37°C for 48 h. Averages of three independent determinations were recorded. Agars were melted and poured in petri dishes according to the Clinical and Laboratory Standards Institute (CLSI, M2-A5 January 2007). Approximately 10^7 cell cultures were spread, and cups were prepared by the sterile borer. The 100 µl compounds were inoculated in each cup. The plates were incubated at 37°C, examined after 24 h, and incubated further for 48 h, where necessary. The zone of inhibition produced by each compound was measured in mm. The results of antibacterial activity are depicted in Table 2.4, and that of antifungal activity are given in Table 2.5. The tested compounds showed slight to moderate antibacterial and antifungal activity.

2.5.3   SAR OF SYNTHESIZED COMPOUNDS

2.5.3.1   ANTIBACTERIAL ACTIVITY

The synthesized new substituted 4,6-dimethoxy-*N*-phenyl-1,3,5-triazin-2-amine derivatives **(2a-l)** were evaluated for their antibacterial activities using Chloramphenicol (250 µg/mL) as standard drugs and DMSO as control. The compounds **2c, 2e, 2f, 2g, 2i,** and **2l** are shown potential antibacterial activities against human pathogenic micro organisms, i.e., Gram-positive, *Staphylococcus aureus* NCIM 2178, *B. subtilis* NCIM 2250, Gram-negative, *Escherichia coli* NCIM 2137 and *Pseudomonas aeruginosa* NCIM 2036. However, the compounds **2e** and **2f** are shown promising antibacterial activity against both Gram-positive and Gram-negative bacteria as compare with Chloramphenicol. Also, remaining **2c, 2g, 2i, 2l** compounds are moderately active against Gram-positive and Gram-negative bacteria. Potency may be increased due to the presence of a fluorine functional group. Also, maybe **2l** compound shows the potency due to the presence of imidazole as a heterocyclic ring in their moiety. Synthesized compounds are shows promising antibacterial activities against Gram-positive, *Staphylococcus aureus* NCIM 2178, *B. subtilis* NCIM 2250 as compared to Gram-negative, *Escherichia coli* NCIM 2137 and *Pseudomonas aeruginosa* NCIM 2036 pathogens. This is due to the presence of methoxy (-OCH$_3$) groups in these compounds [20]. The results of antibacterial activities are summarized in Table 2.4.

TABLE 2.4   Antibacterial Activity Data of Triazine Amine Derivatives (**2a-l**)

Compound (2a-l) 1 mg/mL	Gram Positive Bacteria		Gram Negative Bacteria	
	S. aureus	*B. subtili*	*E. coli*	*P. aeruginosa*
a	16	15	11	15
b	16	13	11	13
c	20	20	19	18
d	16	16	15	14
e	25	24	21	21
f	23	22	20	19
g	19	18	18	17
h	16	17	15	14
i	20	21	19	18
j	16	15	13	14
k	16	15	12	13
l	22	21	20	21
Chloramphenicol (250 μg/mL)	24	25	20	22
DMSO	00	00	00	00

Zone of inhibition (mm).

2.5.3.2   ANTIFUNGAL ACTIVITY

The antifungal activities of synthesized new substituted 4,6-dimethoxy-*N*-phenyl-1,3,5-triazin-2-amines **(2a-l)** are determined by using *Candida* *albicans* MTCC 227, *Candida glabrata* NCIM 3236, *Candida tropicalis* NCIM 3110, and *Aspergillus niger* NCIM 545 pathogens. *Griseofulvin* (250 µg/mL) is used as a standard drug for the comparison of their antifungal activities, and DMSO is used as control. Most of the tested compounds **2c, 2e, 2f, 2g, 2i,** and **2l** are found to exhibit good anti-fungal activity. Out of these compounds, it is observed that compounds **2e** and **2f** are shown promising antifungal activities against all fungi compared with standard *Griseofulvin* drugs. This increased potency may be due to the presence of 4,6-dimethoxy-1,3,5-triazine ring with $-OCF_3$ and $-F$ functional groups that are present in the compound. Also, synthesized compounds are shows promising antifungal activity against *Candida albicans* (MTCC 227), and *Candida tropicalis* (NCIM 3110) compare with test remaining fungi *Candida glabrata* (NCIM 3236) and *Aspergillus niger* (NCIM 545) were observed. This is observed due to the presence of methoxy ($-OCH_3$) group in these triazine amines [20]. The results of antifungal activities are summarized in Table 2.5.

TABLE 2.5 Antifungal Activity Data of Triazine Amine Derivatives **(2a-l):**

Compound (2a-l) 1 mg/mL	C. albicans	C. tropicalis	C. glabrata	A. niger
a	14	15	12	14
b	14	14	13	13
c	19	18	17	16
d	14	16	11	15
e	24	23	21	22
f	23	22	20	21
g	19	17	16	17
h	14	15	17	15
i	18	17	16	17
j	16	15	12	13
k	16	15	11	13
l	21	20	19	18
Griseofulvin (250 µg/mL)	23	24	22	21
Control (DMSO)	00	00	00	00

Zone of inhibition (mm).

2.6 CONCLUSION

In this chapter, we have reported the synthesis of CDMT from cyanuric chloride. It has an advantage of the small reaction time of 30 min giving an excellent yield of 75%. The synthesis of compounds (**2a-l**) using CDMT and substituted anilines/heterocyclic amines (1 mmol) in dry THF offer uniqueness in synthesis in the presence of anhydrous K_2CO_3 at reasonable temperature (70°C) condition, shorter reaction time, good yield (70–75%) of products. The process offers a cleaner reaction profile and an easy workup procedure. All the synthesized derivatives (**2a-l**) were screened for their antibacterial and antifungal activities. Compounds **2c, 2e, 2f, 2g, 2i,** and **2l** shows potential antibacterial activity against human pathogenic microorganisms. Potency may be increased due to the presence of a fluorine functional group and imidazole as a heterocyclic ring in their moiety. Also, compounds **2c, 2e, 2f, 2g, 2i,** and **2l** are found potential anti-fungal against *Candida albicans* MTCC 227, *Candida glabrata* NCIM 3236, *Candida tropicalis* NCIM 3110 and *Aspergillus niger* NCIM 545. This increased potency may be due to the presence of 4,6-dimethoxy-1,3,5-triazine ring with –OCF and –F functional groups are present in the moiety. The synthesized products (**2a-l**) showed promising antibacterial activity (*zone of inhibition*: 11 mm to 25 mm) and antifungal activity (*zone of inhibition*: 11 mm to 24 mm).

KEYWORDS

- 2-chloro-4,6-dimethoxy-1,3,5-triazine
- antifungal activity
- cyanuric chloride
- diluted in dimethyl sulfoxide
- dimethyl sulfoxide
- substituted anilines

REFERENCES

1. Kaswala, P. B., Chikhalia, K. H., Shah, N. K., Patel, D. P., Patel, D. H., & Mudaliar, G. V., (2009). *Arkivoc, Xi, 326.*
2. Raval, J. P., Rai, A. R., Patel, N. H., Patel, H. V., & Patel, P. S., (2009). *Intre. J. Chem. Tech. Research, 3*(1), 616.
3. Bhat, H. R., Singh, U. P., Gahtori, P., Ghosh, S. K., Gogoi, K., Prakashe, A., & Singh, R. K., (2013). *New Journal of Chemistry*, *37*, 2654.
4. Kumar, J. G., Bomma, S., Srihari, E., Shrivastav, S., Naidu, M. G. V., Srinivas, K., & Rao, J. V., (2013). *Med. Chem. Res., 22*(12), 5973.
5. Thurston, J. T., Schaefer, F. C., Dudley, J. R., & Holm, H. D., (1951). *J. Am. Chem. Soc., 73*, 2992.
6. José, R. R., (2015). *ACS Sustainable Chem. Eng., 3*(12), 3405. (b) Antonio, D. L. H., (2014). *Arkivoc, ii*, 308.
7. Scharn, D., Wenschuh, H., Reineke, U., Schneider-Mergener, J., & Germeroth, L. J., (2000). *Comb. Chem.*, *2*, 361.
8. De Hoog, P., Gamez, P., Driessen, W. L., & Reedijk, J., (2002). *Tetrahedron Lett., 43*, 6783.
9. a) Bork, J. T., Lee, J. W., Khersonsky, S. M., Moon, H. M., & Chang, Y. T., (2003). *Tetrahedron Lett., 44*, 6141. (b) Moon, S. H., (2002). *J. Am. Chem. Soc., 124*, 11608.
10. Ronchi, S., Prosperi, D., Compostella, F., & Panza, L., (2004). *Synlett*, 1007.
11. Oliva, J. M., Azenha, E., Burrows, H. D., Coimbra, R., De Melo, J. S. S., Canle, M. L., Fernandez, M. I., Santaballa, J. A., & Serrano-Andres, L., (2005). *Chem. Phy. Chem., 6*, 306.
12. Hu, X. P., Chen, H. L., & Zheng, Z., (2005). *Adv. Synth. Catal., 347*, 541.
13. Pedroso, L. M., Castro, M., Simoes, P., & Portugal, A., (2005). *Polymer, 46*, 1766.
14. (a) De Hoog, P., Gamez, P., Mutikainen, H., Turpeinen, U., & Reedijk, J., (2004). *Angew. Chem. Int. Edit., 43*, 5815. (b) De Hoog, P., Gamez, P., Driessen, W. L., & Reedijk, J., (2002). *Tetrahedron Lett., 43*, 6783.
15. Wise, R., Hart, T., Cars, O., Helmuth, R., Huovinen, P., & Sprenger, M., (1998). Streulens MB., *M. J., 317*, 609.
16. Barker, J., (2006). *Drugs Discov. Today, 11*, 391.
17. Srinivas, K., Srinivas, U., Bhanuprakash, K., Harakishore, K., Murthy, U. S. N., & Rao, V. J., (2006). *Eur. J. Med. Chem., 41*, 1240.
18. Zhou, Y., Sun, Z., Froelich, J. M., Hermann, T., & Wall, D., (2006). *Bioorg. Med. Chem. Lett., 16*, 5451.
19. Barry, A. L., (1977). *The Antimicrobic Susceptibility Test: Principles and Practices*, (IIIus Lea and Febiger: Philadelphia, Pa, USA), 180, *Bio Abstr, 64*, 25183.
20. Parikh, K. S., & Vyas, S. P., (2012). *Am. J. Pharmatech. Res., 2*(1), 570.

CHAPTER 3

AN EFFICIENT GREEN SYNTHESIS OF DIPHENYL PYRAZOL-4-YL-THIO-PYRIDIN-4-YL-1,3,4-OXADIAZOLE DERIVATIVES AND EVALUATION OF THEIR ANTIMICROBIAL AND ANTIOXIDANT ACTIVITY

AJAY N. AMBHORE

Department of Chemistry, Padmabhushan Dr. Vasantraodada Patil College, Tasgaon, Sangli, Maharashtra, India
Email: ambhorevijay1@gmail.com, rss.333@rediffmail.com

ABSTRACT

Design and development of new heterocycles predicting significant thera-peutic values based on molecular hybridization are the main aspects of drug discovery. This may lead to enhance the bioactivity of the hybrid molecule. The development of an eco-friendly route for the synthesis of bioactive compounds is one of the prime goals of a medicinal chemist. The classical method adopted for the synthesis of bioactive hybrid molecules suffers from many serious disadvantages like prolonged reaction time, use of toxic solvents and reagents, expensive ligands, poor yields, and one or more side products. So as to overcome such issues and to make the ideal synthesis, the principle of green chemistry attracted the attention of synthetic chemists. In this section, we report an efficient green method for the synthesis of diphenyl pyrazol-4-yl-thio-pyridin-4-yl-1,3,4-oxadiazole derivatives (**6a-s**) by using Bleaching Earth Clay (pH 12.5) and PEG-400 as green reaction media. It includes the hybridization of two impor-tant pharmacophores, i.e., pyrazole, and 1,3,4-oxadiazole into a single molecular skeleton leading to the new prototype as a better drug possibly having some advantages like improving biological activities as well as to overcome drug resistance. All the synthesized compounds are characterized and screened for their antimicrobial and *in vitro* antioxidant activity in which most of the screened compounds show significant activity.

3.1 INTRODUCTION AND REVIEW OF LITERATURE

The chemistry of heterocyclic compounds attracted much consideration in recent times due to its increasing significance in the field of pharmaceuticals and industrial applications [1, 2]. In fact, the development of simple, elegant, and facile methodologies for the synthesis of heterocycles is one of the most essential aspects of organic synthesis.

Oxadiazoles are the very well inevitable class of heterocyclic compounds with assorted pharmaceutical applications. The 1,3,4-oxadiazoles have emerged as an important class of compound with resourceful applications in the meadow of pharmaceutical, pesticide, and polymer sciences. The synthesis of 1,3,4-oxadiazole and its derivatives have been established scrupulous attention for a long time because of its outstanding biological and pharmacological properties such as, antitubercular [3], anti-HIV [4], antiviral [5], anti-inflammatory [6], antimalarial [7], antioxidant [8–10], antineoplastic [11], and hypoglycemic activity [12]. Thus, the synthesis of oxadiazole offers a great impulsion to research and development of bioactive compounds.

On the other hand, pyrazole and their derivatives have acknowledged standing attention in heterocyclic chemistry and captivate substantial interest because of its versatile biological activities like antimalarial [13], antifungal [14, 15], and anti-inflammatory [16–21]. In recent times, some pyrazoles have been reported for their potential therapeutic bioactivity like antimicrobial, antiviral, and anticancer [22–28].

These virtues of both the oxadiazole and pyrazole scaffold make them very peculiar in the field of medicinal chemistry for the synthesis of various bioactive molecules, as pointed out in Figure 3.1 [29–34], and show widespread therapeutic application beneficial for society.

In the view of above sensible observations and considering the structural diversity plays an important role in combinatorial and pharmaceutical chemistry and our exposure to use of BEC and PEG-400 as green reaction media for the synthesis of bioactive molecules [35–40]. Herein we design and develop some new compounds predicting significant therapeutic values based on molecular hybridization. It includes the hybridization of two important pharmacophores, i.e., pyrazole, and 1,3,4-oxadiazoleinto a single molecular skeleton leading to the new prototype as a better drug possibly having some advantages like improved biological activities [41] as well as to overcome drug resistance [42].

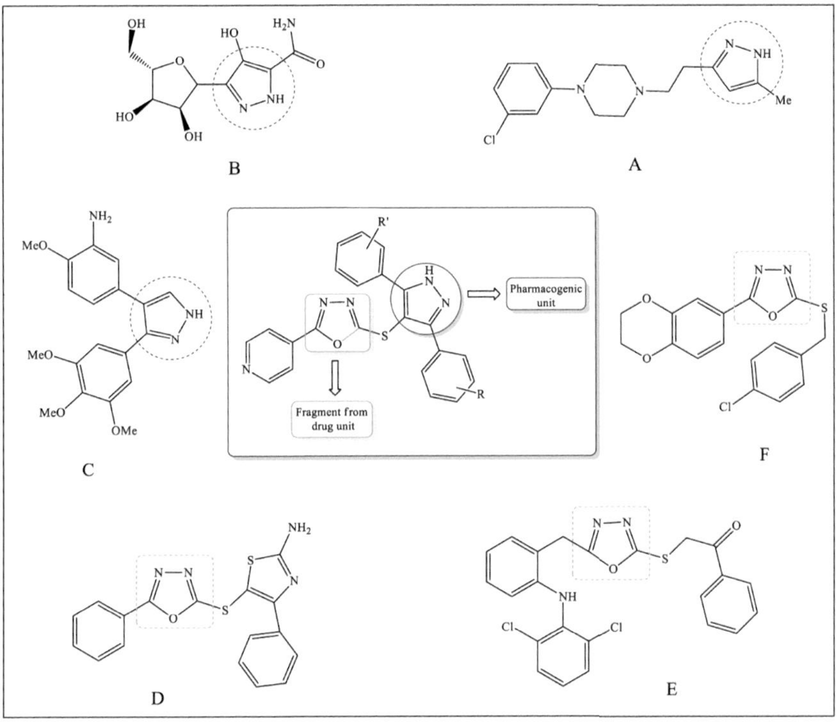

FIGURE 3.1   Bioactive molecules containing 1*H*-pyrazole and 1,3,4-oxadiazole scaffold.

3.2   RESULT AND DISCUSSION

3.2.1   CHEMISTRY

The synthetic route of the title compound *diphenyl pyrazol-4-yl-thio-pyridin-4-yl-1,3,4-oxadiazole derivatives* (**6a–s**) is depicted in Scheme 3.1. According to this scheme, the precursor two was prepared by the reaction of isoniazid with carbon disulfide under the basic medium [43–46]. The structure of compound **2** was confirmed by IR, NMR, and Mass spectral data. IR spectrum of compound **2** gives absorption band at 3273 cm^{-1} for –NH stretching. The absorption band at 1610 cm^{-1} corresponds to >C=N stretching. The C-O-C and >C=S stretching viewed at 1374 cm^{-1} and 1282 cm^{-1}, respectively. The ^{1}H NMR spectrum of compound **2** revealed a singlet at δ 14.66 ppm was attributed to –NH proton. Whereas, remaining protons were observed at their corresponding aromatic region at δ 8.82–7.82 ppm. The molecular ion peak observed at *m/z* 178 corresponds to the molecular mass of the compound. Furthermore, precursor **2** when react with substituted phenacyl bromide (**3a-e**) in the presence of BEC and PEG-400 as green reaction medium to get an intermediate (**4a-e**).

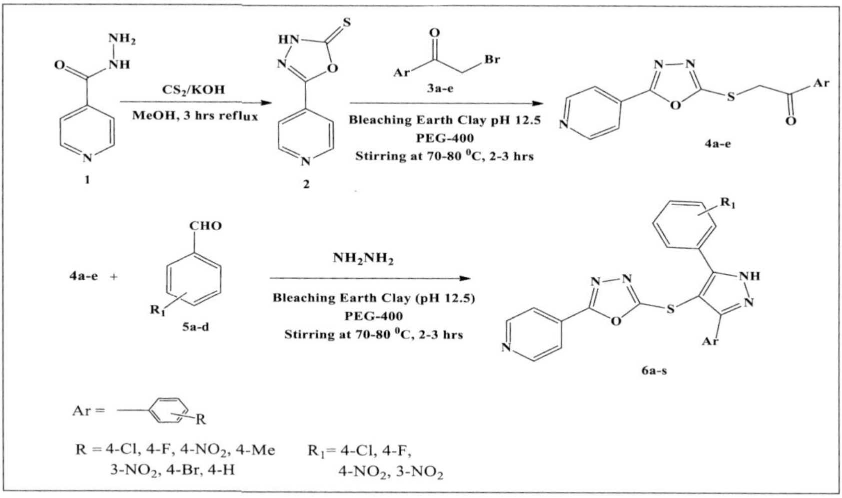

SCHEME 3.1   Synthetic route of diphenyl pyrazol-4-yl-thio-pyridin-4-yl-1,3,4-oxadiazole derivatives (**6a-s**).

The structures of compounds (**4a-e**) were confirmed by the IR, ^{1}H NMR, and Mass spectral analysis. The IR spectrum of compound **4a** shown a characteristic absorption band at 1678 cm^{-1} clearly indicates the presence of >C=O (carbonyl) group. The ^{1}H NMR spectrum of compound **4a** revealed a singlet at δ 5.21 ppm was attributed to aliphatic -CH$_2$ protons, whereas the remaining protons appear in their respective aromatic region at δ 8.82–7.67ppm. The molecular ion peak in the mass spectrum observed at *m/z* 331 corresponds to the molecular mass of the compound.

Furthermore, one-pot condensation of **4a-e** with substituted benzaldehyde (**5a-d**) and hydrazine hydrate in the presence of BEC and PEG-400
offer title compound in good yield. Initially, *in situ* generations of α,
β-unsaturated compounds by the BEC catalyzed Knoevenagel condensation of **4a-e** with substituted benzaldehyde (**5a-d**) followed by the Michael
addition of hydrazine hydrate to give the title compounds (**6a-s**). The
structures of compounds **6a-s** were established by the satisfactory spectral
analysis. In an IR spectrum, the compounds **6a** shown a strong stretching
vibration band at 3180 cm^{-1} indicate the presence of -NH group. A strong
stretching vibration observes at 1625 cm^{-1} due to the presence of >C=N
and a strong stretching vibration at 1090 cm^{-1} confirms the presence of
C-O-C linkage. The ^{1}H NMR spectra of compound **6a** revealed a singlet
at δ 8.65 ppm was attributed to -NH of pyrazole, whereas the remaining
protons are present in their corresponding aromatic region at δ 8.43–7.20
ppm. The compound **6a** in the mass spectrum gave a peak at *m/z* 467 due to
[M+1]. The plausible mechanism was outlined in Scheme 3.2.

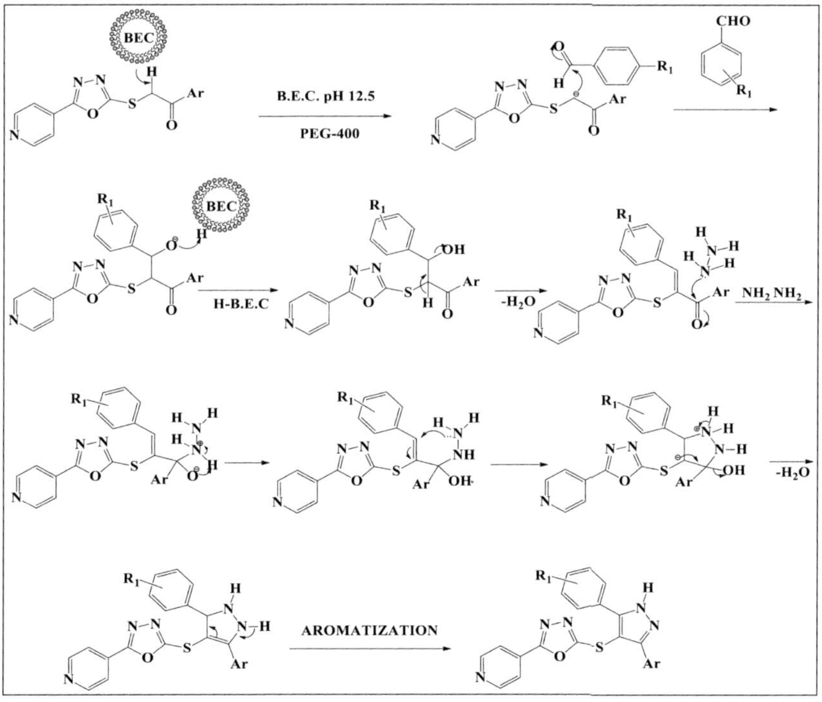

SCHEME 3.2   Possible mechanism of compounds (**6a-s**).

In order to synthesize the title compounds (**6a-s**) in good quantitative yield, the model reaction was studied for the optimization of the newly designed cyclization route. Keeping in mind "Principles of Green Chemistry," initially, the reaction was carried out under solvent-free and catalyst-free condition. We observed that in the absence of catalyst, there was no reaction at room temperature or even at a higher temperature.

Moreover, the model reaction was studied under different basic catalysts such as K_2CO_3, Triethylamine (TEA), Piperidine, Morpholine, and BEC. Among these catalysts, BEC was found to be effective due to their reusability and offer the best yield 90% (entry 9, Table 3.1).

TABLE 3.1   Influence of the Catalyst on the Synthesis of (**6c**)

Entry	Catalyst (mole/wt%)	Temperature (°C)	Time (h)[a]	Yield(%)[b]
1	No Catalyst	RT	7	0
2	No Catalyst	80	7	0
3	K_2CO_3 (mole%)	70	6	60
4	TEA (mole%)	70	6	64
5	Piperidine (mole%)	70	5	65
6	Morpholine (mole%)	70	6	55
7	Bleaching Earth Clay (1 wt%)	80	3	73
8	Bleaching Earth Clay (5 wt%)	80	2.5	85
9	Bleaching Earth Clay (10 wt%)	80	2	90

[a] Reaction progress monitored by thin-layer chromatography (TLC).
[b] Yields refer to isolated yield.

The synthesis is said to be ideal if it is carried out under a solvent-free condition or by adopting the use of a green solvent. Initially, the model reaction was studied under the solvent-free condition in the presence of BEC as a catalyst, and it was observed that the yield of reaction appears at the lower side. In order to enhance the yield of the reaction, the model reaction was carried out in the water, considering water as green reaction media. It revealed that the reaction was not clean and efficient as far as the yield and purity of the product was a concern (Table 3.2, entry1). In recent years PEG-400 attracted much attention to synthetic chemists for its use as green reaction media. Hence, we studied a model reaction in PEG-400 in the presence of BEC as a catalyst, and to our delight, the combination of PEG-400 and BEC was found efficient for the conversion of reactant to a product near about 90% yield. An increase in the yield of the product by the present protocol can be assumed by the fact that PEG-400 can act as a solvent as well as a phase transfer catalyst. With this optimized condition utilizing PEG-400 and BEC as a green catalytic media, we have efficiently synthesized all remaining derivatives in good yield and high purity.

TABLE 3.2 Influence of the Solvent on the Synthesis of **(6c)**

Entry	Solvent	Time(h)[a]	5c(%)[b]
1	Water	6	0
2	EtOH	5	71
3	CH$_3$COOH	6	62
4	DMF	6	67
5	PEG-400	2	85

[a] Reaction progress monitored by thin-layer chromatography (TLC).
[b] Yields refer to isolated yield.

Finally, we focus on the recycling of the catalyst, and it was found that the catalyst BEC shows good catalytic power up to five-run with minimum loss of activity (Figure 3.2). This shows the reusability of the catalyst. Thus, at the end of the model reaction, the catalyst was filtered by simple filtration, washed thoroughly with water, dried at room temperature, and reused for the next reaction (Table 3.3).

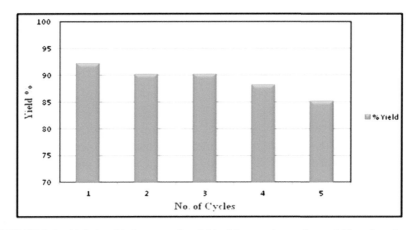

FIGURE 3.2 Relationship between the yield of the reaction and reusability of catalyst.

TABLE 3.3 Synthesis of Compounds (6a-s)

Entry	Product	Ar	R_1	Molecular Formula	Yield (%)	M.P. (°C)
1	6a	4-Cl C_6H_4-	4-Cl	$C_{22}H_{13}Cl_2N_5OS$	87	152–154
2	6b	4-Cl C_6H_4-	4-F-	$C_{22}H_{13}ClFN_5OS$	82	142–145
3	6c	4-Cl C_6H_4-	4-NO_2-	$C_{22}H_{13}ClN_6O_3S$	92	156–158
4	6d	4-Cl C_6H_4-	3-NO_2-	$C_{22}H_{13}ClN_6O_3S$	90	162–164
5	6e	4-F C_6H_4-	4-Cl-	$C_{22}H_{13}ClFN_5OS$	80	148–151
6	6f	4-F C_6H_4-	4-F-	$C_{22}H_{13}F_2N_5OS$	82	138–140
7	6g	4-F C_6H_4-	4-NO_2-	$C_{22}H_{13}FN_6O_3S$	91	156–159
8	6h	4-F C_6H_4-	3-NO_2-	$C_{22}H_{13}FN_6O_3S$	88	162–164
9	6i	4-NO_2 C_6H_4-	4-Cl-	$C_{22}H_{13}ClN_6O_3S$	93	166–168
10	6j	4-NO_2 C_6H_4-	4-F-	$C_{22}H_{13}FN_6O_3S$	89	162–164
11	6k	4-NO_2 C_6H_4-	4-NO_2-	$C_{22}H_{13}N_7O_5S$	92	168–170
12	6l	4-NO_2 C_6H_4-	3-NO_2-	$C_{22}H_{13}N_7O_5S$	92	167–169
13	6m	3-NO_2 C_6H_4-	4-Cl-	$C_{22}H_{13}ClN_6O_3S$	80	159–161
14	6n	3-NO_2 C_6H_4-	4-F-	$C_{22}H_{13}FN_6O_3S$	83	153–155
15	6o	3-NO_2 C_6H_4-	4-NO_2-	$C_{22}H_{13}N_7O_5S$	82	167–169
16	6p	3-NO_2 C_6H_4-	3-NO_2-	$C_{22}H_{13}N_7O_5S$	80	164–167
17	6q	4-Br C_6H_4-	4-Cl-	$C_{22}H_{13}BrClN_5OS$	82	176–178
18	6r	4-Br C_6H_4-	4-F-	$C_{22}H_{13}BrFN_5OS$	81	172–175
19	6s	4-Br C_6H_4-	4-NO_2-	$C_{22}H_{13}BrN_6O_3S$	84	181–183

3.2.2 BIOLOGY

3.2.2.1 ANTIBACTERIAL SCREENING

All the newly synthesized compounds (6a-s) were evaluated for their antibacterial activity (Table 3.4).

Antibacterial activity was carried out against *Bacillus megaterium* (Gram +ve) and *Escherichia coli* (Gram -ve) bacterial species by using the agar diffusion method. This study revealed that all the synthesized compounds show moderate to excellent antibacterial activity in comparison with penicillin as a standard drug, as shown in Table 3.4.

Among the synthesized compounds (6a-s), compound 6s showed excellent activity against *Bacillus megaterium* (MIC = 11.15) and *Escherichia coli* (MIC = 10.21). Compound **6k** had excellent activity (MIC = 30.12) against *Escherichia coli*. These data revealed that compound **6l** was highly active (MIC = 21.40) against *Bacillus megaterium*, and compound **6o** displayed strong activity (MIC = 44.20) against *Escherichia coli*. It is noteworthy that compound **6p** exhibited good activity (MIC = 50.12) against *Bacillus megaterium*. Compound **6c** (MIC = 62.78) and **6m** (MIC = 82.69) showed moderate activity against *Escherichia coli* while compound **6d** (MIC = 78.23) and **6i** (MIC=89.11) displayed good activity against *Bacillus megaterium*. Moreover, the remaining compounds possessed feeble antibacterial activities.

TABLE 3.4 Antibacterial Activities of the Synthesized Compounds (**6a-s**)

Entry	Product	Minimum Inhibition Concentration (MIC) in µg/mL	
		Bacillus megaterium	*Escherichia coli*
1	6a	250	250
2	6b	500	500
3	6c	125	62.78
4	6d	78.23	250
5	6e	500	500
6	6f	500	500
7	6g	250	250
8	6h	250	250
9	6i	89.11	125
10	6j	500	500
11	6k	125	30.12
12	6l	21.40	250
13	6m	250	82.69
14	6n	125	125
15	6o	250	44.20
16	6p	50.12	125
17	6q	125	125
18	6r	500	500
19	6s	11.15	10.21
STD	Penicillin	3.9 µg	3.9 µg

The results summarized are the mean values of the three independent experiments.

3.2.2.2 ANTIOXIDANT SCREENING

From the result depicted in Figure 3.3, it is revealed that all the newly synthesized compounds **(6a-s)** exhibit excellent to moderate antioxidant activities when compared with Ascorbic Acid (AA) as a standard. The DPPH assay has been widely used to study the ability of the compound acts as free radical scavengers or hydrogen donors to evaluate antioxidant activity. Compound **6s** (68.80%), **6k** (58.20%), and **6l** (57.82%) showed excellent DPPH radical scavenging activity as compared to standard AA (76.45%), while the rest compounds show moderate DPPH radical scavenging activity. The overall range of DPPH scavenging activity of all the tested compounds was (43.77–68.80%). OH, radicals are highly hyperactive among the relative oxygen species and play a key role in the physiological regulation and control of cell function [49]. It was observed that compound **6o** (61.25%), **6s** (58.89) and **6p** (55.95) exhibit very good OH radical scavenging activity as compared to standard AA (69.37%) whereas the remaining tested compounds displayed moderate to good radical scavenging activities. The overall range of OH scavenging activity of all the tested compounds was (32.86–61.25%). The profile of SOR radical scavenging activities indicates that compound **6l** (58.40%), **6p** (54.68%), and **6s** (52.02) exhibit very strong SOR radical scavenging activity as compared to standard AA (72.58%) whereas the rest compounds displayed moderate SOR radical scavenging activities. The overall range of SOR scavenging activity of all the tested compounds was (30.97–58.40%).

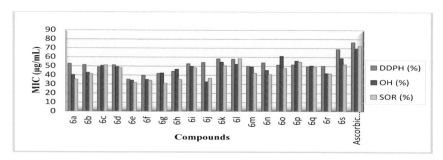

FIGURE 3.3   Graphical representation of Antioxidant screening of diphenyl pyrazol-4-yl-thio-pyridin-4-yl-1,3,4-oxadiazole derivatives **(6a-s)**.

[*The results summarized are the mean values of the three independent experiments*].

3.3   MATERIAL AND METHODS

3.3.1   CHEMISTRY

Melting points were determined by the open capillary method and were uncorrected. The chemicals and solvents used were of laboratory grade and purified prior to use. BEC was a gift from Supreme Silicones, Pune. The completion of the reaction was monitored by thin-layer chromatography (TLC) on pre-coated sheets of silica gel-G (Merck, Germany) using iodine vapors for detection. IR spectra were recorded (in KBR pallets) on the Shimadzu spectrophotometer. ^{1}H NMR and ^{13}C NMR spectra were recorded (in DMSO) d_6 on Bruker Avance-400 MHz spectrometer using TMS as an internal standard. The mass spectra were recorded on the EI-Shimadzu-GC-MS spectrometer.

3.3.2   GENERAL PROCEDURE FOR THE SYNTHESIS OF 5-(PYRIDINE-4-YL)-1,3,4-OXADIAZOLE-2(3H)-THIONE(2)

A mixture of isoniazid (0.005 mol) and carbon disulfide (5ml) in alcoholic KOH (20 ml, 10%) was refluxed for 12 hours. After completion of the reaction (monitored by TLC), the solution was cooled at room temp and poured into ice-cold water (50 ml) and acidified with dil. HCl. The solid product separated out was filtered and recrystallized from aq. acetic acid as white crystals.

IR (KBr) υ cm^{-1}: 3273 (-NH), 1610 (>C=N), 1375 (C-O-C), 1282 (>C=S); ^{1}H NMR (400MHz, DMSO-d$_6$, TMS, δ, ppm): 14.66 (s, 1H, -NH), 8.82 (d, 2H, Ar-H), 7.82 (d,2H, Ar-H).

3.3.3   GENERAL PROCEDURE FOR THE SYNTHESIS OF 1-(SUBSTITUTED PHENYL)-2((5-(PYRIDIN-4-YL))-1,3,4-OXADIAZOLE-2-YL) THIO)ETHANONE (4A-E)

A mixture of **2**(0.015 mol), substituted phenacyl bromide (**3a-e**) (0.015 mol), and BEC (10 wt%) was stirred in PEG-400 at 70–80°C for 2–3 hour. After completion of the reaction (monitored by TLC), the catalyst was separated by simple filtration, and the reaction mixture was poured into ice-cold water (50 ml) and neutralized with dilHCl. The separated solid was filtered and recrystallized by aq. Acetic acid as pink colored crystals.

3.3.3.1   1-(4-CHLOROPHENYL)-2-((5-(PYRIDIN-4-YL)-1,3,4-OXADIAZOL-2-YL)THIO)ETHANONE (4A)

M.P.131–133°C; Yield, 89%; IR (KBr, cm^{-1}): 3088 (Ar-H), 2959 (aliphatic -CH), 1678 (>C=O), 1615 (>C=N), 1312 (>C=S), 1293 (C-O-C oxadiazole), 1185 (C-S-C); ^{1}H NMR (400Mz, DMSO-d$_6$,TMS, δ, ppm): 8.81 (d, 2H, Ar-H), 8.08 (d, 2H, Ar-H), 7.88 (d, 2H, Ar-H), 7.67 (d,2H, Ar-H), 5.21 (s, 2H, CH$_2$); EIMS: 331[M+].

3.3.3.2   1-(4-NITROPHENYL)-2-((5-(PYRIDIN-4-YL)-1,3,4-OXADIAZOL-2-YL)THIO)ETHANONE (4C)

M.P. 136–138°C; Yield, 90%;IR (KBr, cm-1): 3148 (Ar-H), 2996(aliphatic, -CH), 1689 (>C=O), 1620 (>C=N), 1315 (>C=S), 1278 (C-O-C oxadiazole), 1150 (C-S-C); ^{1}H NMR (400Mz, DMSO-d$_6$, TMS, δ, ppm): 8.78 (d, 2H, Ar-H), 7.96 (d, 2H, Ar-H), 7.72 (d, 2H, Ar-H), 7.56 (d, 2H, Ar-H), 5.12 (s, 2H, CH$_2$); EIMS: 342 [M+].

3.3.3.3   1-(3-NITROPHENYL)-2-((5-(PYRIDIN-4-YL)-1,3,4-OXADIAZOL-2-YL)THIO)ETHANONE (4D)

M.P. 129–131°C;Yield, 89%; IR (KBr, cm^{-1}): 3130 (Ar-H), 2990 (CH$_2$), 1682 (>C=O), 1627 (>C=N), 1335 (>C=S), 1240 (C-O-C oxadiazole), 1178 (C-S-C); ^{1}H NMR (400Mz, DMSO-d$_6$,TMS, δ, ppm): 8.92 (d,2H, Ar-H), 8.12 (d, 2H, Ar-H), 7.91 (d, 2H, Ar-H), 7.78 (d, 2H, Ar-H), 5.30 (s, 2H, CH$_2$); EIMS: 342 [M+].

3.3.3.4   1-(4-BROMOPHENYL)-2-((5-(PYRIDIN-4-YL)-1,3,4-OXADIAZOL-2-YL)THIO)ETHANONE (4E)

M.P. 158–160°C; Yield, 87%; IR (KBr, cm^{-1}): 3156 (Ar-H), 2940 (aliphatic, -CH), 1672 (>C=O), 1624 (>C=N), 1332 (>C=S), 1280 (C-O-C oxadiazole), 1192 (C-S-C); ^{1}H NMR(400 Mz, DMSO-d$_6$,TMS, δ, ppm): 8.97 (d,2H, Ar-H), 8.16 (d, 2H, Ar-H), 7.94 (d,2H, Ar-H), 7.89 (d, 2H, Ar-H), 5.38 (s, 2H, CH$_2$); EIMS: 374 [M+].

3.3.4 GENERAL PROCEDURE FOR THE SYNTHESIS OF 2-((3,5 DISUBSTITUTED(4-SUBSTITUTEDPHENYL)-1H-PYRAZOL-4-YL) THIO)-5-(PYRIDIN-4-YL)-1,3,4-OXADIAZOLE (6A-S)

A mixture of **4a-e** (1.00mmol) and substituted benzaldehyde **5a-d** (1.00mmol) was stirred in PEG-400 in the presence of BEC (10% wt) at 70°C for 1 hour. After completion of the reaction (indicated by TLC), hydrazine hydrate (99%) (1.00 mmol) was added to the reaction mixture, and the reaction mixture stirred for 1 hour at 80°C. After completion of the reaction (monitored by TLC), the solid catalyst was separated by simple filtration, and the mother liquor was poured into ice-cold water and then neutralized with dil. HCl. The solid separate out was filtered, washed with 10 ml ice-cold water, and recrystallized by chloroform to get pure product.

3.3.4.1   2-((3,5-BIS(4-CHLOROPHENYL)-1H-PYRAZOL-4-YL) THIO)-5-(PYRIDIN-4-YL)-1,3,4-OXADIAZOLE(6A)

M.P. 152–154°C;Yield, 87%;IR (KBr, cm^{-1}): 3180 (-NH), 1625 (>C=N), 1393 (C-S-C), 1090 (C-O-C); ^{1}H NMR (400 MHz, DMSO-d$_6$, TMS, δ, ppm): 8.65 (s, 1H, -NH), 8.65–7.20 (m, 12H, Ar-H); ^{13}C NMR (100 MHz, DMSO-d$_6$, TMS, δ, ppm): 160.40, 155.06, 150.10, 149.57, 137.21, 136.13, 132.92, 132.43, 131.88, 129.79, 129.29, 129.07, 128.84, 121.28; EIMS: 466 [M+]; Elemental Analysis. Calculated (found) for C$_{22}$H$_{13}$Cl$_2$N$_5$OS;% C, 56.66 (56.63); H, 2.81 (2.85); N, 15.02 (15.05); S, 6.88 (6.91).

3.3.4.2   2-((5-(4-CHLOROPHENYL)-3-(4-FLUOROPHENYL)-1H-PYRAZOL-4-YL)THIO)-5-(PYRIDIN-4-YL)-1,3,4-OXADIAZOLE (6E)

M.P. 148–151°C; Yield, 80%;IR (KBr, cm^{-1}): 3259 (-NH), 1620 (>C=N), 1315(C-S-C), 1080 (C-O-C); ^{1}H NMR (400 MHz, DMSO-d$_6$, TMS, δ, ppm): 8.72 (s, 1H, -NH), 7.96–7.19 (m,12H, Ar-H); ^{13}C NMR (100 MHz, DMSO-d$_6$, TMS, δ, ppm): 160.48, 156.42, 150.97, 149.91, 143.76, 132.54, 131.85,

130.46, 129.94, 128.83, 126.27, 124.67, 122.48, 121.74; EIMS: 449.05 [M+]; Elemental Analysis. Calculated (found) for $C_{22}H_{13}ClFN_5OS$;% C, 58.73 (58.76); H, 2.91 (2.88); N, 15.57 (15.60); S, 7.13 (7.17).

3.3.4.3   2-((3-(4-FLUOROPHENYL)-5-(3-NITROPHENYL)-1H-PYRAZOL-4-YL)THIO)-5-(PYRIDIN-4-YL)-1,3,4-OXADIAZOLE (6H)

M.P. 162–164°C; Yield, 88%; IR (KBr, cm⁻¹): 3215 (-NH), 1606 (>C=N), 1334 (C-S-C), 1130 (C-O-C); ¹H NMR (400 MHz, DMSO-d₆, TMS, δ, ppm): 8.49 (s, 1H, -NH), 7.86–7.17 (m,12H, Ar-H); ¹³C NMR (100 MHz, DMSO-d₆, TMS, δ, ppm): 160.92, 158.67, 156.39, 154.21, 150.34, 149.98, 134.46, 130.25, 129.10, 128.87, 127.89, 126.74, 121.42, 116.56; EIMS: 460[M+]; Elemental Analysis. Calculated (found) for $C_{22}H_{13}FN_6O_3S$;% C, 57.39 (57.35); H, 2.85 (2.87); N, 18.25 (18.27); S, 6.96 (6.92).

3.3.4.4   2-((3,5-BIS(4-NITROPHENYL)-1H-PYRAZOL-4-YL)THIO)-5-(PYRIDIN-4-YL)-1,3,4-OXADIAZOLE (6K)

M.P. 168–170°C; Yield, 92%; IR (KBr, cm⁻¹): 3225 (-NH), 1635 (>C=N), 1233 (C-S-C), 1120 (C-O-C); ¹H NMR (400 MHz, DMSO-d₆, TMS,δ, ppm): 8.77 (s, 1H, -NH), 8.43–8.11 (m, 12H, Ar-H); ¹³C NMR (100 MHz, DMSO-d₆, TMS,δ, ppm): 161.95, 156.77, 152.89, 149.22, 148.34, 146.24, 144.10, 141.85, 140.41, 139.48, 137.54, 135.88, 127.82; EIMS: 487 [M+]; Elemental Analysis. Calculated (found) for $C_{22}H_{13}N_7O_5S$;% C, 54.21 (54.25); H, 2.69 (2.66); N, 20.11 (20.13); S, 6.58 (6.62).

3.3.4.5   2-((3-(3-NITROPHENYL)-5-(4-NITROPHENYL)-1H-PYRAZOL-4-YL)THIO)-5-(PYRIDIN-4-YL)-1,3,4-OXADIAZOLE (6O)

M.P. 167–169°C; Yield, 82%; IR (KBr, cm⁻¹): 3190 (-NH), 1602 (>C=N), 1239 (C-S-C), 1086 (C-O-C); ¹H NMR (400 MHz, DMSO-d₆, TMS, δ, ppm): 8.73 (s, 1H, -NH), 8.12–7.51 (m, 12H, Ar-H); ¹³C NMR (100 MHz, DMSO-d₆, TMS, δ, ppm): 163.95, 156.77, 152.89, 149.22, 148.34, 146.24, 144.10, 141.85, 140.41, 139.48, 137.54, 135.88, 127.82; EIMS: 487 [M+]; Elemental Analysis. Calculated (found) for $C_{22}H_{13}N_7O_5S$;% C, 54.21 (54.25); H, 2.69 (2.67); N, 20.11 (20.14); S, 6.58 (6.60).

3.3.4.6   2-((3-(4-BROMOPHENYL)-5-(4-FLUOROPHENYL)-1H-PYRAZOL-4-YL)THIO)-5-(PYRIDIN-4-YL)-1,3,4-OXADIAZOLE (6R)

M.P. 172–175°C; Yield, 81%; IR (KBr, cm^{-1}): 3242 (-NH), 1600 (>C=N), 1221 (C-S-C), 1055 (C-O-C); ^{1}H NMR (400 MHz, DMSO-d$_6$,TMS, δ, ppm): 8.85 (s, 1H, -NH), 7.98–7.22 (m,12H, Ar-H); ^{13}C NMR (100 MHz, DMSO-d$_6$, TMS, δ, ppm):161.37, 148.85, 146.03, 140.66, 140.16, 130.71, 130.68, 128.08, 127.87, 126.00, 123.62, 118.85, 118.51, 107.63; EIMS: 495 [M+]; Elemental Analysis. Calculated (found) for C$_{22}$H$_{13}$BrFN$_5$OS;% C, 53.45 (53.48); H, 2.65 (2.62); N, 14.17 (14.19); S, 6.49 (6.45).

3.3.5   BIOLOGY

3.3.5.1   ANTIMICROBIAL SCREENING

The anti-microbacterial activities of the synthesized compounds were screened by using the agar diffusion method against two different bacterial species such as *Bacillus megaterium* and *Escherichia coli*. Penicillin was used as a standard drug for antibacterial activities. Dimethyl sulfoxide (DMSO) was used as a solvent. Nutrient agar plates are used for the evaluation of antibacterial activities, which was seeded with respective bacterial culture strain (0.1 ml) of the suspension prepared in sterile saline. All the plates were incubated at 37 ± 0.5 C for 24 h. The minimum inhibitory concentrations (MIC) are noted, and the results are summarized in Table 3.4.

3.3.5.2   ANTIOXIDANT SCREENING

In the present study, we investigate *in vitro* DPPH (1,1-diphenyl-2-picryl-hydrazil), OH, and SOR (superoxide anion) radical scavenging assay [50, 51] to evaluate the antioxidant potential of substituted pyrazolylthiopyr-idinyl 1,3,4-oxadiazole derivatives (**6a-s**) with respect to standard AA using spectrophotometer and the results are summarized in Figure 3.3.

3.3.5.2.1   DPPH Radical Scavenging Assay

The synthesized compound was added to 10^{-4}M ethanol solution of DPPH for the preparation of the solution having an equimolar concentration

(0.5–1mM). After incubation (30 min) at room temperature, the sample absorbance was measured on spectrophotometrically at 517 nm. AA was used as a standard.

3.3.5.2.2   OH Radical Scavenging Assay

For the generation of OH radicals, the ferric ion (Fe^{+3})/AA system was used. The OH radical detection being carried out by measuring the amount of formaldehyde generated from the oxidation of dimethyl sulfoxide (DMSO). The reaction mixture contain 0.1 mM EDTA, 167 mM Fe^{+3}, 33 mM DMSO in phosphate buffer (50 mM pH 7.4), 0.05–0.1mL individual 2(3,5-disubstituted)-1H-pyrazol-4-yl-thio-5-(pyridin-4-yl)1,3,4-oxadiazole derivatives (0.5–1mM) solution. The reaction was initiated by the addition of AA (150 mL, 10 mmole in phosphate buffer). The reaction was terminated by using Trichloroacetic acid (17% w/v). The generated formaldehyde was detected spectrophotometrically at 412 nm. For comparative study AA (1mM) was used as a reference compound.

3.3.5.2.3   Superoxide Anion Radical (SOR) Scavenging Assay

The superoxide anion radical (SOR) was generated by PMS/NADH system. Afterward, the superoxide anion was made to diminish NBT, which yields a chromogenic product withλ_{max}at 560 nm. The radical scavenging activities, which are concentration-dependent were performed separately. The reaction cocktail contain NBT (300mM), NADH (936mM), PMS (120 mM), and individual concentration of substituted pyrazolylthiopyridinyl 1,3,4-oxadiazolederivatives (0.5–1mM) in TrisHCl(buffer 100mM, pH 7.4). The reaction was initiated by the addition of PMS to the reaction mixture. After the incubation period (5 min) at room temperature, the reaction mixture was read at 560 nm by using thermo make the automatic ex-microplate reader (M51118170). The percentage activity of DPPH, OH, and SOR radical scavenging activity was calculated by using the following equation.

$$Activity\,(\%) = 1 - \frac{T}{C}\,X\,100$$

where, T = absorbance of the test sample; and C = absorbance of the standard sample.

3.4   CONCLUSIONS

In conclusion, we have found an efficient, mild, clean, and eco-friendly method for the synthesis of a new series of substituted pyrazolylthiopyridinyl 1,3,4-oxadiazole using BEC and PEG-400. The method offers several rewards, including short reaction time, simple isolation, and reusability of the catalyst, easy work-up. Furthermore, the biological screening result revealed that the newly synthesized compounds exhibited moderate to excellent biological activity. Compounds (**6k, 6l, 6o, 6p, 6s**) displayed excellent antibacterial activity as compared to standard drug penicillin were as compounds (**6s, 6o, 6l**) showed excellent antioxidant activities as compared to standard AA. Thus the present rout of the synthesis expected to contribute for the development of a green strategy for the synthesis of a novel class of antibacterial and antioxidant agents.

3.5   SPECTRA OF REPRESENTATIVE COMPOUNDS

Figures 3.4–3.17 show spectra of representative compounds.

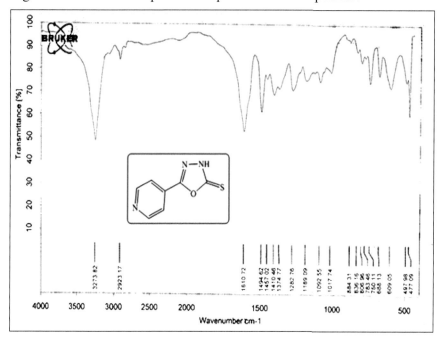

FIGURE 3.4   IR spectra of compound **2**.

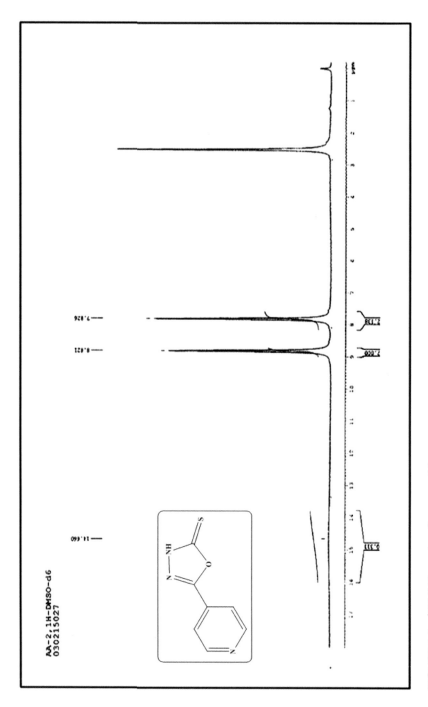

FIGURE 3.5   ¹H NMR spectra of compound **2.**

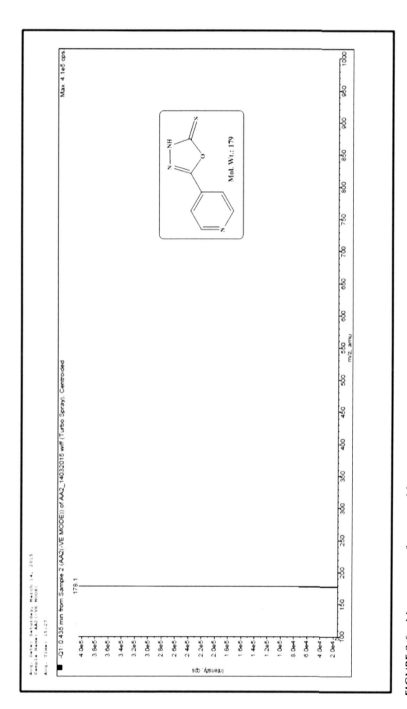

FIGURE 3.6 Mass spectra of compound **2.**

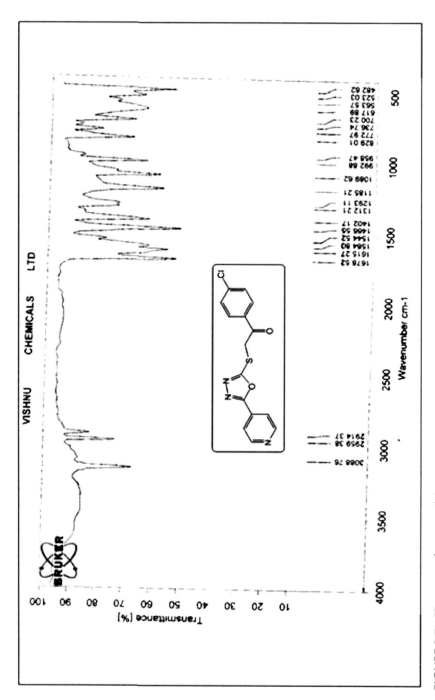

FIGURE 3.7   IR spectra of compound **4a**.

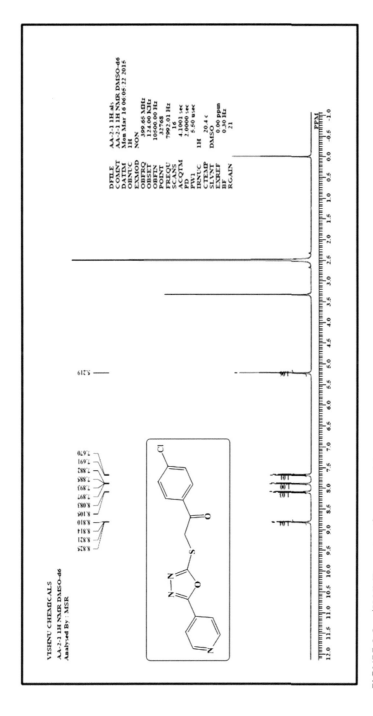

FIGURE 3.8   ¹H NMR spectra of compound **4a**.

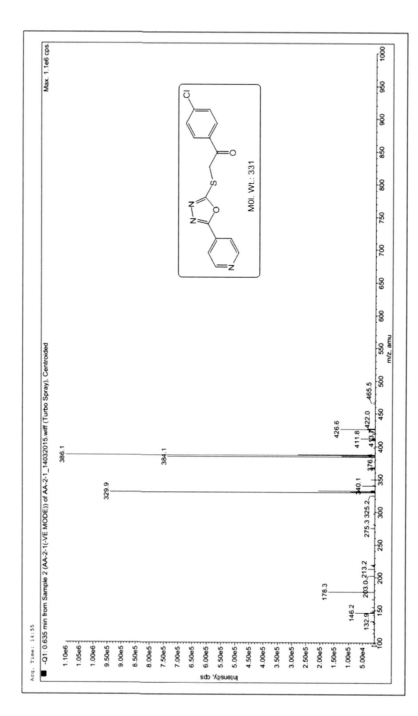

FIGURE 3.9   Mass spectra of compound **4a**.

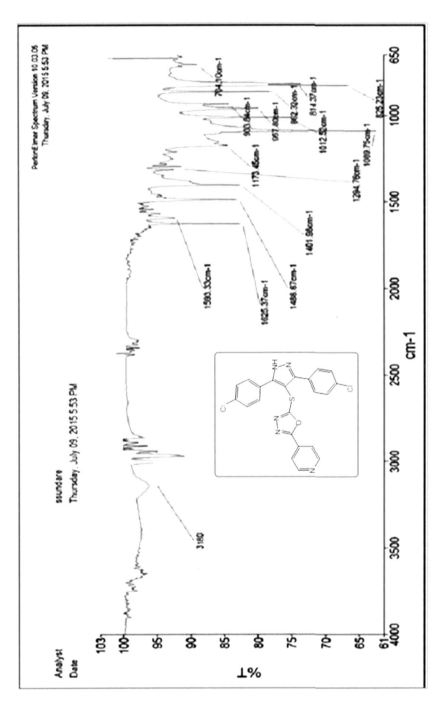

FIGURE 3.10 IR spectra of compound **6a.**

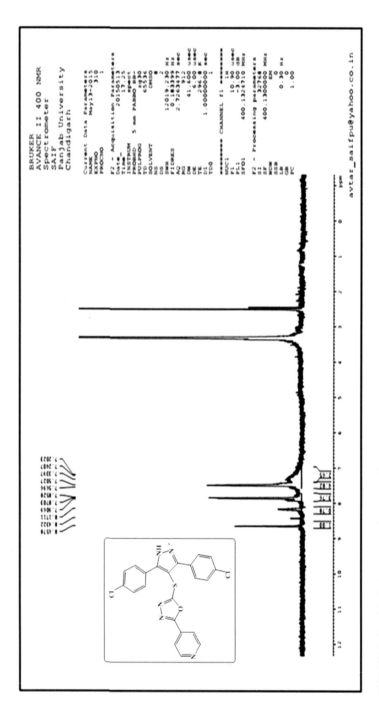

FIGURE 3.11 ^{1}H NMR spectra of compound **6a**.

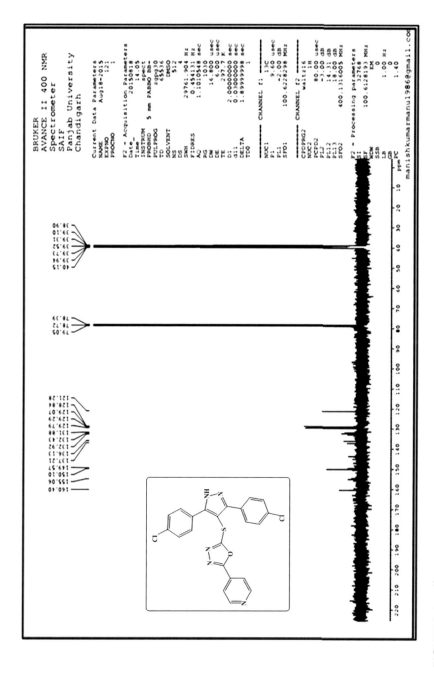

FIGURE 3.12 ^{13}C NMR spectra of compound **6a.**

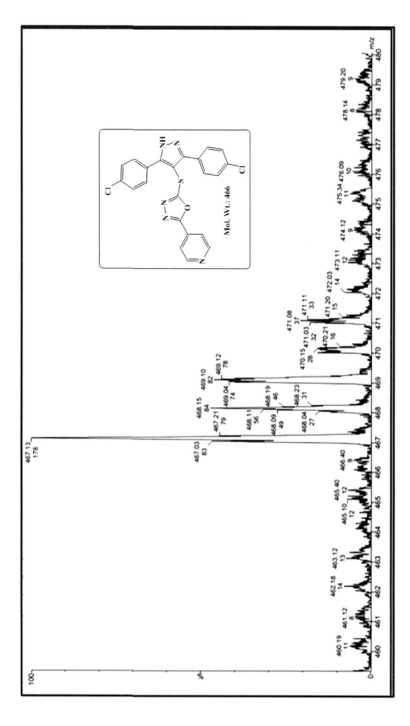

FIGURE 3.13 Mass spectra of compound **6a.**

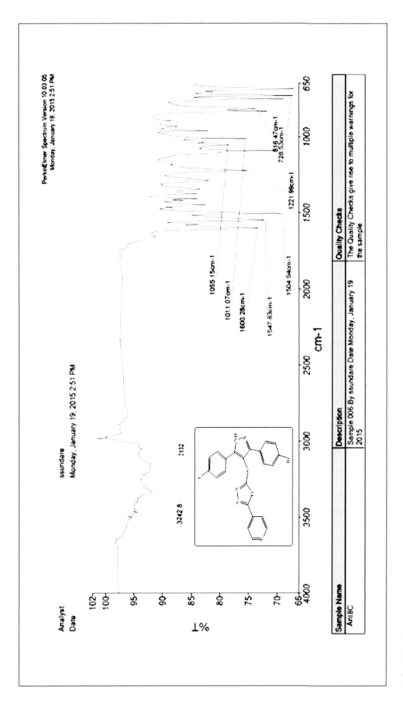

FIGURE 3.14 IR spectra of compound **6r.**

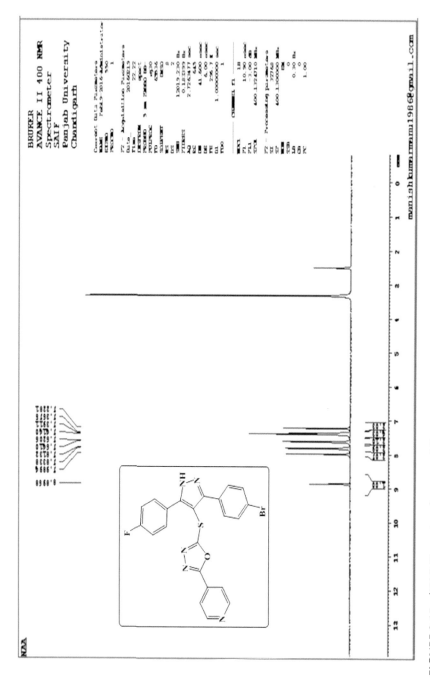

FIGURE 3.15   ¹H NMR spectra of compound **6r**.

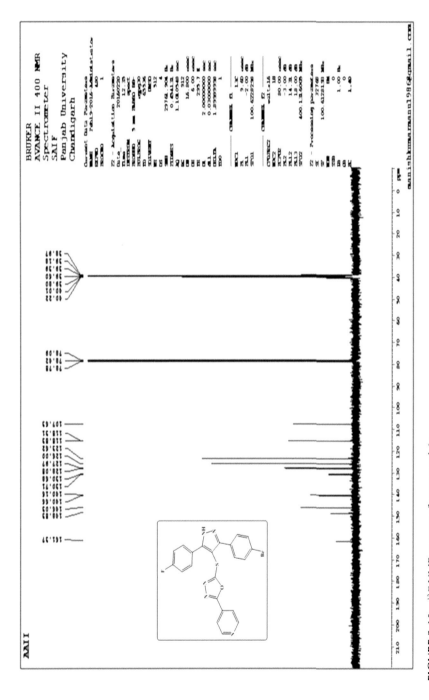

FIGURE 3.16 ¹³C NMR spectra of compound **6r.**

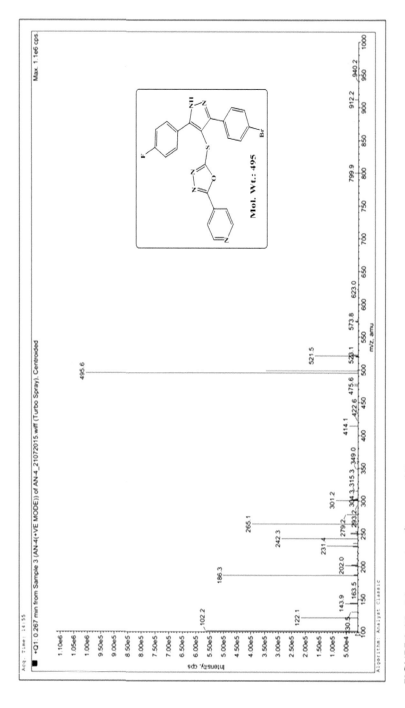

FIGURE 3.17   Mass spectra of compound **6r.**

KEYWORDS

- **1,3,4-oxadiazole**
- **antioxidant activity**
- **dimethyl sulfoxide**
- **minimum inhibition concentration**
- **thin-layer chromatography**
- **triethylamine**

REFERENCES

1. Dua, R., Shrivastava, S., Sonwane, S. K., & Srivastava, S. K., (2011). *Adv Bio Res., 5*, 120.
2. Ponnuswamy, M. N., Gromiha, M. M., Sony, S. M. M., & Saraboji, K., (2006). In: Gupta, R. R., (ed.), *Topics in Heterocyclic Chemistry*. Springer.
3. Kucukguzel, S. G., Oruc, E. E., Rollas, S., Sahin, F., & Ozbek, A. E., (2002). *Eur. J. Med. Chem., 37*(3), 197.
4. EI-Emam, A. A., AI-Deeb, O. A., AI-Omar, M., & Lehmann, J., (2004). *Bioorg. Med. Chem., 12*, 5107.
5. Al-Soud, Y. A., Al-Dweri, M. N., & AI-Masoudi, N. A., (2004). *II Farmaco., 59*, 775.
6. Jayshankar, B., Loknath, R. K. M., Baskaran, N., & Satish, H. S., (2009). *Eur. J. Med. Chem., 44*, 3898.
7. Zareef, M., Iqbal, R., De Dominguez, N. G., Rodrigues, J., Zaidi, J. H., Arfan, M., & Supuran, C. T., (2007). *J. Enzyme Inhib. Med. Chem., 22*(3), 301.
8. Abdu, M. E., Mohamed, R., Saeed, B. A., Vishwanath, B. S., & Rai, K. M., (2011). *Bioorg. Med. Chem. Lett., 21*, 3536.
9. Kumarv, A., D'Souza, S. S., Gaonkar, S. L., Rai, K. M. L., & Salimath, B. P., (2008). *Invest. New Drugs, 26*, 425.
10. George, S., Parameswaran, M. K., Chakraborty, A. R., & Ravi, T. K., (2008). *Acta Pharm., 58*, 119.
11. Aboraia, A. S., Rahman, H. M. A., Mahfouz, N. M., & EI-Gendy, M. A., (2006). *Bioorg. Med. Chem. Lett., 14*, 1236.
12. Michael, S. M., Janet, S., Michael, M., Iwan, G., Brenda, M., & Donald, S., (2001). *Eur. J. Med. Chem., 36*, 31.
13. Acharya, B. N., Saraswat, D., Tiwari, M., Shrivastava, A. K., Ghorpade, R., Bapna, S., & Kaushik, M. P., (2010). *Eur. J. Med. Chem., 45*, 430.
14. Bekhit, A. A., & Abdel-Aziem, T., (2004). *Bioorg. Med. Chem., 12*, 1935.
15. Ali, I., Wani, W. A., Khan, A., Haque, A., Ahmad, A., Saleem, K., & Manzoor, N., (2012). *Microb. Pathog., 53*(2), 66.

16. Bashir, R., Ovais, S., Yaseen, S., Hamid, H., Alam, M. S., Samim, M., Singh, S., & Javed, K., (2011). *Bioorg. Med. Chem. Lett., 21*(14), 4301.

17. Bano, S., Javed, K., Ahmed, S., Rathish, I. G., Singh, S., & Alam, M. S., (2011). *Eur. J. Med. Chem., 46*(12), 5763.

18. Rathish, I. G., Javed, K., Ahmed, S., Bano, S., Alam, M. S., Pillai, K. K., Singh, S., & Bagchi, V., (2009). *Bioorg. Med. Chem. Lett., 19*(1), 255.

19. Joshi, R. S., Mandhane, P. G., Diwakar, S. D., Dabhade, S. K., & Gill, C. H., (2010). *Bioorg. Med. Chem. Lett., 20*(12), 3721.

20. Amir, M., Kumar, H., & Khan, S. A., (2008). *Bioorg. Med. Chem. Lett., 18*(3), 918.

21. Manna, K., & Agrawal, Y. K., (2009). *Bioorg. Med. Chem. Lett., 19*(10), 2688.

22. Ragavan, R. V., Vijayakumar, V., & Kumari, N. S., (2010). *Eur. J. Med. Chem., 45*(3), 1173.

23. Vijesh, A. M., Isloor, A. M., Shetty, P., Sundershan, S., & Fun, H. K., (2013). *Eur. J. Med. Chem., 62*, 410.

24. El-Sabbagh, O. I., Baraka, M. M., Ibrahim, S. M., Pannecouque, C., Andrei, G., Snoeck, R., Balzarini, J., & Rashad, A. A., (2009). *Eur. J. Med. Chem., 44*(9), 3746.

25. Wu, L., Song, B., Bhadury, S. P., Yang, S., Hu, D., & Jin, L., (2011). *J. Heterocyclic. Chem., 48*, 389.

26. Abdel-Aziz, M., Abuo-Rahma, G., Beshr, E. A., & Ali, T. F., (2013). *Bioorg. Med. Chem., 21*, 3839.

27. Zhu, S. L., Wu, Y., Liu, C. J., Wei, C. Y., Tao, J. C., & Liu, H. M., (2013). *Eur. J. Med. Chem., 65*, 70.

28. Parekh, S., Bhavsar, D., Savant, M., Thakrar, S., Bavishi, A., Parmar, M., Vala, H., Radadiya, A., Pandya, N., Serly, J., Molnar, J., & Shah, A., (2011). *Eur. J. Med. Chem., 46*(5), 1942.

29. Bassaco, M. M., Fortes, M. P., Kaufman, T. S., & Silveira, C. C., (2015). *RSC Adv., 5*, 21112.

30. Clercq, E. D., (2016). *J. Med. Chem., 59*(6), 2301.

31. Burja, B., Ciimbora-Zovko, T., Tomic, S., Jelusic, T., Kocevar, M., Polanc, S., & Osmak, M., (2010). *Bioorg. Med. Chem., 18*, 2375.

32. Macaev, F., Rusa, G., Pogrebnoi, S., Gudima, A., Stingaci, E., Vlad, L., Shvets, N., Kandemirli, F., Dimoglo, A., & Reynolds, R., (2005). *Bioorg. Med. Chem., 13*, 4842.

33. Bhandari, S. V., Bothara, K. G., Raut, M. K., Patil, A. A., Sarkate, A. P., & Mokale, V. J., (2008). *Bioorg. Med. Chem., 16*, 1822.

34. Zhang, X. M., Qiu, M., Sun, J., Zhang, Y. B., Yang, Y. S., Wang, X. L., Tang, J. F., & Zhu, H. L., (2011). *Bioorg. Med. Chem., 19*, 6518.

35. Mandawad, G. G., Kamble, R. D., Hese, S. V., More, R. A., Gacche, R. N., Kodam, K. M., & Dawane, B. S., (2014). *Med. Chem. Res., 23*, 4455.

36. Kamble, R. D., Hese, S. V., Meshram, R. M., Kota, J. R., Gacche, R. N., & Dawane, B. S., (2015). *Med. Chem. Res., 24*, 1077.

37. Acharya, A. P., Kamble, R. D., Patil, S. D., Hese, S. V., Yemul, O. S., & Dawane, B. S., (2015). *Res. Chem. Intermed., 41*(5), 2953.

38. Kamble, R. D., Jawadwar, G. V., Patil, S. D., Hese, S. V., Acharya, A. P., Dawane, B. S., & Pekamwar, S. S., (2013). *Org. Commun., 6*, 2, 95.

39. Acharya, A. P., Kamble, R. D., Hese, S. V., Kadam, S. N., Gacche, R. N., & Dawane, B. S., (2014). *Org. Commun., 7*(2), 68.

40. Gaikwad, M. V., Kamble, R. D., Hese, S. V., Acharya, A. P., Mogle, P. P., Kadam, S. N., & Dawane, B. S., (2015). *Res. Chem. Intermed., 41*, 4673.

41. Pingaew, R., Prachayasittikul, S., Ruchirawat, S., & Prachayasittikul, V., (2014). *Med. Chem. Res., 23*(4), 1768.

42. Hubschwerlen, C., Specklin, J. L., Sigwalt, C., Schroeder, S., & Locher, H. H., (2003). *Bioorg. Med. Chem., 11*(10), 2313.

43. Gilani, S. J., Khan, S. A., Alam, O., & Siddiqui, N., (2011). *Acta Pol. Pharma., 68*(2), 205.

44. Moustafa, O. S., (2000). *J. Chi. Chem. Soc., 47*(2), 351.

45. Mansour, A. K., Eid, M. M., & Khalil, N. S. A. M., (2003). *Molecule., 8*(10), 744.

46. Mohamed, B., & Othman, A. A., (2006). *Arkivoc., XI*, 183.

47. Droge, W., (2002). *Physiol. Rev., 82*(1), 47.

48. Kamble, V. T., Sawant, V. S., Pisal, P. M., Gacche, R. N., Kamble, S. S., & Kamble, V. A., (2015). *Arch Pharm. Chem. Life Sci., 348*, 338.

49. Gacche, R. N., Dhole, N. A., Kamble, S. G., & Bandgar, B. P., (2008). *J. EnzInh. Med. Chem., 23*(1), 28.

CHAPTER 4

MULTICOMPONENT SYNTHESIS OF 2-SUBSTITUTED DERIVATIVES OF 6-AMINO-5-CYANO-1,4-DIHYDRO-3-METHYL-1,4-DIPHENYLPYRANO-[2,3-C]-PYRAZOLE USING KNOEVENAGEL AND MICHAEL ADDITION

JAMAN A. ANGULWAR

Department of Chemistry, Dayanand Science College, Latur, Maharashtra, India

ABSTRACT

Clean and simple synthesis of 6-amino-4-aryl-3-methyl-1-phenyl-1,4-di-hydropyrano [2,3-*c*] pyrazole-5-carbonitrile was accomplished in good to excellent yield via the one-pot three-component condensation of 3-methyl-1-phenyl-2-pyrazolin-5-one, an aromatic aldehyde and malononitrile catalyzed by cesium fluoride in ethanol.

4.1 INTRODUCTION

In recent years, pyran, and fused pyran derivatives have attained to great deals of interest due to their various kinds of biological properties. They have been reported for their anticonvulsant [1], antiviral [2], antimicrobial [3–5], cytotoxic [6], and antigenotoxic [7] activities. Pyrazole derivatives have their activities such as antipyretic [8], antidiabetic [9], anti-inflammatory [10], antitumor [11], antihypertensive [12], antidepressant agent

[13], and peptide deformylase inhibitor [14]. Furthermore, Dihydropyrano [2,3-*c*]pyrazole showed molluscicidal activity [15] and was identified as a screening hit for Chkl kinase inhibitor [16]. Here we report another remarkable catalytic activity of Cesium fluoride for the one-pot three-component condensation of malononitrile, an aromatic aldehyde and 3-methyl-1-phenyl-2-pyrazolin-5-one to form a variety of 6-amino-4-aryl-3-methyl-1-phenyl-1,4-dihydropyrano[2,3-*c*] pyrazole-5-carbonitriles.

Pyrano[2,3-*c*] pyrazole is a fused heterocycle comprised of pyrazole and pyran rings, which are known as the sub-structural units of several biologically active compounds [17, 18]. Polyfunctionalized benzopyrans have been widely used as medicinal intermediates due to their biological and pharmacological properties such as antibacterial, molluscicidal, anthelmintic, hypnotic, and insecticidal activity [19–25]. Some 2-amino-4*H*-pyrans can be used as photoactive materials [26]. A 4*H*-pyran ring is also a structural unit of a number of natural products [27–29].

1,4-Dihydropyrano[2,3-*c*]pyrazoles are generally prepared by one-pot three-component condensations of malononitrile, aldehyde, and 3-methyl-1-phenyl-2-pyrazolin-5-one using KF/Al$_2$O$_3$ in DMF at room temperature [30]. The utilization of water as a reaction medium for the synthesis of 1,4-dihydropyrano[2,3-*c*]pyrazoles is demonstrated by using various phase transfer catalysts such as triethyl-benzyl ammonium chloride (TEBA) [31] and hexadecyltrimethylammonium bromide (HTMAB) [32]. Similarly, the use of the neutral organo-catalyst DL-proline using the grinding technique [33] and a surfactant such as *p*-dodecylbenzene sulfonic acid (DBSA) [34] has recently been demonstrated. Solvent-free reaction conditions along with microwave irradiation technique using piperidine as the base have also been introduced for the synthesis of 1,4-dihydropyrano [2,3-*c*]pyrazoles [35]. Clean and simple synthesis of 6-amino-4-aryl-3-methyl-1-phenyl-1,4-dihydropyrano[2,3-*c*] pyrazole-5-carbonitriles was accomplished in good to excellent yields *via* the one-pot three-component condensation of 3-methyl-1-phenyl-2-pyrazolin-5-one, an aromatic aldehyde, and malononitrile catalyzed by sulfamic acid in ethanol [36]. In recent years, the catalytic activity of Cesium fluoride has emerged as a useful acid imparting high regio- and chemoselectivity in various chemical transformations [37–40]. The versatility of sulfamic acid because of its low cost, eco-friendly nature, and ready availability as a common organic chemical encouraged us to explore it in various multicomponent reactions under benign reaction conditions.

The recent fashion in this scenario is the development of multicomponent reaction (MCR) processes. By definition, MCR is reaction processes in which three or more reactants are combined in a single chemical step to produce products that incorporate a substantial portion of all the components reacted.

MCRs are particularly effective at building functionalized drug-like structures from different families of compounds in a single step. Inventing and developing new MCR processes are important pursuits in academic, industrial, and pharmaceutical chemistry. The last few years have seen a revolution in the development of new MCR reactions focused on the use of new reagents and catalysts.

The parallel synthesis of large libraries of pure single compounds has been established in many pharmaceutical and agrochemical companies over the last years. Carbonyl compounds played a crucial role in the early discovery of MCRs. The various MCRs are involved by carbonyl compounds like Biginelli reaction, Bucherer-Bergs reaction, Gewald reaction, and Strecker synthesis, etc.

4.2   PRESENT WORK

The development of the new process, use of cheap catalysts is an important synthetic aspect as they make a vital role for effective greener organic transformation and to minimize the amount of west byproduct from the chemical process.

In this present work, we wish to investigate the greener method for synthesis of 6-amino-1,4-dihydro-3-methyl-4-(4-methoxyphenyl)-1-phenylpyrano [2,3-c] pyrazole-5-carbonitrile (V-04).

A mixture of different substituted aromatic aldehydes like, benzaldehyde, p-methoxy benzaldehyde, p-methyl benzaldehyde, 3,4-dimethoxy benzaldehyde, o-chloro benzaldehyde, p-chloro benzaldehyde, p-nitro benzaldehyde, m-nitro benzaldehyde, m-bromo benzaldehyde, p-bromo benzaldehyde, p-fluoro benzaldehyde, 3-hydroxy-4-hydroxy benzaldehyde, o-hydroxy benzaldehyde, m-hydroxy benzaldehyde, p-hydroxybenzaldehyde (V-0a-o), 3-methyl-1-phenyl-5-pyrazolone (V-02) and malononitrile (V-03) in ethanol and cesium fluoride to isolate 6-amino-1,4-dihydro-3-methyl-4-(phenyl, 4-methoxy phenyl, 4-methyl phenyl, 3,4-dimethoxy phenyl, 2-chlorophenyl, 4-chlorophenyl, 4-nitro phenyl, 3-nitro phenyl, 3-bromo phenyl, 4-fluoro phenyl, 3-hydroxy, 4-methoxy phenyl, 2-hydroxy phenyl, 3-hydroxy phenyl, 4-hydroxy phenyl)-1-phenylpyrano [2,3-c] pyrazole-5-carbonitrile (V-04a-o). The structure of these newly synthesized compounds has been confirmed by elemental analysis and spectral data.

4.2.1   OBJECTIVE

On reviewing the literature, it can be seen that the various methods were reported for the synthesis of pyrano [2,3-*c*] pyrazole and its derivatives. The development of efficient and environment-friendly chemical processes for the preparation of biologically active molecules constitute a major challenge for chemist by organic synthesis.

To find out the ways to overcome the limitation and drawbacks of the reported method such as harsh reaction conditions, use of expensive catalysts, and develop a one-pot synthesis of pyrano [2,3-*c*] pyrazole from aldehyde, malononitrile, and 3-methyl-1-phenyl-5- pyrazolone using a commercially available reagent. To find out the role of catalyst and to depict the mechanistic pathway for the formation of pyrano [2,3-*c*] pyrazole.

4.2.2   RESULT AND DISCUSSION

A mixture of differently substituted like anisaldehyde **(V-01)**, 3-methyl-1-phenyl-5-pyrazolone **(V-02)**, and malononitrile **(V-03)** in ethanol and cesium fluoride was refluxed for 1–5 hours to isolate 6-amino-1,4-dihydro-3-methyl-4-(4-methoxyphenyl)-1-phenylpyrano[2,3-*c*] pyrazole-5-carbonitrile. The progress of the reaction was monitored by TLC (**Scheme-V-17**).

(V- 01a-o) (V- 02)   (V- 03)   (V- 04a-o)

(Scheme-V- 17)

R- different substitutent on aromatic aldehydes.

Structure to these compounds **(VI-4b)** was assigned on the basis of analytical and spectral data. Its IR spectrum shows the absorption band at 3390, 3321, 2190, 1658 cm^{-1} indicating the presence of –NH$_2$,-CN and -C=N- functionalities, respectively **(Spectrum-V-01).**

The ^{1}H-NMR (300) spectrum of the compounds was recorded in DMSO. It displayed a singlet at δ 1.8 due to C$_3$- CH$_3$ singlet at δ 3.75 due to Ar-OCH$_3$ protons. It shows an important peak at δ 4.6 for methine proton. The remaining aromatic protons give multiplet at δ 7.15–7.30 due to N-Ar and aromatic protons gives two doublets at δ 7.5 and 7.8 due to methoxy group at p-position **(Spectrum-V-02).**

The mass spectrum **(Spectrum-V-03)** shows a molecular ion peak at m/z 358, which corresponds to its molecular weight. The structure of the compounds **(VI-4b)** is further confirmed by its ^{13}C-NMR spectrum **(Spectrum-V-04).**

The spectral and physical data of the compound was found to be in agreement with the literature data. Encouraged by this result, we planned to develop the methodology by varying the substitution at the C-4 position of pyrano [2, 3-c] pyrazoles.

4.2.3 MECHANISM

The plausible mechanism involves cesium fluoride catalyzed the formation of cyano olefin [5] through Knovenagel condensation between aryl aldehyde and malononitrile, which occurs due to high acidity of methylene proton of malononitrile as compared to that of pyrazole. Further, Michael addition of enolate ion on an electron-deficient olefinic carbon of cyano olefin to form desired products (Table 4.1).

Mechanism

TABLE 4.1   Reaction Time, Yields, and M.P. of Pyrano [2,3-c] Pyrazole

Entry	Comp. Code	Structure of Compounds	Time (Hrs.)	Yielda%	M.P. Obs.	M.P. (Lit °C)
01	V-04a		06	72	167–169	168–170
02	V-04b		04	81	166–168	167–170
03	V-04c		08	80	168–170	168–170

TABLE 4.1 (Continued)

Entry	Comp. Code	Structure of Compounds	Time (Hrs.)	Yielda%	M.P. Obs.	M.P. (Lit °C)
04	V-04d		03	70	191–193	191–193
05	V-04e		04	65	178–180	178–180
06	V-04f		05	72	175–177	175–177

TABLE 4.1 *(Continued)*

Entry	Comp. Code	Structure of Compounds	Time (Hrs.)	Yielda%	M.P. Obs.	M.P. (Lit °C)
07	V-04g		10	61	235–237	235–238
08	V-04h		03	60	185–187	185–187
09	V-04i		10	64	198–200	198–200

TABLE 4.1 *(Continued)*

Entry	Comp. Code	Structure of Compounds	Time (Hrs.)	Yielda%	M.P. Obs.	M.P. (Lit °C)
10	V-04j		01	66	154–156	155–156
11	V-04k		10	60	162–164	163–164
12	V-04l		10	68	168–170	168–170

TABLE 4.1 *(Continued)*

Entry	Comp. Code	Structure of Compounds	Time (Hrs.)	Yielda%	M.P. Obs.	M.P. (Lit °C)
13	V-04m		10	62	295–297	295–297
14	V-04n		10	65	240–242	243–245
15	V-04o		05	80	208–210	208–209

4.3 EXPERIMENTAL

A mixture of malononitrile (10 mmol), 3-methyl-1-phenyl-2-pyrazolin-5-one (10 mmol) was treated independently with a different substituted aromatic aldehyde in Cesium fluoride and ethanol to afford the 4-substituted derivatives of 6-amino-1,4-dihydro-3-methyl-4-(substituted phenyl)-1-phenyl pyrano [2,3-*c*] pyrazole-5-carbonitrile.

4.4 SPECTRAL ANALYSIS

All the products were characterized by IR, NMR (¹H and ¹³C), and mass spectrum analysis. A detail spectral analysis of compound (V-4a-o) is discussed below.

1. 6-amino-1,4-dihydro-3-methyl-1,4-diphenyl pyrano[2,3-c] pyrazole-5-carbonitrile (V-04a)

IR spectrum of 6-amino-1,4-dihydro-3-methyl-1,4-diphenyl pyrano [2,3-*c*] pyrazole-5-carbonitrile (**V-04a**) in KBr shows asymmetric and symmetric stretching band at 3472 and 3320 cm⁻¹ for primary amino group, medium intensity band at 2195 cm⁻¹ for C-N stretching of –C≡N group and band at 1660 cm⁻¹ for C=N stretching of pyrazolone ring.

The ¹H-NMR (300 MHz) spectrum analysis of the same compound was recorded in DMSO and shows singlet at δ 1.93 for C_3-CH_3 protons, most important singlet at δ 4.68 for C_4-H proton, singlet at δ 6.75 due to –NH₂ protons and multiplet at δ 7.16–7.32 due to aromatic Ar-H protons.

Yield: 72% M.P.: 167–169°C.
Molecular formula: $C_{20}H_{16}N_4O$; and *Molecular weight:* 328.
Elemental analysis: %C%H%N.
Calculated: 73.15, 4.91, 17.06.
Found: 73.15, 4.91, 17.06.

2. 6-amino-1,4-dihydro-3-methyl-4-(4-methoxyphenyl)-1-phenyl pyrano[2,3-c] pyrazole-5-carbonitrile (V-04b).

IR spectrum of 6-amino-1,4-dihydro-3-methyl-4-(4-methoxy phenyl) -1-phenyl pyrano[2,3-*c*] pyrazole-5-carbonitrile **(V-04b)** in KBr shows asymmetric and symmetric stretching band at 3390 and 3321 cm^{-1} for primary amino group, medium intensity band at 2190 cm^{-1} for C-N stretching of –C≡N group and band at 1658 cm^{-1} for C=N stretching of pyrazolone ring **(Spectrum-V-01).**

The ^{1}H-NMR (300 MHz) spectrum analysis of the same compound was recorded in DMSO and shows singlet at δ 1.8 for C_3-CH$_3$ protons, singlet at δ 3.8 for C_4, Ar-OCH$_3$ protons and most important singlet at δ 4.6 for C_4-H proton, singlet at δ 6.9 due to –NH$_2$ protons and multiplet at δ 7.1–7.3 due to N-Ar-H protons and two doublet at δ 7.5 and δ 7.8 due to p-substituted aromatic protons **(Spectrum-V-02).**

The mass spectrum shows a molecular ion peak at (m/e) 358 (M$^+$) The fragments observed in the spectrum at 292, 261, 251, 208, 185, 174, 159 **(Spectrum-V-03).**

The ^{13}C –NMR (300MHz) of same compounds showed signal at 12, 36, 55, 59, 99, 114, 120 (-C≡N), 127, 129, 136, 138, 144, and 159 **(Spectrum-V-04).**

Yield: 81% M.P.: 166–168°C.

Molecular formula: $C_{21}H_{18}N_4O_2$; and *Molecular weight:* 358.
Elemental analysis: %C%H%N.
Calculated: 70.38, 5.06, 15.63.
Found: 70.35, 5.03, 15.61.

3. 6-amino-1,4-dihydro-3-methyl-4-(4-methyl phenyl)-1-phenyl pyrano[2,3-c] pyrazole-5-carbonitrile(V-04c)

IR spectrum of 6-amino-1,4-dihydro-3-methyl-4-(4-methyl phenyl)-1-phenyl pyrano [2,3-*c*] pyrazole-5-carbonitrile **(V-04c)** in KBr shows asymmetric and symmetric stretching band at 3398 and 3444 cm⁻¹ for primary amino group, medium intensity band at 2187 cm⁻¹ for C-N stretching of –C=N group and band at 1647 cm⁻¹ for C=N stretching of pyrazolone ring **(Spectrum-V-05)**.

The ¹H-NMR (300 MHz) spectrum analysis of the same compound was recorded in DMSO and shows singlet at δ 1.9 for C-CH₃ protons, singlet at δ 2.3 for –CH₃ protons and most important singlet at δ 4.6 for C₄-H proton, one broad singlet at δ 7.15 due to –NH₂ protons, multiplet at δ 7.2–7.3 due to N-Ar protons and two doublets at δ 7.5 and 7.8 due to p-substituted aromatic protons **(Spectrum-V-06)**.

The mass spectrum shows the molecular ion peak at (m/e) 342 (M⁺⁺), which is in agreement with its molecular weight. The fragments observed in the spectrum at 342, 292, 276, 261, 185, 251, 185, 168 **(Spectrum-V-07)**.

Yield: 80% M.P.: 168–170°C.
Molecular formula: $C_{21}H_{18}N_4O$; and *Molecular weight:* 342.
Elemental analysis: %C%H%N.
Calculated: 73.67 5.30 16.36.
Found: 73.66 5.30 16.36.

4. 6-amino-1,4-dihydro-3-methyl-4-(3,4-dimethoxy phenyl)-1-phenyl pyrano[2,3-c] pyrazole-5-carbonitrile (V-04d)

IR spectrum of 6-amino-1,4-dihydro-3-6-amino-1,4-dihydro-3-methyl-4-(3,4-dimethoxy phenyl)-1-phenyl pyrano[2,3-*c*] pyrazole-5-carbonitrile **(V-04d)** in KBr shows asymmetric and symmetric stretching band at 3460 and 3328 cm⁻¹ for primary amino group, medium intensity band at 2198 cm⁻¹ for C-N stretching of –C=N group and band at 1658 cm⁻¹ for C=N stretching of pyrazolone ring **(Spectrum-V-08).**

The ¹H-NMR (300 MHz) spectrum analysis of the same compound was recorded in DMSO and shows singlet at δ 1.8 for C-CH₃ protons and singlet at δ 3.75 for C₄ two Ar-OCH₃ protons and most important singlet at δ 4.6 for C₄-H proton and multiplet at δ 6.7–6.9 due to C₄, Ar-H protons, singlet at δ 7.15 due to –NH₂ protons, multiplet at δ 7.3–7.8 due to N-ArH protons **(Spectrum-V-09).**

The mass spectrum shows the molecular ion peak at (m/e) 388 (M⁺), which is in agreement with its molecular weight. The fragments observed in the spectrum at 388, 322, 307, 291, 276, 252,251, 214, 189, 185, 174 **(Spectrum-V-10).**

The ¹³C –NMR (300MHz) of the same compounds showed signal at 13, 37, 56, 58, 99, 112, 120, 126, 129, 136, 145, 149, and 159 **(Spectrum-V-11).**

Yield: 70% M.P.: 191–193°C.
Molecular formula: C₂₂H₂₀N₄O₃; and *Molecular weight:* 388.
Elemental analysis: %C%H%N.
Calculated: 68.03 5.19 14.42.
Found: 68.02 5.18 14.40.

5. 6-amino -1, 4-dihydro-3-methyl-4-(2'-chloro phenyl)-1-phenyl pyrano[2,3-c] pyrazole-5-carbonitrile(V-04e)

IR spectrum of 6-amino-1,4-dihydro-3-methyl-4-(2'-chlorophenyl)-1-phenyl pyrano[2,3-c] pyrazole-5-carbonitrile **(V-04e)** in KBr and shows asymmetric and symmetric stretching band at 3472 and 3324 cm^{-1} for primary amino group, medium intensity band at 2194 cm^{-1} for C-N stretching of –C=N group and band at 1656 cm^{-1} for C=N stretching of pyrazolone ring.

The ^{1}H-NMR (300 MHz) spectrum analysis of the same compound was recorded in DMSO and shows singlet at δ 1.90 for C_3-CH_3 protons and most important singlet at δ 4.62 for C_4-H proton and singlet at δ 6.72 due to –NH_2 protons, multiplet at δ 7.22–7.44 due to N-Ar-H protons, multiplet at δ 7.5–7.8 due to C_4-ArH protons.

Yield: 65% M.P.: 178–180°C.
Molecular formula: $C_{20}H_{15}ClN_4O$; and *Molecular weight:* 363.
Elemental analysis: %C%H%N.
Calculated: 66.21, 4.17, 15.44.
Found: 66.19, 4.16, 15.43.

6. 6-amino-1,4-dihydro-3-methyl-4-(4'-chlorophenyl)-1-phenyl pyrano[2,3-c] pyrazole-5-carbonitrile (V-04f)

IR spectrum of 6-amino-1,4-dihydro-3-methyl-1,4-diphenyl pyrano [2,3-*c*] pyrazole-5-carbonitrile **(V-04f)** in KBr shows asymmetric and symmetric stretching band at 3468 and 3325 cm^{-1} for primary amino group, medium intensity band at 2200 cm^{-1} for C-N stretching of –C=N group and band at 1662 cm^{-1} for C=N stretching of pyrazolone ring.

The ^{1}H-NMR (300 MHz) spectrum analysis of the same compound was recorded in DMSO and shows singlet at δ 1.88 for C$_3$-CH$_3$ protons and most important singlet at δ 4.74 for C$_4$-H proton and singlet at δ 6.32 due to –NH$_2$ protons, multiplet at δ 7.38–7.42 due to N-Ar-H protons, two doublets at δ 7.48–7.52 and δ 7.78–7.86 due to C$_4$-ArH protons.

Yield: 72% M.P.: 175–177°C.
Molecular formula: C$_{20}$H$_{15}$ClN$_4$O; and *Molecular weight:* 363.
Elemental analysis: %C%H%N.
Calculated: 66.21, 4.17, 15.44.
Found: 66.21, 4.17, 15.44.

7. 6-amino-1,4-dihydro-3-methyl-4-(4′-nitrophenyl)-1-phenyl pyrano[2,3-c] pyrazole-5-carbonitrile(V-04g)

IR spectrum of 6-amino-1,4-dihydro-3-methyl-1,4-diphenyl pyrano [2,3-*c*] pyrazole-5-carbonitrile shows the asymmetric and symmetric stretching band at 3430 and 3340 cm^{-1} for primary amino group, medium intensity band at 2192 cm^{-1} for C-N stretching of –C=N group and band at 1665 cm^{-1} for C=N stretching of pyrazole ring.

Yield: 61% M.P.: 235–237°C.
Molecular formula: C$_{20}$H$_{15}$N$_5$O$_3$; and *Molecular weight:* 373.
Elemental analysis: %C%H%N.

Calculated: 64.34, 4.05, 12.86.
Found: 64.34, 4.03, 12.85.

8. 6-amino-1,4-dihydro-3-methyl-4-(3′-nitro phenyl)-1-phenyl pyrano[2,3-c]pyrazole-5-carbonitrile(V-04h)

IR spectrum of 6-amino-1,4-dihydro-3-methyl-1,4-diphenyl pyrano [2,3-*c*] pyrazole-5-carbonitrile shows the asymmetric and symmetric stretching band at 3420 and 3330 cm^{-1} for primary amino group, medium intensity band at 2194 cm^{-1} for C-N stretching of –C≡N group and band at 1675 cm^{-1} for C=N stretching of pyrazolone ring.

Yield: 601% M.P.: 185–187°C.
Molecular formula: $C_{20}H_{15}N_5O_3$; and *Molecular weight:* 373.
Elemental analysis: %C%H%N.
Calculated: 64.34, 4.05, 12.86.
Found: 64.34, 4.03, 12.85.

9. 6-amino-1,4-dihydro-3-methyl-4-(3′-bromo phenyl)-1-phenyl pyrano[2,3-c]pyrazole-5-carbonitrile(V-04i)

IR spectrum of 6-amino-1,4-dihydro-3-methyl-4-(4'-bromo phenyl)-1-phenyl pyrano [2,3-*c*] pyrazole-5-carbonitrile rile shows asymmetric and symmetric stretching band at 3472 and 3330 cm^{-1} for primary amino group, medium intensity band at 2194 cm^{-1} for C-N stretching of –C=N group and band at 1660 cm^{-1} for C=N stretching of pyrazolone ring.

Yield: 64% M.P.: 198–200°C.
Molecular formula: $C_{20}H_{15}BrN_4O$; and *Molecular weight:* 407.
Elemental analysis: %C%H%N.
Calculated: 58.98, 3.17, 13.76.
Found: 58.98, 3.17, 13.76.

10.   *6-amino-1,4-dihydro-3-methyl-4-(4'-bromo phenyl)-1-phenyl pyrano[2,3-c]pyrazole-5-carbonitrile(V-04j)*

IR spectrum of 6-amino-1,4-dihydro-3-methyl-4-(4'-bromo phenyl)-1-phenyl pyrano [2,3-*c*] pyrazole-5-carbonitrile rile shows asymmetric and symmetric stretching band at 3474 and 3325 cm^{-1} for primary amino group, medium intensity band at 2192 cm^{-1} for C-N stretching of –C=N group and band at 1658 cm^{-1} for C=N stretching of pyrazolone ring.

Yield: 66% M.P.: 154–156°C.
Molecular formula: $C_{20}H_{15}BrN_4O$; and *Molecular weight:* 407.
Elemental analysis: %C%H%N.
Calculated: 58.98, 3.17, 13.76.
Found: 58.98, 3.17, 13.76.

11.   6-amino-1, 4-dihydro-3-methyl-4-(4'-fluoro phenyl) -1-phenyl pyrano[2,3-c]pyrazole-5-carbonitrile(V-04k)

IR spectrum of 6-amino-1, 4-dihydro-3-methyl-4-(4'-fluorophenyl)-1-phenyl pyrano [2,3-c] pyrazole-5-carbonitrile shows asymmetric and symmetric stretching band at 3473 and 3320 cm^{-1} for primary amino group, medium intensity band at 2195 cm^{-1} for C-N stretching of –C=N group and band at 1657 cm^{-1} for C=N stretching of pyrazole ring.

Yield: 60% M.P.: 162–164°C.
Molecular formula: $C_{20}H_{15}FN_4O$; and *Molecular weight:* 346.
Elemental analysis: %C%H%N.
Calculated: 69.35, 4.37, 16.18.
Found: 69.35, 4.37, 16.18.

12.   6-amino-1, 4-dihydro-3-methyl-4-(3'-Hydroxy, 4'-methoxy phenyl)-1-phenylpyrano[2,3-c] pyrazole -5-carbonitrile(V-04l)

IR spectrum of 6-amino-1,4-dihydro-3-methyl-4-(3'-hydroxy-4'-methoxyphenyl)-1-phenyl pyrano[2,3-c] pyrazole-5-carbonitrile shows asymmetric and symmetric stretching band at 3474 and 3325 cm^{-1} for primary amino group, medium intensity band at 2192 cm^{-1} for C-N stretching of –C=N group and band at 1659 cm^{-1} for C=N stretching of pyrazole ring.

Yield: 68% M.P.: 168–170°C.
Molecular formula: $C_{21}H_{18}N_4O_3$; and *Molecular weight:* 374.
Elemental analysis: %C%H%N.
Calculated: 67.37, 4.85, 14.96.
Found: 67.37, 4.84, 14.96.

13. 6-amino-1, 4-dihydro-3-methyl-4-(2'-hydroxy phenyl) -1-phenyl pyrano[2,3-c] pyrazole-5-carbonitrile(V-04m)

IR spectrum of 6-amino-1,4-dihydro-3-methyl-4-(2'-Hydroxy phenyl) 1-diphenyl pyrano [2,3-c] pyrazole-5-carbonitrile shows asymmetric and symmetric stretching band at 3475 and 3314 cm^{-1} for primary amino group, medium intensity band at 2195 cm^{-1} for C-N stretching of –C=N group and band at 1658 cm^{-1} for C=N stretching of pyrazolone ring.

Yield: 62% M.P.: 295–297°C.
Molecular formula: $C_{20}H_{16}N_4O_2$; and *Molecular weight:* 344.
Elemental analysis: %C%H%N.
Calculated: 69.76, 4.68, 16.27.
Found: 69.76, 4.68, 16.27.

14. 6-amino -1, 4-dihydro-3-methyl-4-(3'-Hydroxy phenyl) -1-phenyl pyrano[2,3-c] pyrazole-5-carbonitrile(V-04n)

IR spectrum of 6-amino-1,4-dihydro-3-methyl-4-(3'-hydroxy phenyl) 1-diphenyl pyrano [2,3-c] pyrazole-5-carbonitrile shows asymmetric and symmetric stretching band at 3475 and 3314 cm^{-1} for primary amino group, medium intensity band at 2195 cm^{-1} for C-N stretching of –C≡N group and band at 1662 cm^{-1} for C=N stretching of pyrazolone ring.

Yield: 65% M.P.: 240–242°C.
Molecular formula: $C_{20}H_{16}N_4O_2$; and *Molecular weight:* 344.
Elemental analysis: %C%H%N.
Calculated: 69.76, 4.68, 16.27.
Found: 69.76, 4.68, 16.27.

15. 6-amino-1, 4-dihydro-3-methyl-4-(4'-hydroxy phenyl) -1-phenyl pyrano [2,3-c] pyrazole-5-carbonitrile(V-04o)

IR spectrum of 6-amino-1,4-dihydro-3-methyl-4-(4'-hydroxy phenyl) 1-diphenyl pyrano [2,3-*c*] pyrazole-5-carbonitrile shows asymmetric and symmetric stretching band at 3414 and 3315 cm^{-1} for primary amino group, medium intensity band at 2178 cm^{-1} for C-N stretching of –C=N group and band at 1658 cm^{-1} for C=N stretching of pyrazolone ring.

Yield: 80% M.P.: 208–210°C.
Molecular formula: $C_{20}H_{16}N_4O_2$; and *Molecular weight:* 344.
Elemental analysis: %C%H%N.
Calculated: 69.76, 4.68, 16.27.
Found: 69.76, 4.68, 16.27.

4.5 CONCLUSION

We are successful in the developing efficient method for one-pot multi-component synthesis of pyrano [2,3-*c*] pyrazoles at ambient temperature using Cesium fluoride as an inexpensive catalyst. This procedure offers several advantages, including mild condition, high yields and inexpensive catalysts, wide scope of the substrate and operational simplicity, simple workup, and purification of the product by non-chromatographic methods, i.e., by simple recrystallization from ethanol.

4.6 SPECTRA

Spectrum (V-01): 6-amino -1,4-dihydro-3-methyl-4-(4-methoxy phenyl) -1-phenyl pyrano[2,3-*c*] pyrazole -5-carbonitrile **(V-4b).**

KEYWORDS

- aromatic aldehyde
- cesium fluoride
- malononitrile
- multicomponent reactions
- pyrano pyrazole
- triethyl-benzyl ammonium chloride

REFERENCES

1. Aytemir, M. D., Calis, U., & Ozalp, M., (2004). *Arch. Pharm., 337*, 281.
2. Shamroukh, A. H., Zaki, M. E. A., Morsy, E. M. H., Abdel-Motti, F. M., & Abdel-Megeid, F. M. E., (2007). *Arch. Pharm., 340*, 236.
3. Eid, F. A., Abd El-Wahab, A. H. F., El-Hag, A. G. A. M., & Khafagy, M. M., (2004). *Arch. Pharm., 54*, 13.
4. El-Agrody, A. M., Abd-Latif, M. S., Fakery, A. H., & Bedair, A. H., (2001). *Molecule, 6*, 519.
5. Bedair, A. H., El-Hady, N. A., Abd El-Latif, M. S., & El-Agrody, A. M., (2000). *Il Farmaco, 55*, 708.
6. Melliou, A. P., Mitaku, S., Skaltsounis, A. L., Pierre, A., Atassi, G., & Renard, P., (2001). *Bioorg. Med. Chem., 9*, 607.
7. Chabchoub, F., Messaad. M., Mansour, H. B., Chekir-Ghedira, L., & Salem, M., (2007). *Eur. J. Med. Chem., 42*, 715.
8. Shafiee, A., Bgheri, M., Shekarchi, M., & Abdollahi, M., (2003). *J. Pharm. Sci., 6*, 360.
9. Kanwal, P., Gupta, V. K., Brahmbhatt, D. I., & Patel, M. A., (2000). *Analytical Sci., 23*, 237.
10. Ren, X. L., Li, H. B., Wu, C., & Yang, H. Z., (2005). *ARKIVOC, 15*, 59.
11. Park, H. J., Lee, K., Park, S. J., Ahn, B., Lee, J. C., Cho, H., & Lee, K., (2005). *Bioorg. Med. Chem. Lett., 15*, 3307.
12. Almansa, C., Gomez, L. A., Cavalcanti, F. L., De Arriba, A. F., Garcia-Rafanell, J., & Form J., (1997). *J. Med. Chem., 40*, 547.
13. Prasad, Y. R., Rao, A. L., Prasoona, L., Murali, K., & Kumar, P. R., (2005). *Bioorg. Med. Chem. Lett., 15*, 5030.
14. Cali, P., Naerum, L., Mukhija, S., & Hjelmencrantz, A., (2004). *Bioorg. Med. Chem. Lett., 14*, 5997.
15. Abdelrazek, F. M., Metz, P., Kataeva, O., Jaeger, A., & El-Mahrouky, S. F., (2007). *Arch. Pharm., 340*, 543.
16. Foloppe, N., Fisher, L. M., Howes, R., Potter, A., Robertson, A. G. S., & Surgenor, A. E., (2006). *Bioorg. Med. Chem., 14*, 4792.
17. Elnagdi, M. H., Elmoghayar, M. R. H., & Elgemeie, G. E. H., (1987). *Adv. Heterocyclic Chem., 41*, 319.
18. Elnagdi, M. H., Elmoghayar, M. R. H., & Sadek, K. U., (1990). *Adv. Heterocyclic Chem., 48*, 223.
19. Kuo, S. G., Huang, L. J., & Nakamura, H., (1984). *J. Med. Chem., 27*, 539.
20. Adreani, L. L., & Lapi, E., (1961). *Boll. Chim. Farm., 99*, 583, *Chem. Abstr., 1961, 20.* 55, 2668.
21. Zhang, Y. L., Chen, B. Z., Zheng, K. Q., Xu, M. L., & Lei, X. H., (1982). *Acta Pharm. Sinica, 17*, 17, *Chem. Abstr., 96*, 135 383e.
22. Bonsignore, L., Loy, G., Secci, D., & Calignano, A., (1993). *Eur. J. Med. Chem., 28*, 517.
23. Witte, E. C., Neubert, P., & Roesch, A., (1986). *Ger. Offen. DE*, 3(427), 985, *Chem. Abstr., 104*, 224 915f.
24. Wang, J. L., Liu, D., Zhang, Z. J., Shan, S., Han, X., Srinivasula, S. M., Croce, C. M., Alnemri, E. S., & Huang, Z., (2000). *Proc. Natl. Acad. Sci. U.S.A., 97*, 7124.

25. Mohamed, Y. A., Zahran, M. A., Ali, M. M., El-Agrody, A. M., & El-Said, U. H., (1995). *J. Chem. Res. (S), 322.*

26. Armesto, D., Horspool, W. M., Martin, N., Ramos, A., & Seoane, C., (1989). *J. Org. Chem., 54*, 3069.

27. Hatakeyama, S., Ochi, N., Numata, H., & Takano, S., (1988). *J. Chem. Soc., Chem. Commun.,* 1202.

28. Gonzalez, R., Martin, N., Seoane, C., & Soto, J., (1985). *J. Chem. Soc., Perkin. Trans., 1,* 202.

29. Kamaljit, S., Jasbir, S., & Harjit, S., (1996). *Tetrahedron, 52*, 14273.

30. Wang, X. S., Shi, D. Q., Rong, L. C., Yao, C. S., & Dai, G. Y., (2003). *Jiego Huaxue, 22*, 331.

31. Shi, D. Q., Zhang, S., Zhuang, Q. Y., Tu, S. J., & Hu, H. W., (2003). *Chin. J. Org. Chem., 23*, 1314.

32. Jin, T. S., Wang, A. Q., Cheng, Z. L., Zhang, J. S., & Li, T. S., (2005). *Synth. Commun., 35*, 137.

33. Guo, S. B., Wang, S. X., & Li, J. T., (2007). *Synth. Commun., 37,* 2111.

34. Jin, T. S., Zhao, R. Q., & Li, T. S., (2006). *Arkivoc, XI*, 176.

35. Zhou, J. F., Tu, S. J., Gao, Y., & Ji, M., (2001). *Chinese J. Org. Chem., 21*, 742.

36. Sandeep, V. S., Wamanrao, N. J., Jeevan, M. K., Sumit, V. G., & Nandkishor, N. K., (2008). *Journal of Chemical Research, 08*(5203), 278.

37. Jin, T. S., Sun, G., Li, Y. W., & Li, T. S., (2002). *Green Chem., 4*, 255.

38. Bo, W., Ming, Y. L., & Shuan, S. J., (2003). *Tetrahedron Lett., 44*, 5037.

39. Wang, B., Gu, Y. L., Luo, C., Yang, T., Yang, L. M., & Suo, J. S., (2004). *Tetrahedron Lett., 45*, 3369.

40. Singh, P. R., Singh, D. U., & Samant, S. D., (2004). *Synlett, 11*, 1909.

CHAPTER 5

TRIAZOLE-DERIVED, ARTESUNATE, AND METABOLIC PATHWAYS FOR ARTEMISININ

FRANCISCO TORRENS[1] and GLORIA CASTELLANO[2]

[1]*Institute for Molecular Science, University of Valencia, PO Box 22085, E-46071 Valencia, Spain*

[2]*Department of Experimental Sciences and Mathematics, Faculty of Veterinary and Experimental Sciences, Valencia Catholic University Saint Vincent Martyr, Guillem de Castro-94, E-46001 Valencia, Spain*

*Corresponding author. E-mail: torrens@uv.es

ABSTRACT

Artemisinin (ART) is the unique natural product containing the 1,2,4-trioxane annulus. *Artemisia annua* is the unique source of ART. Phytopharmaceutical research of *A. annua* shows many endoperoxides and hydroperoxides, which were not tested for antimalarial activity. Pharmacophoric 1,2,4-trioxolane annulus spiro-conjugated with activated sesquiterpene δ-lactone results the bioactiphore in ART. The α-methylene-γ-lactone moiety results the potential anti-inflammatory group in sesquiterpene lactones (STLs).

5.1 INTRODUCTION

Setting the scene: carvone-derived 1,2,3-triazoles, artesunate, and proposed metabolic pathways for artemisinin (ART). The STLs can react with nucleophilic groups. The sesquiterpene α/β-lactones are more reactive compared with γ/δ ones, because of the greater strain of the α/β-lactones, regarding the less tensioned γ/δ-lactone cycle. Nevertheless, γ-lactones react with proteins, especially whether the ester bond in the lactone cycle is activated.

Despite much research, ART remains the only known natural product to contain a 1,2,4-trioxane ring, and *Artemisia annua* continues to be the only known natural source. Phytochemical investigation of the species revealed an abnormally wide range of other endoperoxides –O–O– and hydroperoxides –O–O–H, many of which were not tested for their antimalarial activity. 1,2,4-Trioxolane cycle spiro-conjugated with STL δ-lactone (activated δ-lactone) is the key pharmacophore fragment in ART. The α-methylene-γ-lactone moiety may be the potential anti-inflammatory group in STLs.

Earlier publications classified 31 STLs [1, 2]. It was informed the tentative mechanism of action, resistance of ART derivatives (ARTDs, *cf.* Figure 5.1) [3], reflections, proposed molecular mechanism of bioactivity, resistance [4], chemical, biological screening approaches, phytopharmaceuticals [5], chemical components from *Artemisia austro-yunnanensis*, anti-inflammatory effects and lactones [6]. The aim of this work is to review the composition and antioxidant activity of *A. austro-yunnanensis* flowers EO, highly oxidized sesquiterpenes from *A. austro-yunnanensis*, chemical components of *A. austro-yunnanensis* and their bioactivities, *A. austro-yunnanensis* 1,10-secoguaianolides and anti-inflammatory effects, and bioactivity of flavonoids and rare STLs isolated from *Centaurea ragusina*. The purpose of this report is to review carvone-derived 1,2,3-triazoles, artesunate, and proposed metabolic pathways for ART.

5.2   CARVONE-DERIVED 1,2,3-TRIAZOLES

Most terpenes exhibit pronounced bioactivity; e.g., the antimalarial drug ART and the anticancer drug paclitaxel (Taxol®) are the two most prominent members of the class of terpenes used in medicine (*cf.* Figure 5.1) [7].

The triazole fragment is an important pharmacophoric unit, and a large number of drugs containing the heterocycle are known (*cf.* Figure 5.2). Because of the commercial success of some pharmaceutical preparations based on the triazole ring, many pharmaceutical companies and academic groups showed interest in developing methods for synthesizing triazole compounds and screening their bioactivity; e.g., antifungal drugs containing triazole rings are known: Itraconazole, Fluconazole, Voriconazole, antiviral Ribavirin and Mubritinib (used to treat breast, bladder, kidney, and prostate cancer). Ribavirin is a drug for the treatment of viral infections (e.g., herpes, hepatitis).

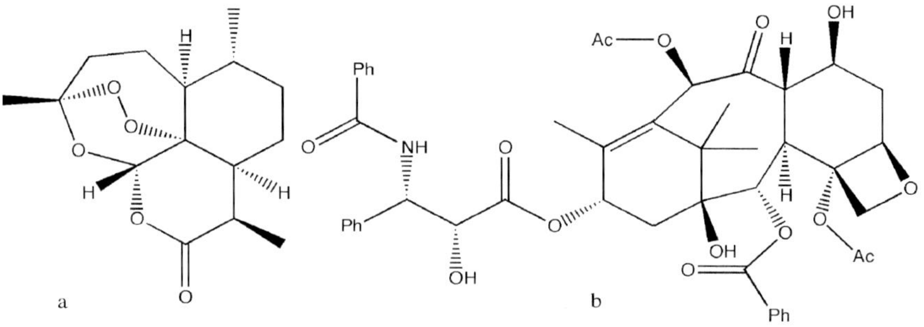

FIGURE 5.1   Structures of: (a) ART and (b) Taxol®.

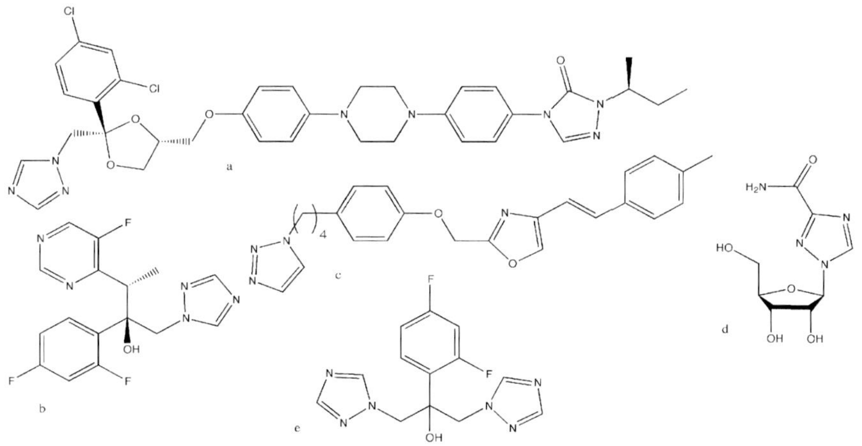

FIGURE 5.2   Triazole-derived drugs: (a) itraconazole; (b) voriconazole; (c) mubritinib; (d) ribavirin; (e) fluconazole.

5.3   ARTESUNATE

Artesunate (Figure 5.3) is a semi-synthetic ARTD isolated from a Chinese plant *Artemisia annua* L. (Asteraceae) medicinal [8]. The ART was synthesized. It was used as an antimalarial drug. Artesunate exhibits activity *vs.* certain types of cancer *via* an anti-angiogenic mechanism. The ART and ARTDs inhibit the growth and proliferation of cells and selectively kill tumor cells. Many ARTDs were described, and it is possible that many will be effective *vs.* cancer. It showed activity *vs.* chronic leukemia *in vitro* and *in vivo*. The ARTDs present low toxicity and are promising agents in antileukemia chemotherapy. The ART is not transported with permeability glycoprotein (P-gp), so it is not involved in multidrug resistance (MDR). After the administration of ART to rats for several weeks, severe adverse effects (AEs) were not found. Other studies compared the efficacy and toxicity of artesunate combined with vinorelbine and *cis*platin, and artesunate alone, in the treatment of advanced non-small cell lung cancer (NSCLC). Artesunate combined with vinorelbine and *cis*platin can elevate the short-term survival rate and prolong the mean survival time of patients, without extra side effects. The ART is cytotoxic to retinoblastoma cell lines with low cytotoxicity on normal retina cell lines. Therapy of ART was used in clinical trial studies without serious AEs. The ART was combined with daunorubicin to produce overall antitumor efficacy without signs of toxicity in mice. No AEs were observed in the treatment of breast cancer (BC). Artesunate exhibited antitumor activity *vs.* human pancreatic cancer (PaC) *via* the induction of apoptosis. The effect depended on the stage of differentiation and was more effective *vs.* less diverse cells. It enhanced the effects of gemcitabine in the control of PaC. Artesunate was effective *vs.* chemoresistant neuroblastoma cells. It induces apoptosis and reactive oxygen species (ROS) in neuroblastoma cells.

5.4   PROPOSED METABOLIC PATHWAYS FOR ARTEMISININ (ART)

A microbial transformation model for simulating mammal metabolism of ART was informed [9]. The proposed metabolic pathways for ART were shown in Figure 5.4.

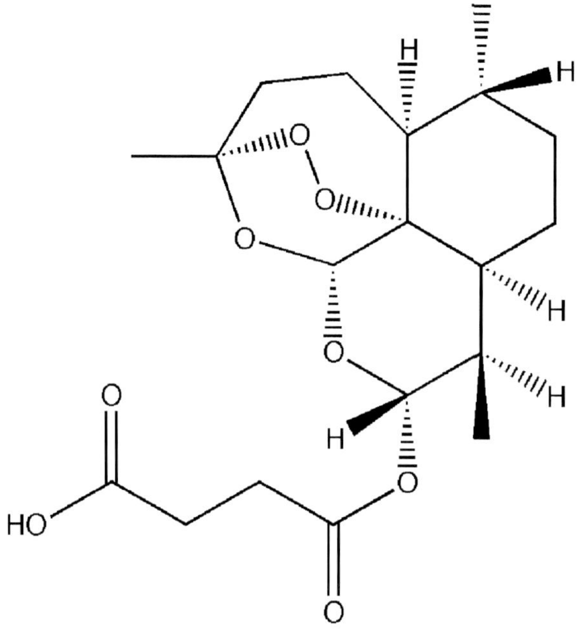

FIGURE 5.3 Molecular structure of artesunate.

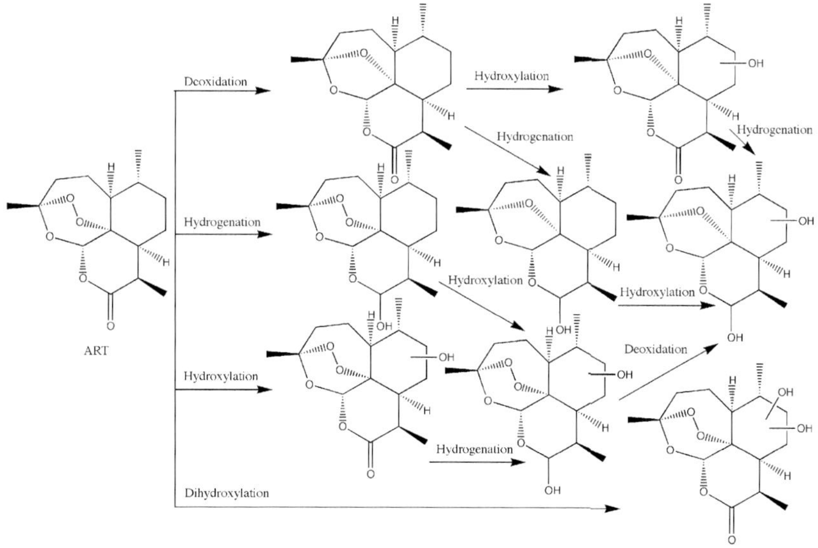

FIGURE 5.4 Proposed metabolic pathways of ART.

5.5 DISCUSSION

The STLs can react with nucleophilic groups [e.g., amino groups of proteins, especially of lysine (Lys, K) amino acids (AAs)]. The STLs with 3- or 4-membered rings (α-lactones and β-lactones, respectively) are more reactive than 5- or 6-atom γ- or δ-lactones, owing to the greater tension strain of the 3-unit α-lactone or 4-membered β-lactone, with regard to the less tensioned 5- or 6-atom γ- or δ-lactone annulus. Notwithstanding, γ-lactones can react with proteins, especially if the ester bond in the lactone ring is activated by additional functional groups, e.g., the activated β-exomethylene of the α-methylene-γ-lactone (ML) group O=C-C=CH_2. The 6-membered δ-lactone ART presents an uncommon characteristic, the 1,2,4-trioxane annulus (pharmacophoric peroxide linkage $-O_1-O_2-$ in endoperoxide ring), which is the basis of its unique antimalarial action.

5.6 FINAL REMARKS

From the preceding results and discussion, the following final remarks can be drawn.

1. Despite much research, ART remains the only known natural product to contain a 1,2,4-trioxane ring, and *Artemisia annua* continues to be the only known natural source. Phytochemical investigation of the species revealed an abnormally wide range of other endoperoxides –O–O– and hydroperoxides –O–O–H, many of which were not tested for their antimalarial activity.
2. 1,2,4-Trioxolane cycle spiro-conjugated with sesquiterpene δ-lactone (activated δ-lactone) is the key pharmacophore fragment in ART.
3. The α-methylene-γ-lactone moiety may be the potential anti-inflammatory group in the STLs.

ACKNOWLEDGMENTS

The authors thank the support from Generalitat Valenciana (Project No. PROMETEO/2016/094) and Universidad Católica de Valencia *San Vicente Mártir* (Project No. 2019-217-001).

KEYWORDS

- **1,2,3-triazole**
- **acetylene**
- **antioxidant activity**
- **bovine serum albumin**
- **carvone**
- **click chemistry**
- *Cunninghamella elegans*
- *in vivo*
- **metabolite**
- **microbial transformation**
- **UNIFI software**
- **UPLC-ESI-Q-TOF-MS[E]**

REFERENCES

1. Castellano, G., Redondo, L., & Torrens, F., (2017). QSAR of natural sesquiterpene lactones as inhibitors of Myb-dependent gene expression. *Curr. Top. Med. Chem.*, *17*, 3256–3268.
2. Torrens, F., Redondo, L., León, A., Castellano, G. Structure-activity relationships of cytotoxic lactones as inhibitors and mechanisms of action. *Curr. Drug Discov. Technol.* (In Press).
3. Torrens, F., Redondo, L., & Castellano, G., (2017). Artemisinin: Tentative mechanism of action and resistance. *Pharmaceuticals*, *10*, Article 20, p. 4.
4. Torrens, F., Redondo, L., & Castellano, G., (2018). Reflections on artemisinin, proposed molecular mechanism of bioactivity and resistance. In: Haghi, A. K., Balköse, D., & Thomas, S., (eds.), *Applied Physical Chemistry with Multidisciplinary Approaches* (pp. 189–215). Apple Academic CRC: Waretown, NJ.
5. Torrens, F., Castellano, G. Chemical/biological screening approaches to phytopharmaceuticals. In: Pourhashemi, A., Deka, S. C., & Haghi, A. K., (eds.), *Research Methods and Applications in Chemical and Biological Engineering*. Apple Academic–CRC: Waretown, NJ (In Press).
6. Torrens, F., & Castellano, G. Chemical components from artemisia austro-yunnanensis: Anti-inflammatory effects and lactones. In: Pogliani, L., Torrens, F., & Haghi, A. K., (eds.), *Molecular Chemistry and Biomolecular Engineering: Integrating Theory and Research with Practice*. Apple Academic–CRC: Waretown, NJ (In Press).

7. Galstyan, A. S., Martiryan, A. I., Grigoryan, K. R., Ghazaryan, A. G., Samvelyan, M. A., Ghochikyan, T. V., & Nenajdenko, V. G., (2018). Synthesis of carvone-derived 1,2,3-triazoles study of their antioxidant properties and interaction with bovine serum albumin. *Molecules*, *23*, Article 2991, p. 12.

8. Lichota, A., & Gwozdzinski, K., (2018). Anticancer activity of natural compounds from plant and marine environment. *Int. J. Mol. Sci.*, *19*, Article 3533, p. 38.

9. Ma, Y., Sun, P., Zhao, Y., Wang, K., Chang, X., Bai, Y., Zhang, D., & Yang, L., (2019). A microbial transformation model for simulating mammal metabolism of artemisinin. *Molecules*, *24*, Article 315, p. 13.

CHAPTER 6

FACILE SYNTHESIS OF SOME 1,3,4 THIADIAZOLE-BASED LIGANDS AND THEIR METAL COMPLEXES AS POTENTIAL ANTIMICROBIAL AGENTS

AJAY M. PATIL,[1] RAVINDRA S. SHINDE,[2] and SUNIL R. MIRGANE[3]

[1]Department of Chemistry, Pratishthan Mahavidyalaya, Paithan, Maharashtra, India

[2]Department of Chemistry, Dayanand Science College, Latur, Maharashtra, India

[3]Department of Chemistry, J.E.S. College, Jalna, Maharashtra, India

*Corresponding author. E-mail: patilan4@gmail.com, rss.333@redifffmail.com

ABSTRACT

The 1,3,4-thiadiazole moieties containing ligand and their metal complex of Cu(II), Zn(II), Cd(II) were prepared by using substituted Salicyladehyde and 5-amino-1,3,4-thiadiazole-2-thiol derivatives. The ligand and its metal complexes were characterized and analyzed by different spectroscopic techniques (UV, ^{1}HNMR, FT-IR, ^{13}CNMR, HRMS), magnetic susceptibility, and molar conductance, elemental analysis. The synthesized transition metal complexes show moderate to excellent antifungal activity against *A. Niger* and *F. Oxysporum* and antibacterial activity against *S. aureus* and *B. subtilis* using Kirby-Bauer disc diffusion method.

6.1 INTRODUCTION

The Schiff base is a condensation of an aldehyde with primary amine important in organic synthesis and pharmacological applications [1]. The 1,3,4-thiadiazole is an important compound because of it's biological, pharmaceutical, and analytical applications [2]. The 1,3,4-thiadiazole acts as ligands. Enhance biological activity by forming complexes [3]. Most of the heterocyclic moieties have biological activity that depends on their orientation and their Structure [4]. The aldehyde is ortho-substituted with (-OH) hydroxyl group, which acts as a bidentate donor ligand for transition metal ions [5]. The Schiff base is very important because of its structural resemblance and flexibility with naturally occurring biological and chemical substances. The imine group >C=N- (azomethine) also helps to determine the transformation and racemization in biological systems [6]. During the last few years, more intensely focus on variable thiadiazole derivative. Because of their potent biological properties like anti-inflammatory [7], analgesic [8], antituberculosis [9], antihypertensive [10], antimicrobial [11], anticonvulsants [12], antioxidant [13], antifungal [14], anticancer [15], and antidepressant [16]. We now report the synthesis and characterization and biological analysis of 1,3,4-thiadiazole containing ligand and its Cu (II), Zn (II), and Cd (II) metal complexes.

6.2 PRESENT WORK

The present scheme involves the synthesis of ligand 2,4-dichloro-6-(((5-mercapto-1,3,4-thiadiazol-2-yl)imino)methyl)phenol illustrated in Scheme 6.1 and its Metal Complexes of Cu(II), Zn(II), Cd(II) shown in Figure 6.1.

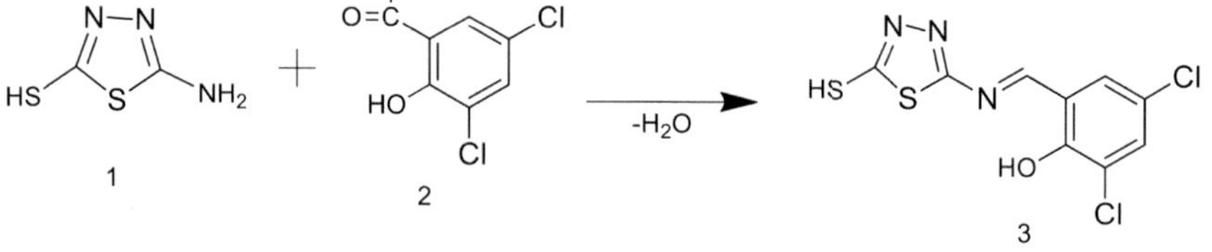

SCHEME 6.1   2,4-dichloro-6-(((5-mercapto-1,3,4-thiadiazol-2-yl)imino)methyl)phenol.

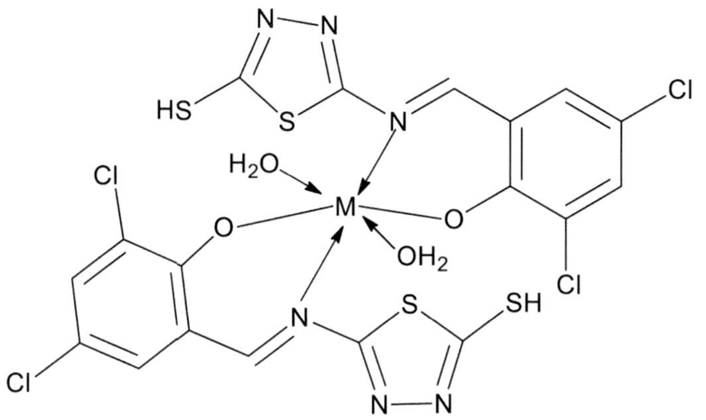

FIGURE 6.1 Proposed Structures of metal complexes M: Cu (II), Zn (II), and Cd (II).

6.3 EXPERIMENTAL

All the chemicals of analytical grade and all the salts are metal nitrates, i.e., $Cu(NO_3)_2.3H_2O$, $Zn(NO_3)_2.6H_2O$, $Cd(NO_3)_2.4H_2O$, etc., were purchased from Sigma-Aldrich and used without further purification. The 3,5-dichloro-2-hydroxybenzaldehyde and 5-amino-1,3,4-thiadiazole-2-thiol from Sigma-Aldrich and Alfa Aesar used without further purification. The distilled ethanol used for the synthesis of metal complexes and ligand diethyl ether (Sigma-Aldrich). The IR Spectra recorded on Perkin Elmer Spectrometer in range 4000–400 cm^{-1} KBr pellets. ^1H and $^{13}CNMR$ Spectra were recorded on BRUKER AVANCE III HD NMR 500 MHz spectrophotometer. The room temperature magnetic moments by Guoy's method in B.M. Electronic Spectra using DMSO on Varian Carry 5000 Spectrometer. The molar Conductance measurements in dry DMSO having 1×10^{-3} concentration on the Systronics conductivity bridge at room temperature. Elemental analysis (C,H,N) was carried out by using Perkin Elmer 2400 elemental analyzer. Mass spectra were recorded on Bruker IMPACT HD.

6.3.1 BIOLOGICAL ACTIVITY

The Schiff base and their metal complexes evaluated in vitro their anti-bacterial activity against two Gram-Positive bacteria, viz, *B. Subtilis, S.*

aureus, two fungal strains *A. niger* and *F. oxysporum* by Kirby-Bauer disc diffusion method [17]. The fungal and bacterial strains sub-cultured on PDA and Nutrient Agar. The stock solution (1mg mL^{-1}) was prepared in DMSO solution. The stock solution again diluted by using sterilized water to dilution in 500 ppm. The bacteria were subculture in agar medium, and disc were kept incubated for 37°C at 24 hrs. The standard antibacterial drug Miconazole and Ciprofloxacin was also screen under the same condition for comparison. The activity was measured and calculated by a zone of inhibition (mm) surrounding discs. The experimental value compares with standard drug value miconazole for the antifungal activity and ciprofloxacin for the antibacterial activity.

6.3.2   SYNTHESIS OF 2,4-DICHLORO-6-(((5-MERCAPTO-1,3,4-THIADIAZOL-2-YL)IMINO) METHYL) PHENOL (HL$_1$)

The target compounds were prepared in the following steps: The mixture of 1:1 3,5-dichloro-2-hydroxybenzaldehyde (1) (1.91 g, 0.01 mol) with 5-amino-1,3,4-thiadiazole-2-thiol (2) (1.33g, 0.01 mol) dissolved in ethanol. Then add few drops of glacial acetic acid was added. The resultant mixture stirred for 3–4 hrs the colored precipitate of ligands was obtained. Then wash with ethanol recrystallized with ethanol and ether then dried in air. The purity of the compound was checked by TLC using the silica gel method (3); scheme 6.1.

> **Yield:** 72% M.P: 118°C.
> **IR(KBr cm^{-1}):** 3319 (vOH/H$_2$O-stretch), 1265 (v C-O), 1645 (**v C=N**), 752 **vC-S-C,**1467(**v -C=N-N=C**)
> ^{1}**H NMR** (500 MHz, DMSO-d_6): δ 11.22 (s,1H,Ar-OH), 8.90(s,1H, CH=N),7.19–7.90 (s,2H,Ar-CH), 13.44 (s,1H,SH).
> **MS(*ESI*) *m/z*:**305 [M+1]$^+$
> **Anal. Data**: Calcd. for C$_9$H$_5$Cl$_2$N$_3$OS$_2$: C, 35.30; H, 1.65; N, 13.72;S, 20.94%. Found: C, 35.89; H, 1.69; N, 13.63;S, 20.21%.

6.3.3   SYNTHESIS OF METAL COMPLEXES

The metal complexes were prepared by mixing of Copper(II) nitrate trihydrate (Cu(NO$_3$)$_2$.3H$_2$O) (0.241g, 0.001 mol) and ethanolic solution of Ligand HL

(0.612g, 0.001mol) (metal: ligand) 1:2 ratio The resulting mixture refluxed on the water bath for 5–6 hr. A colored product obtains washed with ethanol, filtered, and recrystallized with ethanol. Similarly, $Zn(NO_3)_2.6H_2O, Cd(NO_3)_2.4H_2O$ metal complexes were prepared by the same method (Figure 6.1).

6.4   RESULTS AND DISCUSSION

The ligand Scheme 6.1 and its transition metal complexes (Figure 6.1) of 2,4-dichloro-6-(5-mercapto-1,3,4-thiadiazol-2-yl)imino methyl phenol are stable at room temperature in the solid-state. The ligand is soluble in organic solvent DMSO, DMF, and metal complexes are easily soluble in DMSO. The synthesized complexes have 1:2 metal to ligand stoichiometric ratio. The physical and analytical data shown in Table 6.1. The spectral data shows the formation of ligand and its metal complexes.

6.4.1   IR SPECTRA

The IR spectra of 2,4-dichloro-6-(5-mercapto-1,3,4-thiadiazol-2-yl) imino methyl phenol (HL) Schiff base ligand and its complexes are listed in Table 6.2. The Infrared Spectra of the complexes are compared with the free ligand in order to determine the coordination sites that may be involved in a chelation. There are some important peaks in the spectra of the ligand, which is different in metal complexes helps to prove that formation of metal complexes IR spectra of 2,4-dichloro-6-(5-mer- capto-1,3,4-thiadiazol-2-yl)imino methyl phenol (HL) Schiff base ligand having the most characteristic bands at 3316–3330 cm^{-1} (O-H), 1638–1652 cm^{-1} v(C=N, azomethine) and 1258–1272 cm^{-1} v(C-O). The ligand spectra showed bands at 3314–3304 cm^{-1} and 1340–1350 cm^{-1} due to the deformation and stretching of the phenolic –OH [18]. These stretching is not present in the spectra of the complexes indicates that deprotonation of the hydroxyl group (-OH) occurs coordinate through phenolic oxygen atom. The band 1640–1650 cm^{-1} due to the azomethine (-C=N-) group of the Schiff bases ligand have shifted to lower frequency (1612–1636 cm^{-1}) after complexation, indicate that bonding of nitrogen of the azomethine group (-C=N-) of ligand to the metal ions and this can be explained by the donation of electrons from the nitrogen to the empty d-orbital of the metal ion in the complexes

TABLE 6.1 Analytical Data and Physical Properties of Ligand and its Metal Complexes

Comp.	Empirical Formula	Mol. Wt.	Color	M.P (°C)	Yield (%)	Elemental Analysis/ Found (Calc.)				
						C	H	N	S	M
Ligand (HL)	$C_9H_5Cl_2N_3OS_2$	306	Dark Yellow	118°C	72%	35.89 (35.30)	1.69 (1.65)	13.63 (13.72)	20.21 (20.94)	—
Cu(II) Complex	$C_{18}H_{12}Cl_4CuN_6O_4S_4$	709	green	>300	69%	30.10(30.45)	1.78(1.70)	11.80(11.84)	17.98 (18.07)	8.85 (8.95)
Zn(II) Complex	$C_{18}H_{12}Cl_4ZnN_6O_4S_4$	711	Lemon Yellow	>300	71%	30.41 (30.37)	1.65(1.70)	11.75(11.81)	18.12(18.02)	9.23(9.19)
Cd(II) Complex	$C_{18}H_{12}Cl_4CdN_6O_4S_4$	758	Gray	>300	68%	28.40(28.49)	1.65 (1.59)	11.02(11.08)	17.02 (16.90)	14.35(14.81)

[19, 20]. The phenolic λ(C–O) stretching vibration that appeared at 1260–1268 cm^{-1} in Schiff bases shift towards higher frequency (20–32 cm^{-1}) in the metal complexes. This shift confirms the involvement of oxygen in the C–O–M bond. The appearance of broad bands around (3375–3460 cm^{-1}) in the spectra of complexes may be due to water molecules coordinated to the metal in the metal complexes [21]. New bands appearing in the low-frequency range 528–575 cm^{-1} and 464–482 cm^{-1} are due to (M–O) and ν(M–N), respectively. The ν(C–S–C) at 751–758 cm^{-1} of the thiadiazole ring remains unchanged suggested that thiadiazole group does not coordinate to the metal ion by neither sulfur nor nitrogen atom of thiadiazole ring of the ligand [22].

TABLE 6.2   Infrared Spectra of the Schiff Base and Complexes (in cm^{-1})

Compound	νOH/H$_2$O	νC-O	νC=N	νM-N	νM-O	νC-S-C	ν-C=N-N=C	νN-N
Ligand	3319	1265	1645	—	—	752	1467	1028
Cu(II) Complex	3410	1280	1633	470	569	758	1433	1028
Zn(II) Complex	3401	1290	1610	480	575	756	1436	1033
Cd(II) Complex	3460	1274	1611	482	555	755	1443	1030

6.4.2 ^{1}H NMR AND ^{13}C NMR SPECTRA

The ^{1}H-NMR spectra of ligand were recorded in dimethyl sulfoxide (DMSO) solution using TMS as a standard Table 6.3. The spectra of ligand show singlet at δ 7.19–7.90 ppm due to aromatic proton while azomethine (-C=N-) proton resonate at singlet δ 8.90 ppm. The phenolic -OH has show peak singlet at δ 11.22 ppm, and Thiadiazole ring containing thiol (–SH) group shows singlet at δ 13.44 ppm [23]. 13C-NMR of ligand, the peak appeared at 158–164 ppm due to imine group (-C=N-), peak appearing at 187.52 ppm due to carbon-sulfur C-SH bonding in Thiadiazole. 121.96–135.53 ppm peak because of aromatic carbon, 158–172 ppm peak because of the Ar-OH group [24].

TABLE 6.3 ^{1}H NMR Signals (δ, ppm) and Their Assignments

Compound	^{1}H NMR Signals (δ, ppm) and their assignments
Ligand (HL)	11.22 (s,1H,Ar-OH), 8.90(s,1H,CH=N), 7.19–7.90 (s,2H,Ar-CH), 13.44 (s,1H,SH)

6.4.3   MASS SPECTRA

Mass spectra of ligands shows a peak at m/z 305, which is M+H peak at 100% intensity. This peak support to the structure formation of the ligand.

6.4.4   MAGNETIC SUSCEPTIBILITY AND MOLAR CONDUCTANCE

The magnetic susceptibility was seen at room temperature. Synthesized metal complexes of copper(II) is paramagnetic in nature, zinc(II) and cadmium(II) is diamagnetic in nature Table 6.4. Molar conductance of metal complexes was observed at room temperature at 1×10^{-3}M DMSO solution. The studies show negligible molar conductance value in range $8–12$ $ohm^{-1}cm^2mol^{-1}$; results shown in Table 6.4. It is observed that all metal complexes are non-electrolytic in nature [25, 26].

6.4.5   ELECTRONIC ABSORPTION SPECTRA

The electronic spectral data of the ligands and metal complexes in DMSO sol. are given in Table 6.4. The geometry and nature of the ligand field around the metal ion has been concluded from the electronic spectral data of metal complexes and ligand. The band appearing at 220–312 nm is due to the transition of the benzene ring of the ligand. The other band due to free ligands 320–382 nm due to transition for phenolic -OH and azomethine moieties (-C=N-). This band shifts longer wavelengths due to the formation of ligand to metal complexes [27, 28]. The spectra of the complexes display band 424–500 nm assigned to charge transfer transition from ligands to metal [23]. The magnetic moment value for Cu(II) complexes is 1.80 B.M is near to octahedral complex spectra shows two-band at 360 nm, and 560 nm shows that octahedral geometry of Cu (II) complex [29]. Electronic spectra of Zn (II) complexes show band 265 nm, 370–430 nm did not show d-d transition suggest octahedral geometry [30]. Electronic spectra of Cd(II) show two peaks at 325 nm and 307–360 nm ligand to metal donation with diamagnetic suggest octahedral geometry [31].

TABLE 6.4 Electronic Spectral Magnetic and Molar Conductance Data

Compounds	Wavelength in nm	Magnetic Moment μeff (BM)	Molar Conductance (ohm^{-1} cm^2 mol^{-1})
Ligands (HL)	280, 372	—	6.68
$C_{18}H_{12}Cl_4CuN_6O_4S_4$	270–320, 360, 560	1.80	8.2
$C_{18}H_{12}Cl_4ZnN_6O_4S_4$	265, 370–430	Diamagnetic	10.2
$C_{18}H_{12}Cl_4CdN_6O_4S_4$	265, 307–360	Diamagnetic	12

6.5 ANTIMICROBIAL ACTIVITY

The antimicrobial activity *in vitro* of the ligand and their corresponding metal complexes on two-gram positive bacteria (*S. aureus* and *B. Subtlis*) and two fungi (*A. niger* and *F. Oxysporum*) was carried out. All of the tested compounds showed good to moderate biological activity against test microorganisms. The bactericidal and fungicidal investigation data of the ligand and metal complexes are summarized in Table 6.5. The investigation shows that Cu(II) shows more bactericidal and fungicidal activity than Zn(II) and Cd(II) complexes and ligand. Hence, the activity of metal complexes increases due to chelation increase in delocalization of π electron on chelating ring and enhance the penetration of complexes in lipid membrane, and blocks the binding site enzymes of microorganism. There are other factors, i.e., solubility, lipophilicity/hydrophilicity, conductivity, and M-L bond length that increases the activity of complexes [32–37].

6.6 CONCLUSION

In the present work, we have synthesized and characterized some novel metal complexes from conventional methods. These ligands and metal complexes were characterized by physicochemical and spectral analyses. The synthesized Schiff base ligand binds metal ions in a bidentate manner, with the N and O donor site of azomethine-N and deprotonated phenolic-O. The antimicrobial activity data showed that most of the metal complexes are more biologically active compared to those parent ligand against all pathogenic bacteria and fungi. Such studies may help to decrease emerging problems in drug resistance in health sciences over the world.

TABLE 6.5 Antimicrobial Activity of Ligand and its Metal Complexes

| Compounds | Antibacterial Activity | | | | Antifungal Activity | | | |
| | S. aureus | | B. subtilis | | A. niger | | F. oxysporum | |
	Diameter of inhibition zone in mm	% Activity Index	Diameter of inhibition zone in mm	% Activity Index	Diameter of inhibition zone in mm	% Activity Index	Diameter of inhibition zone in mm	% Activity Index
	500 ppm	500 ppm	500 ppm	500 ppm	500 ppm	500 ppm	500 ppm	500 ppm
Ligands (HL)	22	65	21	64	20	65	18	67
Cu	26	76	25	76	23	74	22	81
Zn	21	62	23	70	18	58	16	59
Cd	20	59	22	67	19	61	14	52
Ciprofloxacin (Standard)	34	100	33	100	—	—	—	—
Miconazole (Standard)	—	—	—	—	31	100	27	100

KEYWORDS

- **1,3,4-thiadiazole**
- **antibacterial activity**
- **antifungal activity**
- **hydrophilicity**
- **magnetic susceptibility**
- **metal complexes**

REFERENCES

1. Elzahany, E., Hegab, K., Khalil, S., & Youssef, N., (2008). Synthesis, characterization and biological activity of some transition metal complexes with Schiff bases derived from 2-formylindole, salicylaldehyde and N-amino rhodanine. *Aust. J. Basic Appl. Sci., 2*(2), 210–220.
2. Hadizadeh, F., & Vosoogh, R., (2008). Synthesis of a-[5-(5-amino-1,3,4-thiadiazol-2-yl)-2 imidazolylthio]-acetic acids. *J. Heterocycl. Chem., 45*, 1–3.
3. Lu, S., & Chen, R., (2008). Facial and efficient, synthesis aminophosphate derivatives of 1,3,4-oxadiazole and 1,3,4-thiadizaole. *Org. Prep. Proced. Int., 32*, 302–306.
4. Ugras, H., Basaran, I., Kilic, T., & Cakir, U., (2006). Synthesis, complexation and anti-fungal, antibacterial activity studies of a new macrocyclic Schiff bases. *J. Heterocycl. Chem., 43*, 1679–1684.
5. Wadher, S., Puranik, M., Karande, N., & Yeole, P., (2009). Synthesis and bio-logical evaluation of Schiff base of dapsone and their derivativeas antimicrobial agents. *Int. J. Pharm. Tech. Res., 1*, 22–33.
6. Rajavel, P., Senthil, M., & Anitha, C., (2008). Synthesis, physical characterization and biological activity of some Schiff bases complexes. *E. J. Chem., 5*, 620–626.
7. Barreiro, E. J., Varandas, L. S., & Fraga, C., (2005). Design, synthesis and pharmaco-logical evaluation of new non steroidal anti-inflammatory 1,3,4-thiadiazole derivatives. *Letters in Drug Design and Disco, 2*, 62–67.
8. Arvind, K. S., Mishra, G., & Kshitiz, J., (2011). Review on biological activities of 1, 3, 4-thiadiazole derivatives. *Jou. of Applied Pharmaceutical Sci., 1*, 44–49.
9. Karigar, A., Himaja, M., & Sunil, V., (2011). One pot synthesis and antitubercular activity of 2-amino-5-aryl-5h-thiazole [4,3-b]-1,3,4-thiadiazoles. *Inter. Research Journal of Pharm, 2*, 153–158.
10. Singaravel, M., Sarkkarai, A., & Kambikudi, R. M., (2010). Synthesis, characterization and biological activity of some novel sulfur bridged pyrazoles. *International Journal of Pharma Sci. and Res., 1*, 391–398.

11. Vasoya, S. L., Paghdar, D. J., Chovatia, P. T., & Joshi, H. S., (2005). Synthesis of some New thiosemicarbazide and 1,3,4-thiadiazole heterocycles bearing benzo[b] thiophene nucleus as a potent antitubercular and antimicrobial agents. *J. Sci. Islamic Republic Iran, 16*, 33–36.

12. Turner, S., Myers, M., Gadie, B., Nelson, A. J., Pape, R., Saville, J. F., Doxey, J. C., & Berridge, T. L., (1988). Synthesis of some 2-aryl-5-hydrazino-1,3,4-thiadiazoles with vasodilator activity. *J. Med. Chem., 31*, 902–906.

13. Cressier, D., Prouillac, C., Hernandez, P. A., Mourette, C., Diserbo, M., Lion, C., & Rima, G., (2009). Thiadiazoles: Progress report on biological activities. *Bio. Med. Chem.,* 17, 5275–5284.

14. Kumar, S., Rajendraprasad, G. V., Mallikarjuna, Y., Chandrashekar, B. P., & Kitayama, S. M., (2010). Synthesis of some novel 2-substituted-5-[isopropylthiazole] clubbed 1,2,4-triazole and 1,3,4-oxadiazoles as potential antimicrobial and antitubercular agents. *Eur. J. Med. Chem., 45*, 2063–2066.

15. Swamy, S. N., Basappa, B. S., Priya, B., Prabhuswamy, B. H., Doreswamy, J. S., Prasad, K. S., & Rangappa, (2009). Synthesis, characterization and anticancer activity of 1,2,4-Triazolo[3,4-b]-1,3,4-thiadiazoles on Hep G2 cell lines. *Eur. J. Med. Chem., 41*, 531–538.

16. Yusuf, M., & Ahmed, R., (2008). Syntheses and anti-depressant activity of 5-amino-1, 3, 4-thiadiazole-2-thiol imines and thiobenzyl derivatives. *Bioorg. Med. Chem., 17*, 8029–8034.

17. Bauer, A. W., & Perry, D. M., (1959). Kirby single-disk antibiotic-sensitivity testing of staphylococci: An analysis of technique and results. *AMA Arch Intern Med., 104*, 208–216.

18. Nakamoto, K., (1998). *Infrared and Raman Spectra of Inorganic and Coordination Compounds* (5th edn.). John Wiley and Sons, Part A & B, New York.

19. Temel, H., Ilhan, S., Aslanoglu, M., Kilic, A., & Tas, E., (2006). Synthesis, spectroscopic and electrochemical studied of novel transitionmetal complexes with quadridentate Schiff base. *J. Chin. Chem. Soc., 53*, 1027–1031.

20. Shukla, D., Gupta, L. K., & Chandra, S., (2008). Spectroscopic studies onchromium(III), manganese(II), cobalt(II), nickel(II) and copper(II) complexes with hexadentate nitrogen-sulfur donor [N_2S_4] macrocyclic ligand. *Spectrochim. Acta., 71A*, 746–750.

21. Mohamed, G. G., Omar, M. M., & Hindy, A. M., (2008). Metal complexes of Schiff bases: Preparation, characterization and biological activity. *Turk J. Chem., 30*, 361–382.

22. Neelakantan, M. A., Marriappan, S. S., Dharmaraja, J., Jeyakumar, T., & Muthuku-mara, K., (2008). Spectral, XRD, SEM and biological activities of transition metal complexes of polydentate ligands containing thiazole moiety. *Spectrochim Acta., 71A*, 628–635.

23. Rastogi, R. B., Yadav, M., & Singh, K., (2001). Synthesis and characterization of molybdenum and tungsten complexes of 1-Aryl-2,4-dithiobiurets. *Synth. React. Inorg. Met.-Org. Chem., 31*, 1011–1022.

24. AbdElzaher, M. M., Moustafa, S. A., Labib, A. A., Mousa, H. A., Ali, M. M., & Mahmoud, A. E., (2012). Synthesis, characterization and anticancer studies of ferrocenyl complexes containing thiazole moiety. *Applied Organometallic Chemistry, 26*, 230–236.

25. Geary, W. J., (1971). *Coord. Chem. Rev., 7*, 81.

26. Sampal, S. N., Thakur, S. V., Rajbhoj, A. S., & Gaikwad, S. T., (2017). Synthesis, characterization and antimicrobial screening of 1,3-dione with their metal complexes. *Asian J. Chem., 30*, 398–400.

27. Ucan, S. Y., & Ucan, M., (2005). Synthesis and characterization of new Schiff bases and their cobalt(II), nickel(II), copper(II), zinc(II), cadmium(II) and mercury(II) complexes. *Synth. React. Inorg. Met. Org. Nano-Metal Chem., 35*, 417–421.

28. Turan, N., & Sekerci, M., (2009). Metal complexes of Schiff base derived from terephthalaldehyde and 2-amino-5-ethyl-1,3,4-thiadiazole synthesis, spectral and thermal characterization. *Synthesis and Reactivity in Inorganic, Metal-Organic, and Nano-Metal Chem., 39*, 651–657.

29. Khedr, A. M., & Marwani, H. M., (2012). Synthesis, spectral, thermal analyses and molecular modeling of bioactive Cu(II)-complexes with 1,3,4-thiadiazole Schiff base derivatives. Their catalytic effect on the cathodic reduction of oxygen. *Int. J. Electrochem. Sci., 7*, 10074–10093.

30. Turan, N., & Şekerci, M., (2010). Synthesis, characterization and thermal behavior of some Zn(II) complexes with ligands having 1,3,4-thiadiazole moieties. *Heteroatom Chem., 21*, 14–23.

31. Turan, N., & Şekerci, M., (2009). Synthesis and spectral studies of novel Co(II), Ni(II), Cu(II), Cd(II), and Fe(II) metal complexes with N-[5′-amino-2,2′-bis(1,3,4-thiadiazole)-5-yl]-2-hydroxybenzaldehyde IMINE (HL). *Spectroscopy Letters, 42*, 258–267.

32. Neelakantan, M. A., Marriappan, S. S., Dharmaraja, J., Jeyakumar, T., & Muthuku-maran, K., (2008). Spectral, XRD, SEM and biological activities of transition metal complexes of polydentate ligands containing thiazole moiety. *Spectrochimica Acta Part A: Molecular and Bimolecular Spectroscopy, 7*, 628–635.

33. Chohan, Z. H., Munawar, A., & Supuran, C. T., (2001). Transition metalion complexes of Schiff bases synthesis, characterization and antibacterial properties. *Metal Based Drugs, 8*, 137–143.

34. Hanna, W. G., & Moawad, M. M., (2005). Synthesis, characterization and antimicrobial activity cobalt(II), nickel(II) and copper(II) complexes with new asymmetrical Schiff base ligands derived from 7-formalin-substituted diamine-sulfoxine and acety-lacetone. *Transit Metal Chem., 26*, 644–651.

35. 35. Singh, V. P., & Katiyar, A., (2008). Synthesis, characterization of some transition metal(II) complexes of acetone p-amino acetophenone salicyloyl hydrazone and their antimicrobial activity. *BioMet., 21*, 491–501.

36. Azam, F., Singh. S., Khokhra, S. L., & Prakash, O., (2007). Synthesis of Schiff bases of naphtha [1,2-d] thiazol-2-amine and metal complexes of 2-(20-hydroxy) benzylidene amino naphthothiazole as potential antimicrobial agent. *J. Zhejiang Univ. Sci., 8*, 446–452.

37. Chohan, Z. H., (1999). Ni (II), Cu (II) and Zn (II) metal chelates with some thiazole derived Schiff-bases: Their synthesis, characterization and bactericidal properties. *Metal-Based Drugs, 6*, 75–79.

CHAPTER 7

AN EFFICIENT AND GREEN SYNTHESIS OF 2,3-DIHYDROQUINAZOLIN-4 (1H)-ONE DERIVATIVES CATALYZED BY {[BMIM]METHANESULFONATE} IONIC LIQUID

SHREYAS S. MAHURKAR,[1,*] RAVINDRA S. SHINDE,[1] and SANGITA S. MAKONE[2]

[1]*Department of Chemistry, Dayanand Science College, Latur, Maharashtra, India*

[2]*School of Chemical Sciences, Swami Ramanand Teerth Marathwada University, Nanded, Maharashtra, India*

Corresponding author. E-mail: mahurkar.shrayas1@gmail.com, rss.333@rediffmail.com

ABSTRACT

1-butyl-3-methyl imidazolium methanesulfonate ([Bmim] $CH_3SO_3^-$) ionic liquid catalyzed, an efficient method for the preparation of 2-phenyl-2,3-dihydroquinazolin-4(1H)-ones by the one-pot three-component cyclo condensation of isatoic anhydride, ammonium acetate and aromatic aldehydes in ethanol: water solvent system. This procedure has several advantages such as short reaction time, easy workup, excellent yields, and reuse of ionic liquid.

7.1 INTRODUCTION

Quinazoline derivatives belong to the N-containing heterocyclic compounds, have caused worldwide concerns due to their wide and distinct biopharmaceutical activities. Quinazolinone is classified into the following five categories based on the substitution patterns of the ring system:

1. 2-substituted -4 (3H)-quinazolinones;
2. 3-substituted-4(3H)- quinazolinones;
3. 4-substituted quinazolines;
4. 2,3-disubstituted-4(1H)- quinazolinones; and
5. 2,4-disubstituted-4(3H)- quinazolinones.

Depending upon the position of the keto or oxo group, these compounds are classified into four types, as shown in Figure 7.1.

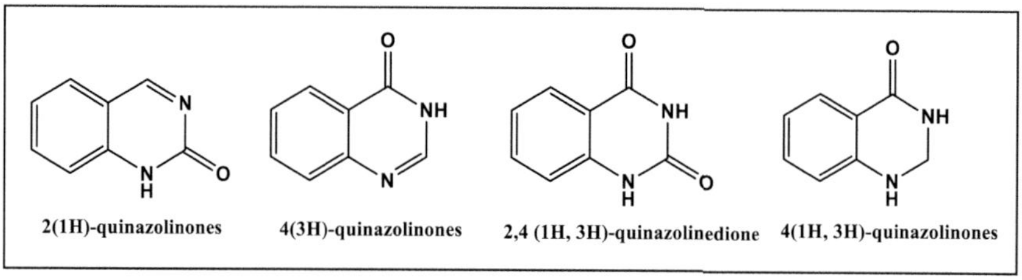

2(1H)-quinazolinones   4(3H)-quinazolinones   2,4 (1H, 3H)-quinazolinedione   4(1H, 3H)-quinazolinones

FIGURE 7.1   Classification of quinazoline compounds.

Out of these four quinazolinone structures, 4(3H)-quinazolinone and 4(1H, 3H)-quinazolinone are most prevalent either as intermediates or as natural products in many proposed biosynthetic pathways. This is partly due to the structure being derived from the anthranilates such as anthranilic acid or various ester, isatoic anhydride, anthranilamide, and anthranilonitrile. While the 2(1H)-quinazolinone is predominantly a product of anthranilonitrile or benzamide with nitriles.

Heterocycles form by far the largest of the classical division of organic chemistry. Moreover, they are of immense importance not only both biologically and industrially but to the functioning of any developed human society as well. Their participation in a wide range of areas cannot be underestimated. The majority of the pharmaceutical products that mimic natural products with biological activity are heterocycles. Most of the significant advances against disease have been made by designing and testing new structures, which are often heteroaromatic derivatives.

Quinazoline is a heterocyclic compound made up of two fused six-member simple aromatic rings, a benzene ring and a pyrimidine ring. Its chemical formula is $C_8H_6N_2$ (Figure 7.2).

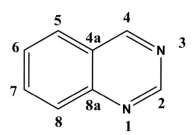

FIGURE 7.2   Structure of the quinazoline compound.

Quinazoline is a solid compound. It is isomeric with other napthyridine, including quinaxaline, phthalazine, and cinnoline. Derivatives of quinazoline are called quinazolines. Medicinally it has been used in various areas, especially as an antimalarial agent and in cancer treatment. One example of a compound containing the quinazoline structure is doxazosin mesylate.

The ring system is typically prepared by heating 2-acylanilides in the presence of ammonia or amines [1]. The attempt was made to prepare the synthesis of quinazoline derivatives by Niementowski in 1895. This involves the reaction of anthranilic acids with amides to form 4-oxo-3,4-dihydroquinazolines or also known as quinazolinone derivative [2].

Heterocyclic chemistry occupies an important place in organic chemistry research worldwide [1–4] and forms the basis of many pharmaceutical, agrochemical, and veterinary products. In the broad class of heterocyclic compounds, the nitrogen heterocycles play an important role. One of such systems is quinazolinone as a class of N-heterocycles having an important place in medicinal and biological chemistry [5]. One of the main groups of quinazolinones, are 2,3-dihydroquinazolin-4(1H)-ones, with various biological activities, and are also key intermediates for the synthesis of quinazoline-4(3H)-ones as another member of this biologically important family [6–8]. These exhibit broad spectrums of pharmacological and biological activities, such as anti-cancer [9–12], anti-inflammation [13, 14], anti-bacterial [15–18], analgesic [13, 17], anti-virus [19], anti-cytotoxin [20], anti-spasm [17, 21], anti-tuberculosis [22], anti-oxidation [23], antimalarial [24], anti-hypertension [25], anti-obesity [26], anti-psychotic [27], anti-diabetic [28], etc., as well as plant growth regulation [29]. Some representative examples of drug molecules having a quinazolinone skeleton are given in Figure 7.3.

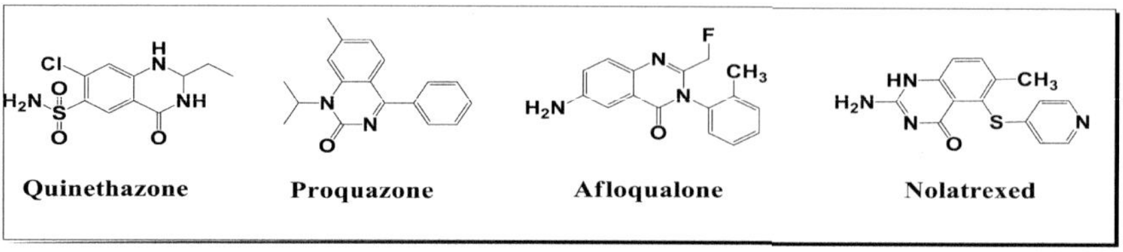

FIGURE 7.3   Representative examples of drug molecules having a quinazolinone skeleton.

Also, the quinazolinone moiety is a building block for approximately 150 naturally occurring alkaloids [30], such as glycosminine [31], luotonin [32], deoxyvasicinone [33], and drugs like methaqualone [34, 35] and piriqualone [36] (Figure 7.4).

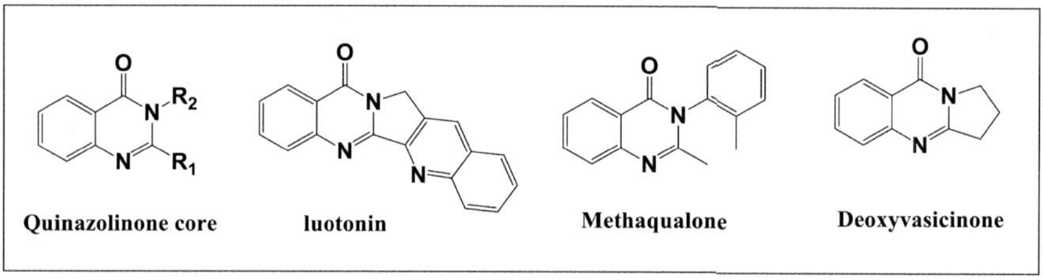

FIGURE 7.4   Quinazolinone core and some well-known quinazolinone derivatives.

In view of these useful properties, various catalyst and reaction conditions used for synthesis of 2,3-diphenyl-2,3-dihydroquinazolin-4(1H)-ones have been reported includes TBAB (Tetra-n-butyl ammonium bromide) [37], Silica supported pressler nanoparticles [38], Potassium carbonate Triphenyl (prpoyl-3-sulfonyl) phosphonium toulenesulfonate [39], Cellulose sulfonic acid [40], Cellulose sulfonic acid [41], Phosphoric acid supported on alumina (H_3PO_4-Al_2O_3) [42], β-cyclodextrin in water [43], Copper benzenesulfonate [44], Aluminium methanesulfonate [45], Cation exchange resin [46], 1-(4-sulfonic acid) butyl pyridinium [HSO_4]-2-amino benzamide [47], L-proline [48], Silica bonded N-propyl sulfamic acid [49], Strontium chloride [50], Silica bonded S-sulfonic acid [51], Zirconium chloride [52], Acetic acid [53], p-TSA/ HCHO [54], Fe_3O_4 [55], Al $(H_2PO_4)_3$ [56], [Bmim]HSO_4 [57], I_2/AcOH [58], Silica sulfuric acid [59], Amberlyst-15 [60], K-10 [61], [Bmim]BF_4 [62], $KAl(SO_4)_2 \cdot 12H_2O$ [63], L-pyrrolidine-2-carboxylic acid-4-hydrogen sulfate [64], Solid phase synthesis [65], Sc (III) inda-pybox [66].

However, many of these methods have their own advantages and disadvantages. Taking into consideration of disadvantages, such as long reaction time, low yields multistep procedure, and use of a large amount of catalyst, therefore, there is a need to develop a method for one-pot synthesis of 2,3-diphenyl-2,3-dihydroquinazolin-4(1H)-ones. As ionic liquids are designer molecules that can efficiently replace the conventional organic solvents used in chemical processes and operations. The thermodynamics and reaction kinetics of processes carried out in ionic liquids are different from those in conventional media. This creates new opportunities for catalytic reactions and separations processes in organic synthesis.

7.2 PRESENT WORK

The present scheme involves the synthesis of 2,3-diphenyl-2,3-dihydroquinazolin-4(1H)-ones by the reaction of isatoic anhydride, amine, and aromatic aldehyde, as shown in Scheme 7.1.

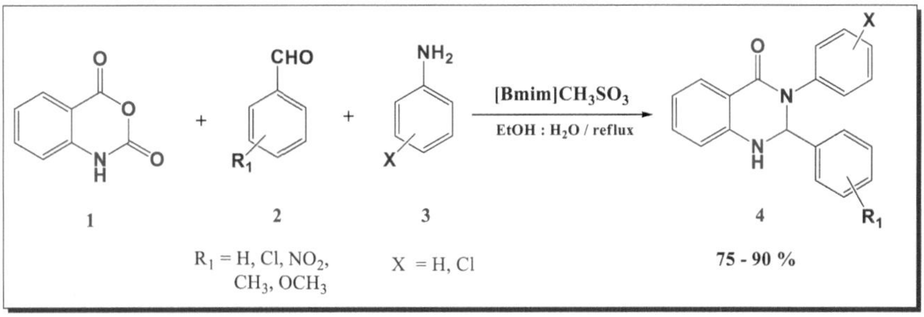

SCHEME 7.1 Synthesis of 2,3-diphenyl-2,3-dihydroquinazolin-4 (1H)-ones.

7.2.1 MECHANISM FOR SYNTHESIS OF 2,3-DIPHENYL-2,3-DIHYDROQUINAZOLIN-4(1H)-ONES

A tentative mechanism for the formation of 2,3-diphenyl-2,3-dihydroquinazolin-4(1H)-ones was proposed, as shown in Scheme 7.2. At the first step, the reaction starts with the condensation of isatoic anhydride **1** activated by acidic H$^+$ of ionic liquid followed by the N-nucleophilic attacks of amine **3** on the carbonyl unit. After the loss of carbon dioxide, N-substituted

2-aminobenzamide **5** is generated. Meanwhile, acidic H^+ of the ionic liquid increases the electrophilic character of the aldehydes **2**. Subsequently, the activate aldehyde reacts with compound **5** to afford the intermediate **6**. The imine fragment in intermediate **6** is activated by acidic proton from ionic liquid. Thus intermediate **6** gets converted into intermediate **7** by intermolecular cyclization. Finally, 2,3-diphenyl-2,3-dihydroquinazolin-4(1H)-ones **4** is formed by a 1,5-proton transfer of compound **7**.

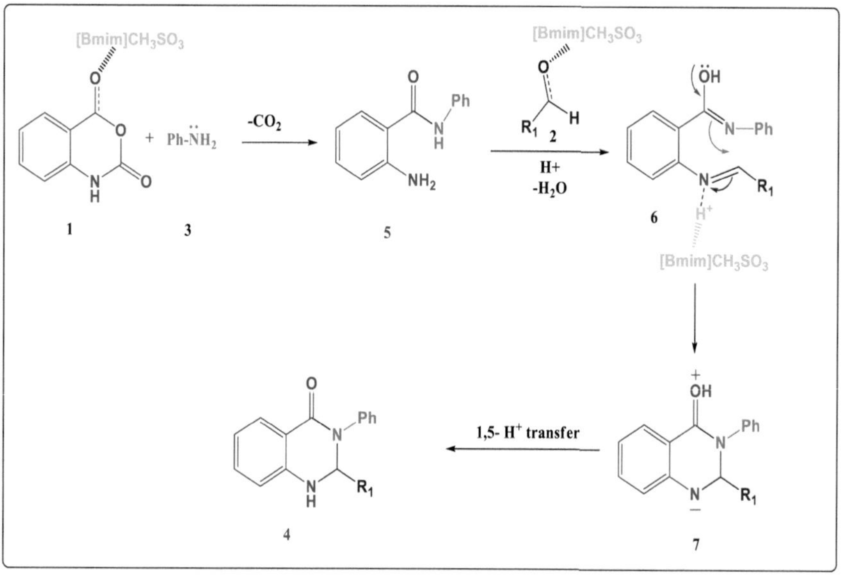

SCHEME 7.2 Mechanism of synthesis of 2,3-diphenyl-2,3-dihydroquinazolin-4(1H)-ones using the ionic liquid.

7.3 EXPERIMENTAL

All the chemicals were purchased from Aldrich, Spectro-chem, Merck chemicals, and were used without further purification, unless otherwise stated. All melting points were measured on Veego digital melting point apparatus and are uncorrected. IR spectra were measured as KBr pellets on a Perkin Elmer spectrum RX FTIR spectrophotometer. The NMR spectra were recorded on a Bruker Avance II 400 MHz instrument. The spectra were measured in either $CDCl_3$ or DMSO-d_6 as a solvent relative to TMS (0.00 ppm). Chemical shifts (δ) are referred to in terms of ppm.

7.3.1 GENERAL PROCEDURE

A mixture of isatoic anhydride (5 mmol), aldehyde (5 mmol), aniline (5 mmol) and 1-butyl, 3-methyl imidazolium methanesulfonate ([Bmim] $CH_3SO_3^-$) ionic liquid (20 mol%) in 7 ml ethanol: water solvent system (1:1) was heated under reflux condition for appropriate time reported in Table 7.1. The progress of the reaction was monitored by TLC (Pet ether: ethyl acetate [7:3]). After completion of the reaction, the mixture was cooled and solid formed was filter and recrystallized with ethanol to afford the desired compound in pure form. The ionic liquid was recovered and reused four times. All the compounds are known compounds and were characterized by spectral data and comparison of their physical data with literature data.

7.4 RESULTS AND DISCUSSION

The one-pot synthesis of 2,3-diphenyl-2,3-dihydroquinazolin-4(1H)-ones was achieved by the three-component condensation reaction of isatoic anhydride, aromatic aldehyde and aniline in the presence of 1-butyl, 3-methyl imidazolium methanesulfonate ([Bmim] $CH_3SO_3^-$) ionic liquid as a catalyst (Scheme 7.1). At first, the synthesis of compound 2,3-diphenyl-2,3-dihydroquinazolin-4(1H)-one was selected as a model reaction to optimize the reaction conditions. The reaction was carried out by heating a mixture of isatoic anhydride, benzaldehyde, and aniline under various conditions.

Initially, a systematic study was carried out for catalytic evaluation of [Bmim]CH_3SO_3 ionic liquid for the synthesis of 2,3-diphenyl-2,3-dihydroquinazolin-4(1H)-one. The three-component reaction between isatoic anhydride, benzaldehyde, and aniline for the synthesis of 2,3-diphenyl-2,3-dihydroquinazolin-4(1H)-one compound was performed in the presence of 5, 10, 15, 20 & 25 mol% of the catalyst using aqueous ethanol at reflux condition. The results were described in Table 7.2.

From the observation, it is clear that the reaction does not take place without a catalyst. The yield of the 2,3-diphenyl-2,3-dihydroquinazolin-4(1H)-one compound was very poor with 5 mol% catalyst, and there was a gradual increase in the yield of the product with an increase in the catalyst loading. The maximum yield was obtained when the catalyst loading was 20 mol%.

TABLE 7.1 Synthesis of 2,3-Diphenyl-2,3-Dihydroquinazolin-4(1H)-Ones Using Ionic Liquid[a]

Sr. No.	Aldehyde	Aniline	Product[b]	Time (h)	Yield[c] (%)	Mp. (°C)	Lit. [Ref.]
1	CHO (phenyl)	NH_2 (phenyl)	(2,3-diphenyl product)	2.30	85	215–216	214–215 [40]
2	CHO (phenyl)	NH_2 (4-Cl-phenyl)	(product)	3.0	82	217–218	219–220 [56]
3	CHO (4-Cl-phenyl)	NH_2 (phenyl)	(product)	3.20	90	214–216	219–220 [40]
4	CHO (4-Cl-phenyl)	NH_2 (4-Cl-phenyl)	(product)	3.30	83	245–247	250–251 [57]
5	CHO (3-NO_2-phenyl)	NH_2 (phenyl)	(product)	3.0	82	182–184	186–188 [46]

TABLE 7.1 (Continued)

Sr. No.	Aldehyde	Aniline	Product[b]	Time (h)	Yield[c] (%)	Mp. (°C)	Lit. [Ref.]
6	CHO, OCH₃, OCH₃	NH₂	(quinazolinone, OCH₃, OCH₃, phenyl)	3.10	75	240–242	244–246 [66]
7	CHO, CH₃	NH₂	(quinazolinone, CH₃, phenyl)	2.45	80	193–195	196–199 [41]
8	CHO, OCH₃	NH₂	(quinazolinone, OCH₃, phenyl)	3.0	82	201–203	203–205 [44]
9	CHO, OCH₃	NH₂, Cl	(quinazolinone, Cl, OCH₃)	3.50	78	231–233	238–239 [57]

TABLE 7.1 (Continued)

Sr. No.	Aldehyde	Aniline	Product[b]	Time (h)	Yield [c] (%)	Mp. (°C)	Lit. [Ref.]
10	CHO, Cl	NH₂	(structure)	3.25	82	213–215	214–217 [24]

[a]Reaction condition: isatoic anhydride (5 mmol), aniline (5 mmol), aromatic aldehydes (5 mmol), and [Bmim]CH₃SO₃ ionic liquid (20 mol%).
[b]All the product were characterized by IR spectral data and comparison of their melting point with those of the authentic samples. Also, the structures of some products were confirmed by ¹H NMR spectral data.
[c]Isolated yield.

TABLE 7.2 The Catalytic Study for the Synthesis of 2,3-Diphenyl-2,3-Dihydroquinazolin-4(1H)-One Compound

Entry	Catalyst (mol%)	Time (h)	Yield (%) [a]
1	0	5	– [b]
2	5	5	Trace
3	10	4	58
4	15	3	71
5	20	2.5	85
6	25	2.5	85

Reaction conditions: Isatoic anhydride (2 mmol), benzaldehyde (2 mmol), aniline (2 mmol), in 7ml of aqueous ethanol (1:1) at 80°C, [a]Isolated yield, [b]No reaction.

After optimizing the catalytic condition for the 2,3-diphenyl-2,3-dihydro-quinazolin-4(1H)-one reaction, we examined [Bmim]CH_3SO_3 ionic liquid catalyzed the synthesis of 2,3-diphenyl-2,3-dihydroquinazolin-4(1H)-one from isatoic anhydride, benzaldehyde, and aniline in various solvents, the results are tabulated in Table 7.3. The best results are observed in aqueous ethanol as compared to the other solvents.

TABLE 7.3 Optimization of Reaction Solvent and Reaction Conditions for the Synthesis of 2,3-Diphenyl-2,3-Dihydroquinazolin-4(1H)-One

Entry	Solvent	Temperature (°C)	Time (h)	Yield (%) [a]
1	Water	RT	8	– [b]
2	Ethanol	RT	8	– [b]
3	Acetonitrile	RT	8	– [b]
4	Methanol	RT	8	– [b]
5	Water	80	5	– [b]
6	Ethanol	78	5	57
7	Methanol	64	5	52
8	Water + Ethanol (1:1)	80	2.30	85
9	Water + Ethanol (2:1)	80	2.30	74
10	Water + Ethanol (1:2)	80	2.30	80
11	Acetonitrile	80	3	45
12	Dichloromethane	40	3	24
13	Chloroform	61	3	38
14	DMF	80	3	59
15	[Bmim]CH_3SO_3	80	3	Trace
16	–	80	8	– [b]

Reaction conditions: Isatoic anhydride (2 mmol), benzaldehyde (2 mmol), aniline (2 mmol), [Bmim]CH_3SO_3 Ionic liquid (20 mol%); [a]Isolated yield; [b]No reaction.

The comparison of the variously reported catalyst with its condition and the time required for the completion of reaction with the obtained yield for the synthesis of 2,3-diphenyl-2,3-dihydroquinazolin-4(1H)-one is shown in Table 7.4.

TABLE 7.4   Comparison Table With Various Reported Catalyst

Sr. No.	Catalyst	Condition	Time (h)	Yield (%)	References
1	β-cyclodextrin	H_2O/ 60–65°C	6.0 h	80%	[43]
2	$Al(MS)_3.4H_2O$	$EtOH:H_2O$	2.0 h	88%	[45]
3	Silica sulfuric acid	Solvent-free, 80°C	5.0 h	80%	[59]
4	K-10	EtOH/ reflux	6.5 h	80%	[61]
5	[Bmim]BF_4 (3 ml)	H_2O	1.0 h	87%	[62]
6	$KAl(SO_4)_2.12H_2O$	EtOH/ reflux	4.0 h	78%	[63]
7	[Bmim]CH_3SO_3	$EtOH:H_2O$	2.5 h	85%	Present work

To evaluate the scope of this reaction, a range of 2,3-diphenyl-2,3-di-hydroquinazolin-4(1H)-one derivatives were prepared by the reaction of isatoic anhydride, aromatic aldehydes, and aniline under optimized reaction conditions. The results are summarized in Table 7.1. Various aromatic aldehydes with electron-withdrawing as well as electron-donating substituents reacted efficiently and quickly with isatoic anhydride and aniline to give corresponding 2,3-diphenyl-2,3-dihydroquinazolin-4(1H)-one derivatives in high yields over short reaction times.

7.4.1   STRUCTURAL DETERMINATION OF ISOLATED COMPOUND

Primary elucidation of the structure for the optimized reaction isolated product starts with FT-IR spectra. A broadband obtained at 3294 cm^{-1} represents the –NH stretch, a medium band obtained at 3058 and 3008 cm^{-1} represents the aromatic CH stretch, a strong band at 1633 cm^{-1} represents the presence of carbonyl group (C=O stretch) a medium band at 1360 cm^{-1} for alkanes (C-H bending) a medium band at 1051 and 1115 cm^{-1} confirms the presence of amine (C-N stretching). The determination of the structure for the product was further confirmed by ^{1}H NMR spectra. A singlet obtained at 6.19 (s, 1H, -CH) and 7.51 (bs, 1H, -NH) confirm the formation of the product. Also, the mass of the product is confirmed by the LC-MS spectra indicating the line at 300.2 giving (M^+) peak authenticates the formation product.

7.4.1.1 IMPORTANT FEATURES OF THIS METHOD

- Use of ionic liquid as a catalyst.
- Only 20 mol% of the catalyst is sufficient for transformation.
- Use of ionic liquid in water: ethanol system as a solvent is an excellent feature of this method.
- Short reaction time.
- Easy workup procedure; the product is simply filtered and purified by recrystallization using ethanol.
- Reuse of ionic liquid.
- High to excellent yield makes this procedure economically useful.
- Both electron-withdrawing, as well as an electron-donating substituent, can easily proceed under this reaction condition.

7.5 CONCLUSION

In conclusion, simple, convenient, and efficient procedures for the syntheses of 2,3-diphenyl-2,3-dihydroquinazolin-4(1H)-one derivative by the condensation of isatoic anhydride, aniline, and aromatic aldehydes in the presence of the catalytic amount of [Bmim]CH_3SO_3 ionic liquid under reflux condition have been developed. The procedure offers several advantages, including cleaner reaction profiles, use of ionic liquid as catalyst, high yields in short reaction time, simple experimental and work-up procedures, as well as recycle and reuse of ionic liquid four times.

7.6 SPECTRAL DATA

Some synthesized 2,3-diphenyl-2,3-dihydroquinazolin-4(1H)-ones derivatives are:

2.3-diphenyl-2,3-dihydroquinazolin-4(1H)-one (Table 7.1, entry 1):

IR (KBr, cm⁻¹): 3294, 3034, 1633, 1509, 1390, 1311, 1158, 1115, 1051,751, 695, 919, 541.

¹H NMR (DMSO-d₆, 400MHz) δ: 6.19 (s, 1H), 6.68–6.76 (m, 2H), 7.15 (t, 1H), 7.17–7.32 (m, 8H), 7.39 (d, 2H), 7.51 (s, 1H), 7.76 (d, 1H), 8.13 (s, 1H) ppm.

¹³C NMR (DMSO-d₆, 400MHz) δ: 74.64, 114.8, 116.89, 119.55, 126.78, 126.84, 126.99, 127.02, 127.04, 128.71, 128.91, 128.96, 129.03, 133.87, 139.89, 140.61, 145.38, 163.15.

m/z: 300.2

2-(3,4-dimethoxyphenyl)-3-phenyl-2,3-dihydroquinazolin-4(1H)-one (Table 7.1, entry 6):

IR (KBr, cm⁻¹): 3291, 3001, 2931, 2832, 1610, 1632, 1509, 1485, 1388, 1265, 1237, 1164, 1028, 852, 747, 694.

¹H NMR (DMSO-d$_6$, 400MHz) δ: 3.70 (s, 3H), 3.73 (s, 3H), 6.12 (s, 1H), 6.69–6.77 (m, 3H), 6.87 (dd, 1H), 6.99 (s, 1H), 7.16–7.32 (m, 6H), 7.38 (bs, 1H), 7.76 (d, 1H) ppm;

¹³C NMR (DMSO-d$_6$, 400MHz) δ: 163.33, 152.51, 145.5, 145.32, 141.39, 133.72, 133.6, 128.87, 126.34, 125.5, 123.9, 119.21, 119.14, 116.51, 114.82, 112.93, 112.18, 69.99, 60.8, 55.7.; **m/z:** 360.4

3-phenyl-2-p-tolyl-2,3-dihydroquinazolin-4(1H)-one (Table 7.1, entry 7):

IR (KBr, cm⁻¹): 3299, 3036, 1634, 1590, 1507, 1489, 1392, 1261, 1159, 1024, 750, 695.

¹H NMR (CDCl$_3$, 400MHz) δ: 2.27 (s, 3H), 4.81 (bs, 1H), 6.04 (s, 1H), 6.60 (d, 1H), 6.86 (t, 1H), 7.06 (d, 2H), 7.11–7.19 (m, 2H), 7.21–7.38 (m, 6H), 8.01 (d, 1H)

m/z: 315.1 (M+1)

7.7 SPECTRA OF REPRESENTATIVE COMPOUNDS

Figures 7.5–7.7 show spectra of representative compounds.

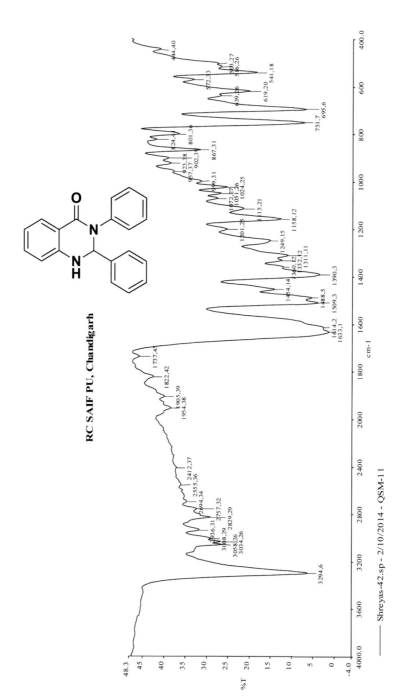

FIGURE 7.5   IR spectra of 2,3-diphenyl-2,3-dihydroquinazolin-4(1H)-one.

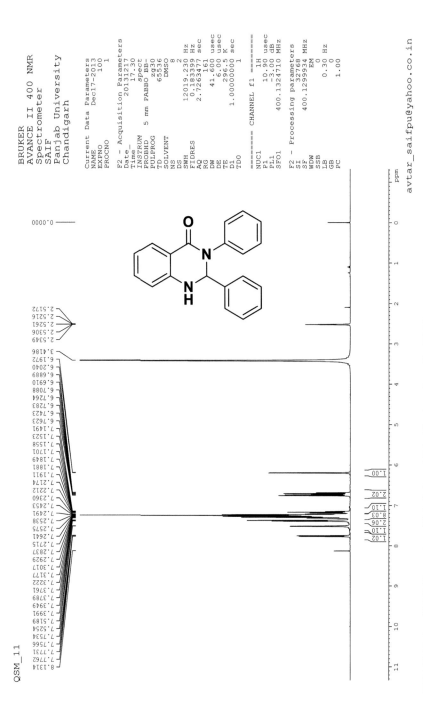

FIGURE 7.6. ^{1}H NMR spectra of 2,3-diphenyl-2,3-dihydroquinazolin-4(1H)-one.

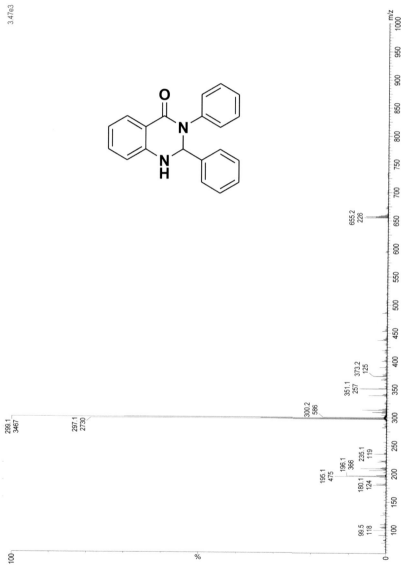

FIGURE 7.7 LC-MS spectra of 2,3-diphenyl-2,3-dihydroquinazolin-4(1H)-one.

KEYWORDS

- **2,3-dihydroquinazolin-4(1H)**
- **green chemistry**
- **heterocyclic chemistry**
- **ionic liquid**
- **isatoic anhydride**
- **reflux condition**

REFERENCES

1. Larksarp, C., & Alper, H., (2000). Palladium-catalyzed cyclocarbonylation of o-iodo-anilines with heterocumulenes: Regioselective preparation of 4(3H)-quinazolinone derivatives. *Org. Chem., 65*, 2773–2777.
2. Krchnak, V., & Holladay, M. W., (2002). Solid phase heterocyclic chemistry. *Chem. Rev., 102*, 61–91.
3. Tour, B. B., & Hall, D. G., (2009). Natural product synthesis using multi-component reaction strategies. *Chem. Rev., 109*, 4439–4486.
4. Roopan, S. M., Khan, F. N., & Mandal, B. K., (2010). Fe nano particles mediated C–N bond-forming reaction: Regioselective synthesis of 3-[(2-chloroquinolin-3-yl) methyl]pyrimidin-4(3H)ones. *Tetrahedron Lett., 51*, 2309–2311.
5. Farghaly, A. M., Soliman, R., Khalil, M. A., Bekhit, A. A., El-Din, A., & Bekhit, A., (2002). Thioglycolic acid and pyrazole derivatives of 4(3H)-quinazolinone: Synthesis and antimicrobial evaluation. *Bull. Chem. Farm., 141*, 372–378.
6. Hour, M., Huang, L., Kuo, S., Xia, Y., Bastow, K., Nakanishi, Y., Hamel, E., & Lee, K., (2000). 6-Alkylamino- and 2,3-dihydro-3-methoxy-2-phenyl-4-quinazolinones and related compounds: Their synthesis, cytotoxicity, and inhibition of tubulin polymerization. *J. Med. Chem., 43*, 4479–4487.
7. Lopez, S. E., Rosales, M. E., Urdaneta, N., Godoy, M. V., & Charris, J. E., (2000). The synthesis of substituted 2-aryl 4(3H)-quinazolinones using NaHSO3/DMAc. Steric effect upon the cyclization-dehydrogenation step. *J. Chem. Res., 6*, 258–259.
8. Connolly, D. J., Cusack, D., O'Sullivan, T. P., & Guiry, P. J., (2006). Synthesis of quinazolinones and quinazolines. *Tetrahedron., 61*, 10153–10202.
9. Chandregowda, V., Kush, A. K., & Chandrasekara, R. G., (2009). Synthesis and *in vitro* antitumor activities of novel 4-anilinoquinazoline derivatives. *Eur. J. Med. Chem., 44*, 3046–3055.
10. Al-Rashood, S. T., Aboldahab, I. A., Nagi, M. N., Abouzeid, L. A., Abdel-Aziz, A. A., Abdel-Hamide, S. G., Youssef, K. M., Al-Obaid, A. M., & El-Subbagh, H. I., (2006). Synthesis, dihydrofolate reductase inhibition, antitumor testing, and molecular

modeling study of some new 4(3H)-quinazolinone analogs. *Bioorg. Med. Chem., 14*, 8608–8621.

11. Vasdev, N., Dorff, P. N., Gibbs, A. R., Nandanan, E., Reid, L. M., Neil, J. P. O., & Van Brocklin, H. F., (2005). Synthesis of 6-acrylamido-4-(2-[^{18}F] fluoroanilino) quinazoline: A prospective irreversible EGFR binding probe. *J. Labeled Compd. Rad., 48*, 109–115.

12. Wakeling, A. E., Guy, S. P., Woodburn, J. R., Ashton, S. E., Curry, B. J., Barker, A. J., & Gibson, K. H., (2002). ZD1839 (Iressa): An orally active inhibitor of epidermal growth factor signaling with potential for cancer therapy. *Cancer Res., 62*, 5749–5754.

13. Alagarsamy, V., Solomon, V. R., & Dhanabal, K., (2007). Synthesis and pharmacological evaluation of some 3-phenyl-2-substituted-3*H*-quinazolin-4-one as analgesic, anti-inflammatory agents. *Bioorg. Med. Chem., 15*, 235–241.

14. Baba, A., Kawamura, N., Makino, H., Ohta, Y., Taketomi, S., & Sohda, T., (1996). Studies on disease-modifying antirheumatic drugs: Synthesis of novel quinoline and quinazoline derivatives and their anti-inflammatory effect. *J. Med. Chem., 39*, 5176–5182.

15. Rohini, R., Muralidhar, R. P., Shanker, K., Hu, A., & Ravinder, V., (2010). Antimicrobial study of newly synthesized 6-substituted indolo[1,2-c]quinazolines. *Eur. J. Med. Chem., 45*, 1200–1205.

16. Antipenko, L., Karpenko, A., Kovalenko, S., Katsev, A., Komarovska-Porokhnyavets, E., Novikov, V., & Chekotilo, A., (2009). Synthesis of new 2-thio-[1,2,4]triazolo[1,5-c] quinazoline derivatives and its antimicrobial activity. *Chem. Pharm. Bull., 57*, 580–585.

17. Jatav, V., Kashaw, S., & Mishra, P., (2008). Synthesis, antibacterial and antifungal activity of some novel 3-[5-(4-substituted phenyl) 1,3,4-thiadiazole-2-yl]-2-styryl quinazoline-4(3H)-ones. *Med. Chem. Res., 17*, 205–211.

18. Aly, A. A., (2003). Synthesis of novel quinazoline derivatives as antimicrobial agents. *Chin. J. Chem., 21*, 339–346.

19. Li, H., Huang, R., Qiu, D., Yang, Z., Liu, X., Ma, J., & Ma, Z., (1998). *Prog. Nat. Sci., 8*, 359–365.

20. Chandrika, P. M., Yakaiah, T., Narsaiah, B., Sridhar, V., Venugopal, G., Rao, J. V., Kumar, K. P., Murthy, U. S. N., & Rao, A. R. R., (2009). Synthesis leading to novel 2,4,6-trisubstituted quinazoline derivatives, their antibacterial and cytotoxic activity against THP-1, HL-60 and A375 cell lines. *Indian J. Chem., 48B*, 840–847.

21. Paneersalvam, P., Raj, T., Ishar, P. S. M, Singh, B., Sharma, V., & Rather, B. A., (2010). Anticonvulsant activity of Schiff bases of 3-amino-6,8-dibromo-2-phenyl-quinazolin-4(3*H*)-ones. *Indian J. Pharm. Sci., 72*, 375–378.

22. Nandy, P., Vishalakshi, M. T., & Bhat, A. R., (2006). Synthesis and antitubercular activity of Mannich bases of 2-methyl-3H-quinazolin-4-ones *Indian J. Heterocycl. Chem., 15*, 293–294.

23. Saravanan, G., Alagarsamy, V., & Prakash, C. R., (2010). Synthesis and evaluation of antioxidant activities of novel quinazolinone derivatives. *Int. J. Pharm. Pharm. Sci., 2*, 83–86.

24. Lakhan, R., Singh, O. P., & Singh, J. R. L., (1987). *J. Indian Chem. Soc., 64*, 316–318.

25. Hess, H. J., Cronin, T. H., & Scriabine, A., (1968). Antihypertensive 2-amino-4(3H)-quinazolinones. *J. Med. Chem., 11*, 130–136.

26. Sasmal, S., Balaji, G., Kanna, R. H. R., Balasubrahmanyam, D., Srinivas, G., Kyasa, S., Sasmal, P. K., et al., (2012). Design and optimization of quinazoline derivatives

as melanin concentrating hormone receptor 1 (MCHR1) antagonists. *Bioorg. Med. Chem. Lett., 22*, 3157–3162.

27. Alvarado, M., Barceló, M., Carro, L., Masaguer, C. F., & Raviña, E., (2006). Synthesis and biological evaluation of new quinazoline and cinnoline derivatives as potential atypical antipsychotics. *Chem Biodivers., 3*, 106–117.

28. Malamas, M. S., & Millen, J., (1991). Quinazolineacetic acids and related analogs as aldose reductase inhibitors. *J. Med. Chem., 34*, 1492–1503.

29. Hamel, E., Lin, C. M., Plowman, J., Wang, H., Lee, K., & Paull, K. D., (1996). Antitumor 2,3-dihydro-2-(aryl)-4(1*H*)-quinazolinone derivatives: Interactions with tubulin. *Biochem. Pharmacol., 51*, 53–59.

30. Mhaske, S. B., & Argade, P., (2006). The chemistry of recently isolated naturally occurring quinazolinone alkaloids. *Tetrahedron, 62*, 9787–9826.

31. Kametani, T., Loc, C. V., Higa, T., Koizumi, M., Ihara, M., & Fukumoto, K. J., (1977). Iminoketene cycloaddition. 2. Total syntheses of arborine, glycosminine, and rutecarpine by condensation of iminoketene with amides. *J. Am. Chem. Soc., 99*, 2306–2309.

32. Mason, J. J., & Bergman, J., (2007). Total synthesis of luotonin A and 14-substituted analogues. *Org. Biomol. Chem., 5*, 2486–2490.

33. Liu, J. F., Ye, P., Sprague, K., Sargent, K., Yohannes, D., Baldino, C. M., Wilson, C. J., & Ng, S. C., (2005). Novel one-pot total syntheses of deoxyvasicinone, mackinazolinone, isaindigotone, and their derivatives promoted by microwave irradiation. *Org. Lett., 7*, 3363–3366.

34. Chenard, B. L., Menniti, F. S., Pagnozzi, M. J., Shenk, K. D., Ewing, F. E., & Welch, W. M., (2000). Methaqualone derivatives are potent noncompetitive AMPA receptor antagonists. *Bioorg. Med. Chem. Lett., 10*, 1203–1205.

35. Bhogal, N., & Balls, M., (2008). Translation of new technologies: From basic research to drug discovery and development. *Curr. Drug Disc. Tech., 5*, 250–262.

36. Wolfe, J. F., Rathman, T. L., Sleevi, M. C., Campbell, J. A., & Greenwood, T. D., (1990). Synthesis and anticonvulsant activity of some new 2-substituted 3-aryl-4(3H)-quinazolinones. *J. Med. Chem., 33*, 161–166.

37. Fard, M. A. B., Mobenikhaledi, A., & Hamidinasab, M., (2014). An efficient one-pot synthesis of 2,3-dihydroquinazolin-4(1H)-ones in green media. *Synthesis and Reactivity in Inorganic, Metal-Organic and Nano Metal Chemistry, 44*, 567–571.

38. Gharib, B. R. H., Khorasani, M., Jahangir, M., & Roshani, R., (2013). Safaee. Synthesis of bis-2,3-dihydroquinazolin-4(1H)-ones and 2,3-dihydroquinazolin-4(1H)-ones derivatives with the aid of silica-supported preyssler nanoparticles. *Org. Chem. International.* http://dx.doi.org/10.1155/2013/848237 (Accessed on 13 November 2019).

39. Sharma, M., Mahar, R., Shukla, S. K., Kant, R., & Chauhan, P. M. S., (2013). Potassium carbonate mediated unusual transformation of 2,3-dihydroquinazolinone via cascade reaction. *Tetrahedron Lett., 54*(46), 6171–6177.

40. Toosi, F. S., & Khakzad, M., (2013). A new and facile synthesis 2,3-dihydroquinazolin-4(1H)-ones. *Res. on Chem. Intermediates.* doi: 10.1007/s11164–013–1193–1.

41. Shaterian, H. R., & Rigi, F., (2013). New applications of cellulose-SO_3H as a bio-supported and biodegradable catalyst for the one-pot synthesis of some three-component reactions. *Research on Chemical Intermediates.* doi: 10.1007/s11164–013–1145–9.

42. Shaterian, H. R., Fahimi, N., & Azizi, K., (2013). New applications of phosphoric acid supported on alumina ($H_3PO_4–Al_2O_3$) as a reusable heterogeneous catalyst for

preparation of 2,3-dihydroquinazoline- 4(1H)-ones, 2H-indazolo[2,1-b]phthalazinetri-ones, and benzo[4,5]imidazo[1,2-a]pyrimidines. *Research on Chemical Intermediates.* doi: 10.1007/s11164–013–1087–2.

43. Ramesh, K., Karnakar, K., Satish, G., Reddy, K. H. V., & Nageswar, Y. V. D., (2012). Tandem supramolecular synthesis of substituted 2-aryl-2,3-dihydroquinazolin-4(1H)-ones in the presence of β-cyclodextrin in water. *Tetrahedron Lett., 53*, 6095–6099.

44. Wang, M., Zhang, T. T., Liang, Y., & Gao, J. J., (2012). Efficient synthesis of mono- and disubstituted 2,3-dihydroquinazolin-4(1H)-ones using copper benzenesulfonate as a reusable catalyst in aqueous solution. *Monatsh. Chem., 143*, 835–839.

45. Song, Z., Liu, L., Wang, Y., & Sun, X., (2012). Efficient synthesis of mono- and disubstituted 2,3-dihydroquinazolin-4(1H)-ones using aluminum methanesulfonate as a reusable catalyst. *Res. on Chem. Intermediates., 38*, 1091–1099.

46. Wang, M., Zhang, T. T., Gao, J. J., & Liang, Y., (2012). Cation-exchange resin as an efficient heterogeneous catalyst for one-pot three-component synthesis of 2,3-dihydro-4(1h)-quinazolinones. *Chemistry of Heterocyclic Compounds, 48*, 897–902.

47. Yassaghi, G., Davoodnia, A., Allameh, S., Zare-Bidaki, A., & Tavakoli-Hoseini, N., (2012). Preparation, characterization and first application of aerosil silica supported acidic ionic liquid as a reusable heterogeneous catalyst for the synthesis of 2,3-dihy-droquinazolin-4(1H)-ones. *Bulletin of the Korean Chemical Society, 33*, 2724–2730.

48. Kumari, K., Raghuvanshi, D. S., & Singh, K. N., (2012). Microwave assisted eco-friendly protocol for one pot synthesis of 2,3-dihydroquinazolin-4(1H)-ones in water. *Ind. J. of Chemistry Sect.: B organic Chemistry Including Medicinal Chemistry, 51B*(6), 860–865.

49. Niknam, K., Jafarpour, N., & Niknam, E., (2011). Silica-bonded N-propylsulfamic acid as a recyclable catalyst for the synthesis of 2,3-dihydroquinazolin-4(1H)-ones. *Chinese Chemical Letters, 22*(1), 69–72.

50. Wang, M., Zhang, T. T., Liang, Y., & Gao, J. J., (2011). Strontium chloride-catalyzed one-pot synthesis of 2, 3-dihydroquinazolin-4(1H)-ones in protic media. *Chinese Chemical Letters, 22*(12), 1423–1426.

51. Niknam, K., Mohammadizadeh, M. R., & Mirzaee, S., (2011). *Chinese Chemical Letters, 29*(7), 1417–1422.

52. Mohammad, A. A., & Elahe, S., (2011). Synthesis of 2,3-dihydroquinazolin-4(1H)-ones catalyzed by zirconium (IV) chloride as a mild and efficient catalyst. *Chinese Chemical Letters, 22*, 10, 1163–1166.

53. Zahed, K. J., & Reza, A., (2011). Acetic acid-promoted, efficient, one-pot synthesis of 2,3-dihydroquinazolin-4(1 H)-ones, *Monatsh. Chem., 142*, 631–635.

54. Saffar, T. A., & Bolouk, S., (2010). One-pot, three-component synthesis of 2,3-dihy-droquinazolin-4(1H)-ones using p-toluenesulfonic acid-paraformaldehyde copolymer as an efficient and reusable catalyst. *Manatshefte fur Chemie., 141*, 1113–1115.

55. Zhang, Z. H., Lu, H. Y., Yang, S. H., & Gao, J. W. J., (2010). Synthesis of 2,3-dihy-droquinazolin-4(1H)-ones by three-component coupling of isatoic anhydride, amines, and aldehydes catalyzed by magnetic Fe(3)O(4) nanoparticles in water. *Combinatorial Chemistry, 12*, 643–646.

56. Shaterian, H. R., Oveisi, A. R., & Honarmand, M., (2010). Synthesis of 2,3-dihydro-quinazoline-4(1H)-ones. *Synthetic Comm., 40*, 1231–1242.

57. Darvatkar, N. B., Bhilare, S. V., Deorukhkar, A. R., Raut, D. G., & Salunkhe, M. M., (2010). [bmim]HSO$_4$: An efficient and reusable catalyst for one-pot three-component synthesis of 2,3-dihydro-4(1*H*)-quinazolinones. *Green Chemistry Letters and Reviews, 3*, 301–306.

58. Dabiri, M., Salehi, P., Bahramnejad, M., & Alizadeh, M., (2010). A practical and versatile approach toward a one-pot synthesis of 2,3-disubstituted 4(3*H*)-quinazolinones. *Monatsh Chem., 141*, 877–881.

59. Dabiri, M., Salehi, P., Baghbanzadeh, M., Zolfigol, M., Agheb, M., & Heydari, S., (2008). Silica sulfuric acid: An efficient reusable heterogeneous catalyst for the synthesis of 2,3-dihydroquinazolin-4(1*H*)-ones in water and under solvent-free conditions. *Catalysis Comm., 9*, 785–788.

60. Surpur, M. P., Singh, P. R., Patil, S. B., & Samant, S. D., (2007). Expeditious one-pot and solvent-free synthesis of dihydroquinazolin-4(1H)-ones in the presence of microwaves. *Synthetic Comm., 37*, 1965–1970.

61. Salehi, P., Dabirri, M., Baghbanzadeh, M., & Bahramnejad, M., (2006). One-pot, three-component synthesis of 2,3-dihydro-4(1*H*)-quinazolinones by montmorillonite K-10 as an efficient and reusable catalyst. *Synthetic Comm., 36*, 2287–2292.

62. Dabiri, M., Salehi, P., & Baghbanzadeh, M., (2007). Ionic liquid promoted eco-friendly and efficient synthesis of 2,3-dihydroquinazolin-4(1*H*)-ones. *Monatshefte fur Chemie., 138*, 1191–1194.

63. Dabiri, M., Salehi, P., Otokesh, S., Baghbanzadeh, M., Kozehgary, G., & Mohammadi, A. A., (2005). Efficient synthesis of mono- and disubstituted 2,3-dihydroquinazolin-4(1*H*)-ones using KAl(SO$_4$)$_2$·12H$_2$O as a reusable catalyst in water and ethanol. *Tetrahedron Lett., 46*, 6123–6126.

64. Ghorbani, C. A., & Zamani, P., (2012). Synthesis of 2,3-dihydroquinazolin-4(1H)-ones via one-pot three-component reaction catalyzed by l-pyrrolidine-2-carboxylic acid-4-hydrogen sulfate (supported on silica gel) as novel and recoverable catalyst. *Journal of Iranian Chemical Society, 9*, 607–613.

65. Liu, Z., Ou, L., Giulianotti, M. A., & Houghten, R. A., (2011). Solid-phase synthesis of N-substituted 3,4-dihydroquinazolinone derivatives. *Tetrahedron Lett., 52*, 2627–2628.

66. Muthuraj, P., Samydurai, J., & Venkitasamy, K., (2013). Investigation of the enantioselective synthesis of 2,3-dihydroquinazolinones using Sc(III)-*inda*-pybox. *Synthesis, 45*(16), 2265–2272.

CHAPTER 8

SYNTHESIS, CHARACTERIZATION, AND BIOLOGICAL EVALUATION OF SUBSTITUTED 2-PHENOXYNICOTINALDEHYDES AS α-AMYLASE INHIBITOR

KISHAN PRABHU HAVAL

Department of Chemistry, Dr. Babasaheb Ambedkar Marathwada University, Sub-Campus, Osmanabad, Maharashtra, India

*Corresponding author. E-mail: havallpp11@gmail.com, rss.333@rediffmail.com

ABSTRACT

Diabetes mellitus is a chronic endocrine disorder that affects the metabolism of carbohydrates, proteins, fat, electrolytes, and water. α-Amylase and α-glucosidase are the important enzymes required for the digestion of the carbohydrate. These enzymes play a vital role in the breakdown of starch in the diet, and its activity has been correlated to postprandial blood glucose levels, the control of which is essential for maintaining quality of life for diabetic patients. Herewith, we are reporting the synthesis, characterization, and biological evaluation of substituted 2-phenoxynicotinaldehydes as α-amylase inhibitors.

8.1 INTRODUCTION

Diabetes mellitus (DM) is an extended metabolic disease of several etiologies characterized by chronic hyperglycemia with the disorder of carbohydrate, fat, and also protein metabolism. It includes a group of metabolic diseases characterized by hyperglycemia, in which blood sugar levels are elevated either from defects in insulin secretion, insulin action, or both of them [1]. Therefore, it is necessary to decrease post-prandial hyperglycemia to treat diabetes [2]. This can be achieved by the inhibition of carbohydrate hydrolyzing enzymes like α-amylase and α-glucosidase [3]. α-Amylase is responsible for the breakdown of long-chain carbohydrates, and α-glucosidase breaks down starch and disaccharides to glucose. They serve as the major digestive enzymes and support in intestinal absorption. Both these enzymes are the potential targets in the development of lead compounds for the treatment of diabetes [4]. Many natural products from plants have been used for the treatment of diabetes [5]. Various drugs are available for the cure of Type 2 diabetes-like acarbose, biguanides, sulphonylureas, thiazolidinediones, etc. [6]. But they have also exhibited a number of undesired side effects like gastrointestinal side effects and thus signifying other effective substitutes [7].

The pyridine substructure is one of the most predominant heterocycles found in natural products, pharmaceuticals, and functional materials [8]. In the recent past, novel derivatives of pyridine have been developed and found to have a large number of biological activities [9]. The pyridine structure is found in natural compounds like nicotinic acid (vitamin B_3) and pyridoxine (vitamin B_6). Over 100 medications on the market today include pyridine rings, such as Lunesta (commonly used to treat insomnia), Singulair (commonly used to treat asthma), Nexium (commonly used to treat acid reflux), and Actos (commonly used to treat Type II diabetes) (Figure 8.1) [10]. The pyridine moiety is also found in structurally simple drugs like isoniazid [11] and ethionamide [12] (both prodrugs for inhibitors of inter alia enoyl-acyl carrier protein reductase; tuberculosis), amrinone (phosphodiesterase 3 inhibitor; heart failure) and bupicomide (dopamine β-hydroxylase inhibitor; hypertension). The high reactivity of pyridine allows for many possible chemical reactions [13].

8.2 PRESENT WORK

In continuation of our efforts on the synthesis of bioactive heterocyclic compounds [14], the present study was carried out to investigate the inhibitory potentials of substituted 2-phenoxynicotinaldehydes (Scheme 8.1).

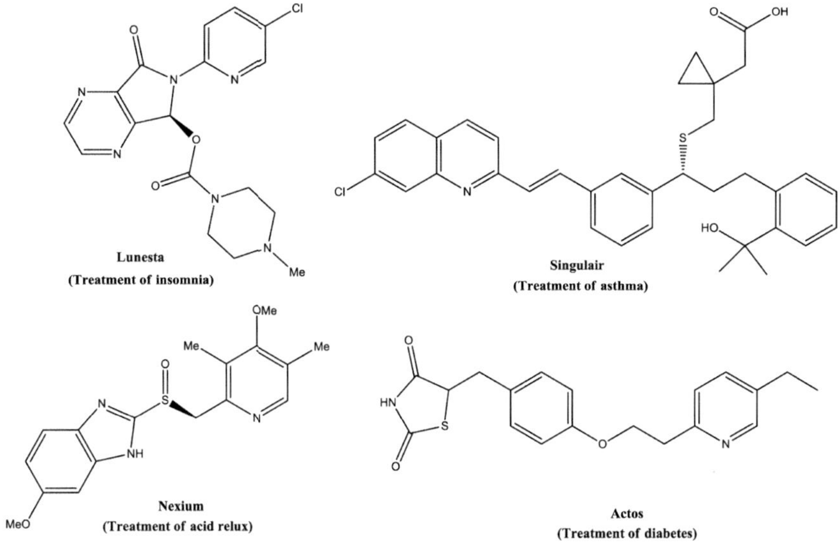

FIGURE 8.1   Commercially available pyridine ring containing drugs.

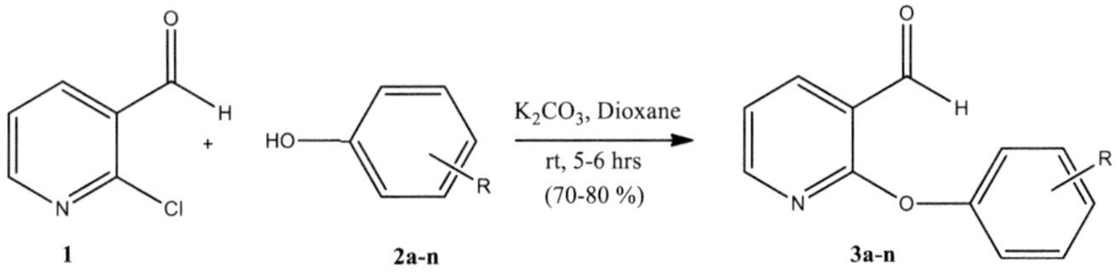

3a : R = 4-Cl; 3b : R ≈ 2, 4-Cl, Cl; 3c : R = 2, 5-Cl, Cl; 3d : R = 4-CH₃; 3e : R = 2-Br;
3f : R = 2-CH₃; 3g : R = 3, 4-Cl, Cl; 3h : R = 3-CH₃; 3i : R = 2-CF₃; 3j : R = 3, 5-Cl, Cl;
3k : R = 2-CF3; 3l : R = H; 3m : R = 2-Cl; 3n : R = 3-Cl

SCHEME 8.1   Synthesis of substituted 2-phenoxynicotinaldehydes.

8.3   EXPERIMENTAL

8.3.1   GENERAL PROCEDURE FOR THE SYNTHESIS SUBSTITUTED 2-PHENOXYNICOTINALDEHYDES

2-Chloronicotinaldehyde (10 mmol), substituted phenols (10 mmol) and potassium carbonate (15 mmol) in dioxane was stirred at room tempera-ture. The progress of reaction was monitored by TLC. After completion of reaction, the solvent was evaporated on rotary evaporator. The reaction mixture was extracted by ethyl acetate. The crude product obtained was purified by recrystallization in ethanol to furnish the corresponding substituted 2-phenoxynicotinaldehydes with 70–80% yields.

- **2-(4-chlorophenoxy)nicotinaldehyde (3a):** Yield: 74%; M.P.: 80–82°C; **^{1}H NMR** (CDCl$_3$, 400 MHz): δ ppm = 7.15–7.19 (m, 3H), 7.41–7.45 (m, 2H), 8.27 (dd, J = 8 & 2Hz, 1H), 8.36 (dd, J = 7 & 2Hz, 1H), 10.56 (s, 1H); **^{13}C NMR** (CDCl$_3$, 100 MHz): δ ppm = 119.32, 119.52, 123.12, 129.80, 130.83, 138.34, 151.46, 152.99, 163.72, 188.52.

- **2-(2,4-dichlorophenoxy)nicotinaldehyde (3b):** Yield: 70%; M.P.: 122–124°C; **^{1}H NMR** (CDCl$_3$, 400 MHz): δ ppm = 7.17–7.20 (m, 1H), 7.26–7.28 (m, 1H), 7.34–7.37 (m, 1H), 7.51–7.52 (m, 1H), 8.28 (dd, J = 8 &2Hz, 1H), 8.31 (dd, J = 7 & 2Hz, 1H), 10.60 (s, 1H); **^{13}C NMR** (CDCl$_3$, 100 MHz): δ ppm = 119.10, 119.58, 125.15, 128.18, 128.32, 130.41, 131.65, 138.41, 147.71, 152.85, 163.05, 188.33.

- **2-(2,5-dichlorophenoxy)nicotinaldehyde (3c):** Yield: 70%; M.P.: 88–90°C; **^{1}H NMR** (DMSO-d$_6$, 400 MHz): δ ppm = 7.38 (dd, J = 8 & 5Hz, 1H), 7.44 (dd, J = 8 & 2Hz, 1H), 7.66–7.68 (m, 2H), 8.30 (dd, J = 8 & 2Hz, 1H), 8.40 (dd, J = 5 & 2Hz, 1H), 10.44 (s, 1H).

- **2-(p-tolyloxy)nicotinaldehyde (3d):** Yield: 80%; M.P.: 78–80°C; **^{1}H NMR** (CDCl$_3$, 400 MHz): δ ppm = 2.41 (s, 3H), 7.10–7.14 (m, 3H), 7.26–7.28 (m, 2H), 8.26 (dd, J = 8 & 2Hz, 1H), 8.37 (dd, J = 5 & 2Hz, 1H), 10.59 (s, 1H); **^{13}C NMR** (CDCl$_3$, 100 MHz): δ ppm =20.94, 118.79, 119.45, 121.45, 130.31, 135.13, 138.04, 150.73, 153.19, 164.36, 188.94.

- **2-(2-bromophenoxy)nicotinaldehyde (3e):** Yield: 76%; M.P.: 83–85°C; **^{1}H NMR** (CDCl$_3$, 400 MHz): δ ppm = 7.15–7.22 (m, 2H), 7.23–7.34 (m, 1H), 7.42–7.46 (m, 1H), 7.68–7.70 (m, 1H), 8.28–8.34 (m, 2H), 10.65 (s, 1H); **^{13}C NMR** (CDCl$_3$, 100 MHz): δ ppm =116.68, 119.23, 119.29, 124.38, 127.14, 128.67, 133.72, 138.21, 150.18, 152.95, 163.36, 188.68.

- **2-(o-tolyloxy)nicotinaldehyde (3f):** Yield: 78%; M.P.: Thick oil; **^{1}H NMR** (CDCl$_3$, 400 MHz): δ ppm = 2.23 (s, 3H), 7.10–7.20 (m, 2H), 7.22–7.34 (m, 3H), 8.27 (dd, J = 8 & 2Hz, 1H), 8.34 (dd, J = 5 & 2Hz, 1H), 10.64 (s, 1H); **^{13}C NMR** (CDCl$_3$, 100 MHz): δ ppm = 16.51,

118.74, 119.13, 122.13, 125.86, 127.20, 130.75, 131.46, 138.17, 151.44, 153.30, 163.98, 188.77.

- **2-(3,4-dichlorophenoxy)nicotinaldehyde (3g):** Yield: 72%; M.P.: 82–84°C; ^{1}**H NMR** (CDCl$_3$, 400 MHz): δ ppm = 7.09–7.20 (m, 1H), 7.20–7.22 (m, 1H), 7.37 (d, J = 2Hz, 1H),7.52 (d, J = 8Hz, 1H), 1H), 8.28 (dd, J = 8 & 2Hz, 1H), 8.36 (dd, J = 5 & 2Hz, 1H), 10.53 (s, 1H); ^{13}**C NMR** (CDCl$_3$, 100 MHz): δ ppm = 119.51, 119.72, 121.45, 124.04, 129.32, 130.97, 133.23, 138.52, 151.68, 152.92, 163.23, 188.18.

- **2-(m-tolyloxy)nicotinaldehyde (3h):** Yield: 75%; M.P.: 54–56°C; ^{1}**H NMR** (CDCl$_3$, 400 MHz): δ ppm = 2.42 (s, 3H), 7.01–7.10 (m, 2H), 7.12–7.16 (m, 2H), 7.34–7.38 (m, 1H), 8.26 (dd, J = 8 & 2Hz, 1H), 8.37 (dd, J = 5 & 2Hz, 1H), 10.58 (s, 1H); ^{13}**C NMR** (CDCl$_3$, 100 MHz): δ ppm = 21.43, 118.59, 118.91, 119.57, 122.19, 126.33, 129.46, 138.06, 140.00, 153.07, 153.23, 164.23, 188.90.

- **2-(3-(trifluoromethyl)phenoxy)nicotinaldehyde (3i):** Yield: 70%; M.P.: 50–52°C; ^{1}**H NMR** (CDCl$_3$, 400 MHz): δ ppm = 7.19–7.22 (m, 1H), 7.29–7.62 (m, 4H), 8.29 (dd, J = 8 & 2Hz, 1H), 8.37 (dd, J = 5 & 2Hz, 1H), 10.57 (s, 1H); ^{13}**C NMR** (CDCl$_3$, 100 MHz): δ ppm =118.92, 119.00, 119.60, 119.63, 122.17, 122.24, 125.26, 130.24, 138.47, 152.94, 153.13, 163.36, 188.31.

- **2-(3,5-dichlorophenoxy)nicotinaldehyde (3j):** Yield: 70%; M.P.: 110–112°C; ^{1}**H NMR** (CDCl$_3$, 400 MHz): δ ppm = 7.17–7.22 (m, 2H), 7.23–7.24 (m, 1H), 7.29–7.30 (m, 1H), 8.28 (dd, J = 8 & 2Hz, 1H), 8.39 (dd, J = 5 & 2Hz, 1H), 10.51 (s, 1H); ^{13}**C NMR** (CDCl$_3$, 100 MHz): δ ppm = 119.62, 119.95, 120.83, 125.84, 135.50, 138.57, 152.96, 153.80, 162.98, 188.04.

- **2-(2-(trifluoromethyl)phenoxy)nicotinaldehyde (3k):** Yield: 77%; M.P.: 50–52°C; ^{1}**H NMR** (CDCl$_3$, 400 MHz): δ ppm = 7.17–7.21 (m, 1H), 7.39–7.43 (m, 2H), 7.65–7.67 (m, 1H), 7.69–7.78 (m, 1H), 8.29 (dd, J = 8 & 2Hz, 1H), 8.34 (dd, J = 5 & 2Hz, 1H), 10.58 (s, 1H); ^{13}**C NMR** (CDCl$_3$, 100 MHz): δ ppm = 119.57, 121.76, 124.47, 125.52, 127.18, 127.23, 127.28, 133.03, 138.24, 150.32, 152.77, 163.43, 188.47.

- **2-phenoxynicotinaldehyde (3l):** Yield: 75%; M.P.: 58–60°C; ^{1}**H NMR** (CDCl$_3$, 400 MHz): δ ppm = 7.11–7.14 (m, 1H), 7.18–7.19 (m, 1H), 7.20–7.21 (m, 1H), 7.26–7.30 (m, 1H), 7.44–7.48 (m, 2H), 8.25 (dd, J = 8 & 2Hz, 1H), 8.35 (dd, J = 5 & 2 Hz, 1H), 10.57 (s, 1H).

- **2-(2-chlorophenoxy)nicotinaldehyde (3m):** Yield: 70%; M.P.: 63–65°C; **^{1}H NMR** (CDCl$_3$, 400 MHz): δ ppm = 7.13–7.16 (m, 1H), 7.23–7.27 (m, 1H), 7.27–7.32 (m, 1H), 7.35–7.38 (m,1H), 7.50–7.52 (m, 1H), 8.27 (dd, $J = 8$ & 2Hz, 1H), 8.31 (dd, $J = 5$ & 2Hz, 1H), 10.62 (s, 1H).
- **2-(3-chlorophenoxy)nicotinaldehyde (3n):** Yield: 70%; M.P.: 56–58°C; **^{1}H NMR** (CDCl$_3$, 400 MHz): δ ppm = 7.01–7.13 (m, 1H), 7.15–7.19 (m, 1H), 7.23–7.25 (m, 1H), 7.26–7.27 (m, 1H), 7.35–7.40 (m, 1H), 8.26 (dd, $J = 8$ & 2Hz, 1H), 8.36 (dd, $J = 5$ & 2Hz, 1H), 10.53 (s, 1H).

8.4 RESULTS AND DISCUSSION

We have synthesized a series of substituted 2-phenoxynicotinaldehyeds by developing new reaction conditions. In the literature, various methods are reported for the aromatic nucleophilic substitution of 2-chloronicotinaldehydes by substituted phenols [15]. All these reported methods have some limitations. It requires a high temperature and longer reaction time. Hence there was a need to develop better reaction conditions for the synthesis of substituted 2-phenoxynicotinaldehydes from 2-chloronicotinaldehydes. In accordance with our aim, we performed the reaction of 2-chloronicotinaldehyde (**1**, 10 mmol) with phenol (**2l**, 10 mmol) in the presence of anhydrous K$_2$CO$_3$ (15 mmol) in dioxane at room temperature and exclusively obtained the corresponding 2-phenoxynicotinaldehyde (**3l**) with 75% yield. In the same conversion, the use of 10 mmol (1 Equiv.) of K$_2$CO$_3$ also furnished the 2-phenoxynicotinaldehyde (**3l**) but less than 60% yield, revealing that 15 mmol (1.5 Equiv.) of K$_2$CO$_3$ is necessary for the quantitative conversion of 2-cholronicotinaldehydes to corresponding substituted 2-phenoxynicotinaldehydes. To establish the generality of this new set of reaction conditions, we performed the aromatic nucleophilic substitution reactions of 2-chloronicotinaldehyde with different substituted phenols in the presence of K$_2$CO$_3$ in dioxane furnished the corresponding substituted 2-phenoxynicontinaldehydes with 70–80% yields (Scheme 8.1). The structures of all the synthesized substituted 2-phenoxynicontinaldehydes were confirmed by ^{1}H and ^{13}C NMR spectral data.

8.5 BIOLOGICAL EVALUATION

The enzyme inhibition activity was studied by the agar diffusion method with some modifications [16]. For evaluating the enzyme inhibitory activity, a commercially available α-amylase sample (from Hi media laboratory) was used. The synthesized compounds were dissolved in DMSO at 25 mg per ml concentration. A paper disc of 6 mm diameter from Hi media was impregnated with 10 microliters of 1% α-amylase solution. Subsequently, 10 microliters of the test compound solution were also impregnated to the enzyme discs. Control discs were prepared by adding 10 microliters of DMSO only. Control and test discs were placed on 1% starch-containing Agar gel plates (pH 6.5). These plates were incubated at 37°C for 24 hours. After 24 hours, the plates were developed by Gram's iodine solution to observe the zone of clearance. Each zone was measured in millimeters (Table 8.1).

TABLE 8.1 Disc and Medium Preparation

Sr. No.	Parameter	Magnitude
1	Concentration of enzyme	10 mg/1000 mm^3 (@1%)
2	Concentration of test compound	25 mg/1000 mm^3
3	Concentration of starch (substrate)	10 mg/1000 mm^3 (@1%)
4	Volume of substrate in each plate	8 ml (8000 mm^3)
5	Amount of substrate in each plate	80 mg
6	Diameter of zone (mm) for blank without enzyme with DMSO	Nil

(1000 mm^3 = 1 ml).

The zone of control was used to calculate the amount of starch hydrolyzed. The amount of starch hydrolyzed was calculated, as shown in Table 8.2. The zone of clearance indicated the amount of starch hydrolyzed in milligrams. The amount of starch hydrolyzed by control was considered as 100% activity, and accordingly, a % change in activity was measured.

From Table 8.3, it is observed that all the tested compounds showed anti−α-amylase activity in the range from 25% to 59%. Among these compounds, **2i** showed the least inhibition at 25.33%, while compounds **2a**, **2e**, and **2g** showed higher inhibition of more than 59%.

TABLE 8.2 Calculation for Substrate Consumed by Control

1	Value of pi	3.14
2	Thickness of medium (mm)	1.01
3	Diameter of zone (mm) for control (with only amylase and DMSO)	22
4	Radius of zone (mm)	11
5	Volume of reaction zone (mm^3) [πr^2*h (thickness of medium)]	383.7394
6	Amount of substrate consumed in control (mg)	3.837394

TABLE 8.3 Calculation of Percent Reduction in α-Amylase Activity

Entry	Diameter of Zone (mm)	Subst. Consumed (mg)	% Activity	% Reduction Activity
Control	22	3.83	100	0.00
2a	14	1.54	40.2	59.8
2b	15.5	1.89	49.34	50.66
2c	15.5	1.89	49.34	50.66
2d	16	2.01	52.48	47.52
2e	14	1.54	40.2	59.8
2f	16.5	2.14	55.87	44.13
2g	14	1.55	40.47	59.53
2h	15.5	1.9	49.6	50.4
2i	19	2.86	74.67	25.33
2j	15.5	1.89	49.34	50.66
2k	16.5	2.14	55.87	44.13
2l	17	2.27	59.26	40.74
2m	18.2	2.6	67.88	32.12
2n	17.6	2.43	63.44	36.56

8.6 CONCLUSION

We have reported a new method for aromatic nucleophilic substitution of 2-cholronicotinaldehyde by substituted phenols to furnish the corresponding substituted 2-phenoxynicoyinaldehydes. All the synthesized compounds showed anti-α-amylase activity. Among these compounds **2a**, **2e**, and **2g** showed higher inhibition of more than 59%. These three compounds can be subjected to *in-vivo* studies.

8.7 SPECTRA OF REPRESENTATIVE COMPOUNDS

Figures 8.2–8.25 show spectra of representative compounds.

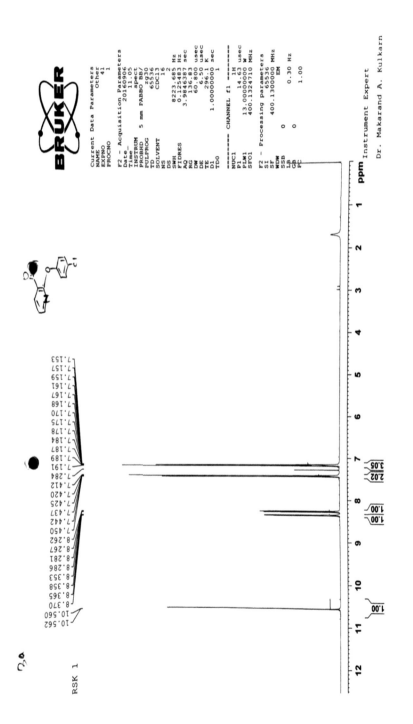

FIGURE 8.2 ¹H NMR spectrum of **3a**.

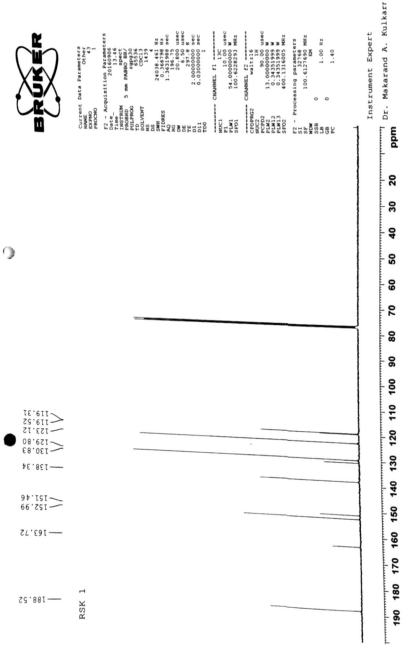

FIGURE 8.3   ¹³C NMR spectrum of **3a.**

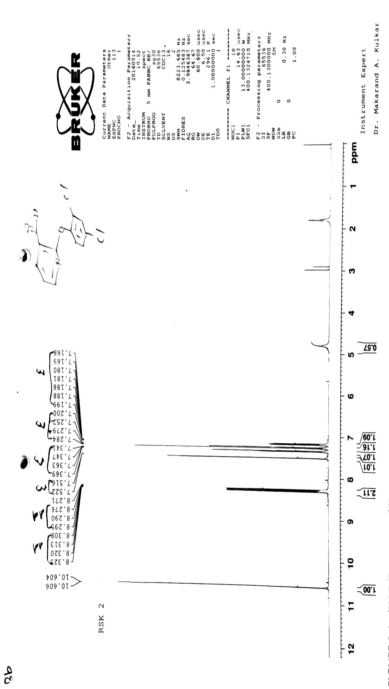

FIGURE 8.4 ¹H NMR spectrum of **3b.**

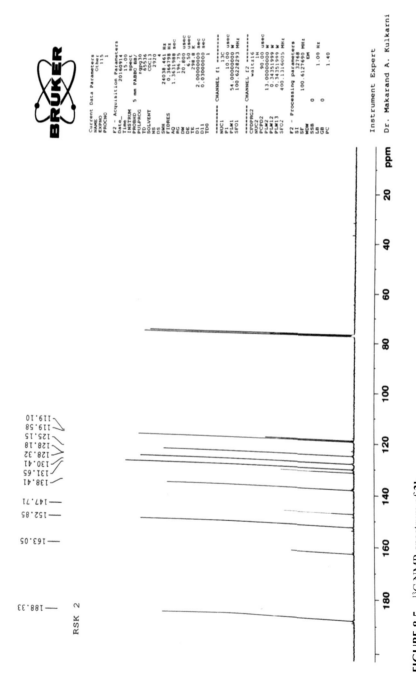

FIGURE 8.5 ^{13}C NMR spectrum of **3b.**

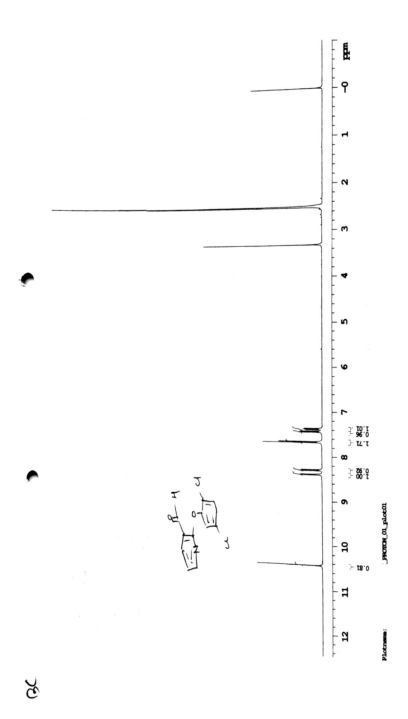

FIGURE 8.6   ¹H NMR spectrum of **3c.**

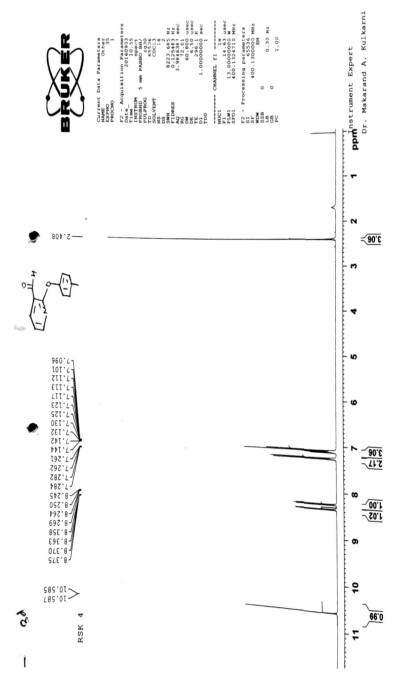

FIGURE 8.7   ¹H NMR spectrum of **3d.**

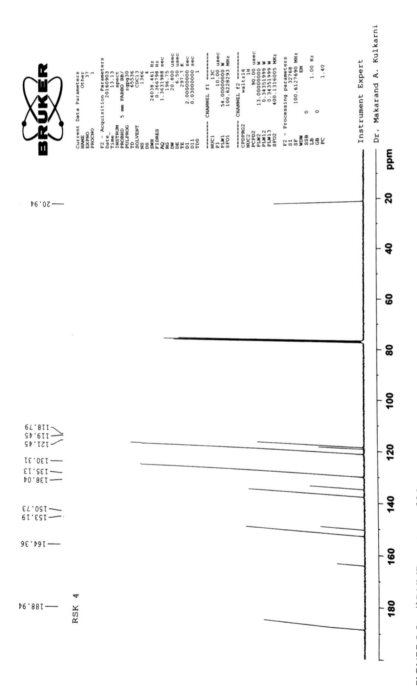

FIGURE 8.8. ^{13}C NMR spectrum of **3d.**

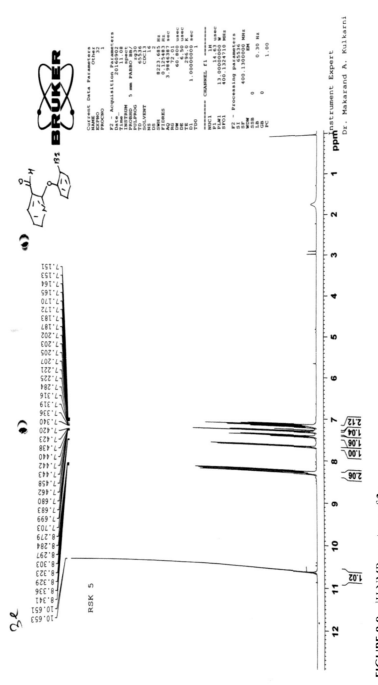

FIGURE 8.9   ¹H NMR spectrum of **3e**.

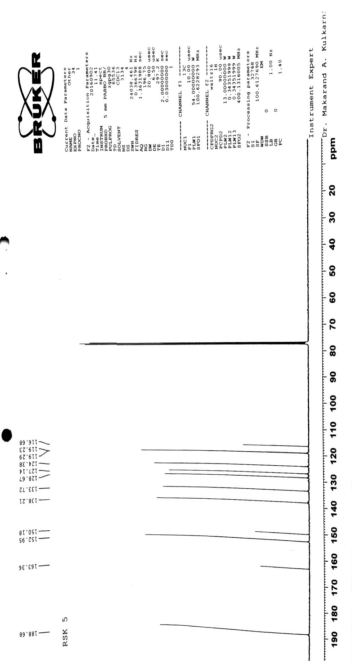

FIGURE 8.10 ^{13}C NMR spectrum of **3e**.

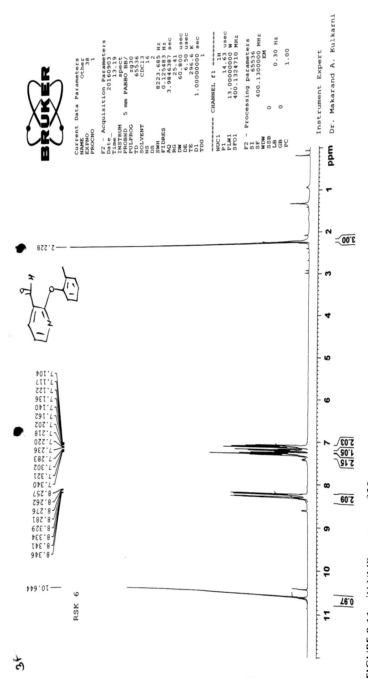

FIGURE 8.11　^{1}H NMR spectrum of **3f.**

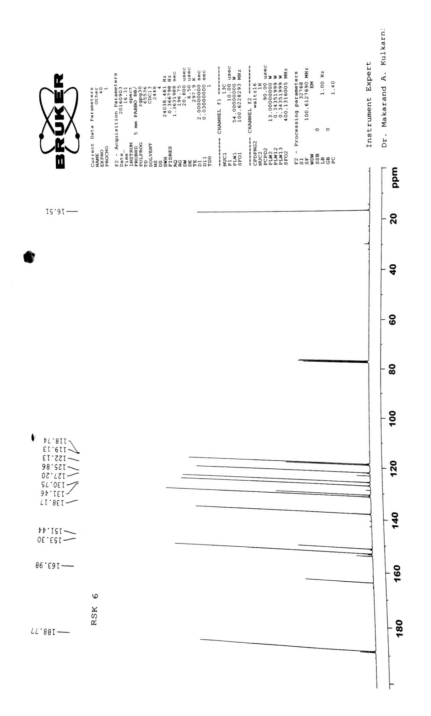

FIGURE 8.12 ^{13}C NMR spectrum of **3f.**

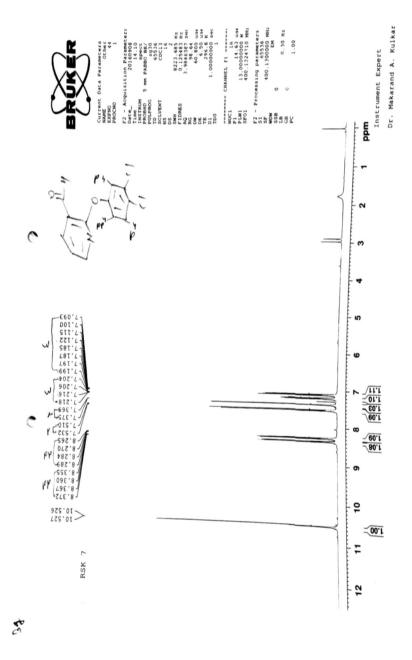

FIGURE 8.13 ¹H NMR spectrum of **3g**.

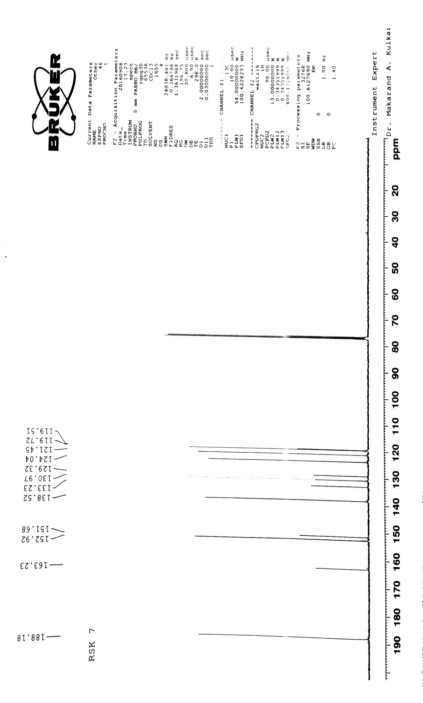

FIGURE 8.14 ^{13}C NMR spectrum of **3g**.

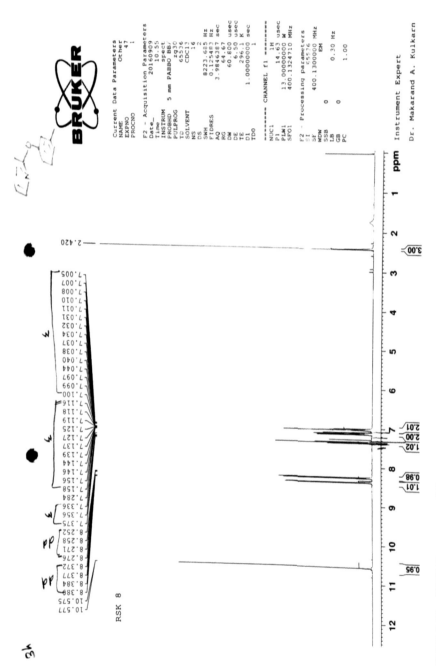

FIGURE 8.15　^{1}H NMR spectrum of **3h.**

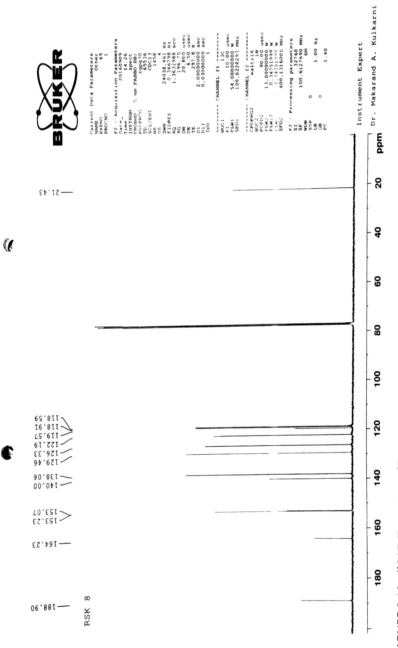

FIGURE 8.16 ¹³C NMR spectrum of **3h.**

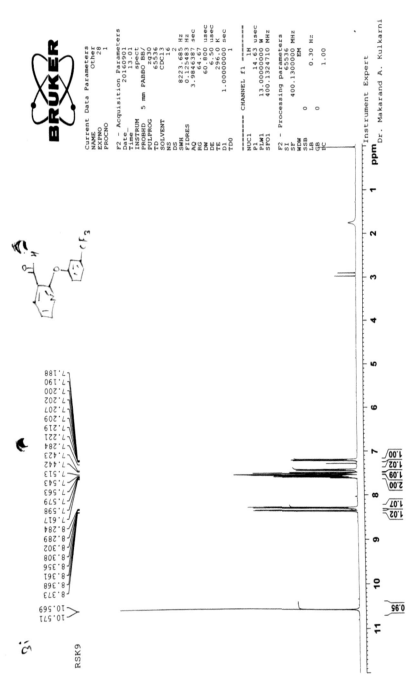

FIGURE 8.17 ¹H NMR spectrum of **3i.**

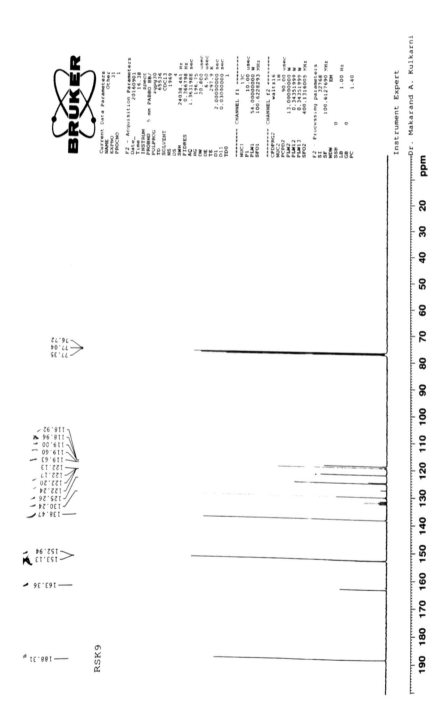

FIGURE 8.18 ^{13}C NMR spectrum of **3i**.

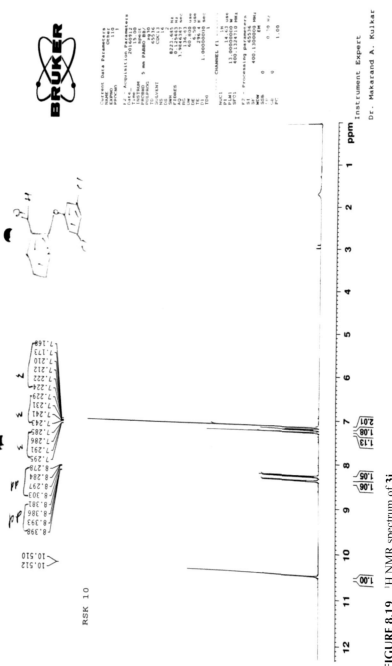

FIGURE 8.19 ¹H NMR spectrum of **3j**.

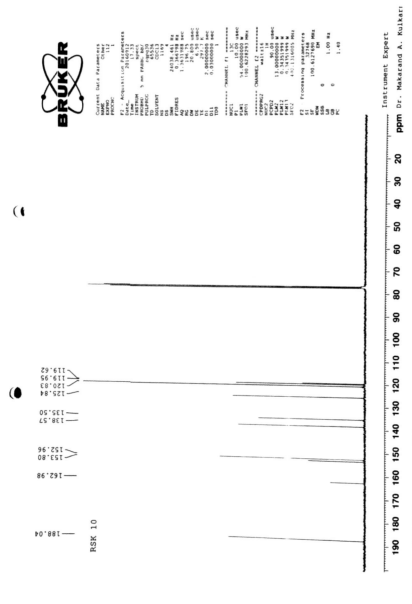

FIGURE 8.20 ¹³C NMR spectrum of **3j**.

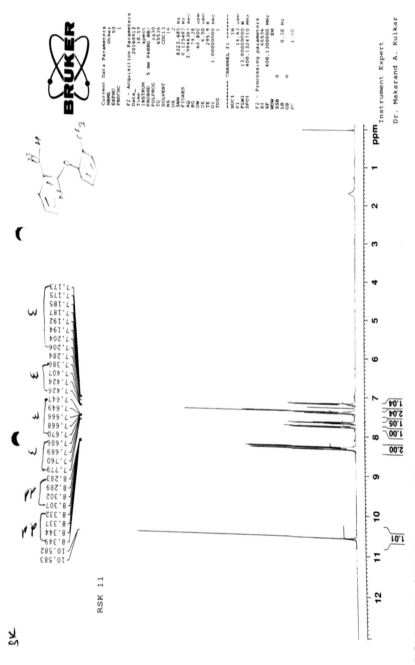

FIGURE 8.21 ^{1}H NMR spectrum of **3k**.

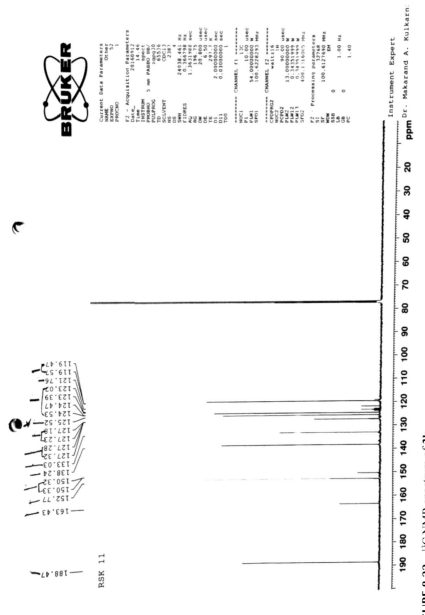

FIGURE 8.22 ¹³C NMR spectrum of **3k.**

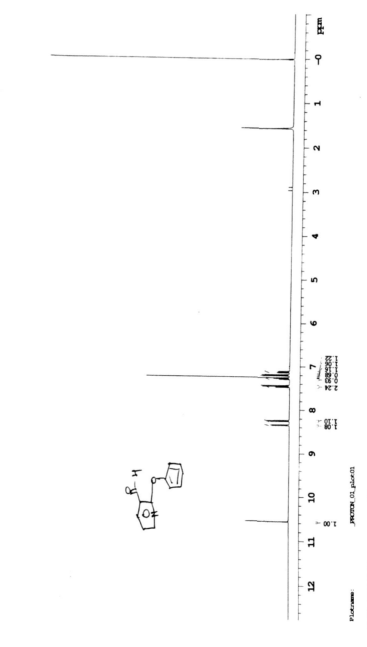

Figure 8.23. ¹H NMR spectrum of **3l**.

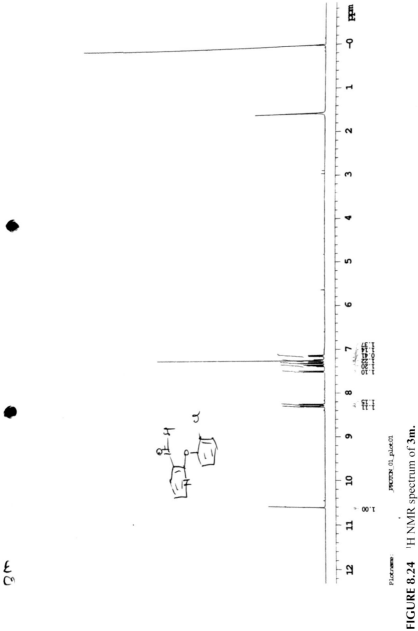

FIGURE 8.24 ¹H NMR spectrum of **3m.**

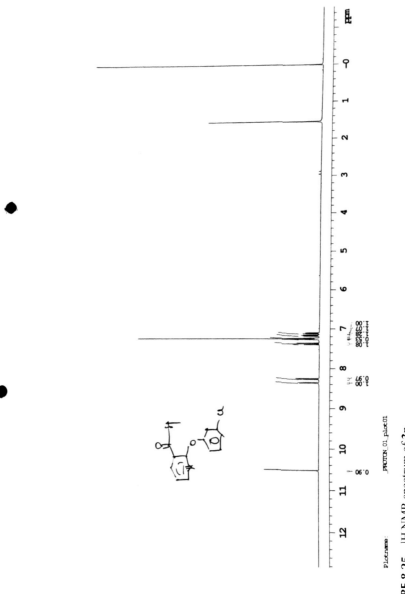

FIGURE 8.25   ¹H NMR spectrum of **3n**.

KEYWORDS

- 2-phenoxynicotinaldehydes
- diabetes
- diabetes mellitus
- inhibitory activity
- α-amylase
- α-glucosidase

REFERENCES

1. West, I. C., (2000). *Diabet. Med.*, *17*, 171.
2. Chakrabarti, R., & Rajagopalan, R., (2002). *Curr. Sci.*, *83*, 1533.
3. Bhosale, U. P., & Hallale, B. V., (2011). *Asian J. Plant Sci. Res.*, *1*, 96.
4. Subramanian, R., Asmawi, A. Z., & Sadikun, A., (2008). *J. Pol. Biochem. Soc.*, *55*, 391.
5. (a) Nickavar, B., & Yousefian, N., (2009). *Iran J. Pharmaceut. Res.*, *8*, 53. (b) Nair, S. S., Kavrekar, V., & Mishra, A., (2013). *Euro. J. Exp. Bio.*, *3*, 128. (c) Dineshkumar, B., Mitra, A., & Manjunatha, M., (2010). *Int. J. Green Pharm.*, *4*, 115. (d) Dastjerdi, Z. M., Namjoyan, F., & Azemi, M. E., (2015). *Europ. J. Biol. Sci.*, *7*, 26.
6. (a) Cheng, A. Y. Y., & Fantus, I. G., (2005). *Can. Med. Assoc. J.*, *172*, 213. (b) Upadhyay, R. K., & Ahmad, S., (2011). *World J. Agric. Sci.*, *7*, 527.
7. Fowler, M. J., (2007). *Clin. Diabetes*, *25*, 131.
8. Lin, Y., Yang, X., Pan, W., & Rao, Y., (2016). *Org. Lett.*, *18*, 2304.
9. (a) Bernardino, A. M. R., & Castro, H. C., (2006). *Bioorg. and Med. Chem.*, *14*, 5765. (b) Attia, A. M., Mansour, H. A., Almehdi, A. A., & Abasi, M. M., (1999). *Nucleos. Nucleot.*, *18*, 2301. (c) Bekhit, A. A., Hymete, A., Damtew, A., Mohamed, A. M. I., & Bekhit, A. A., (2012). *J. Enzyme Inhib. Med. Chem.*, *27*, 69. (d) Rodrigues, T., Guedes, R. C., Dos Santos, D. J., Carrasco, M., Gut, J., Rosenthal, P. J., Moreira, R., & Lopes, F., (2009). *Bioorg. Med. Chem. Lett.*, *19*, 3476. (e) Min, L. J., Shi, Y. X., Yang, M. Y., Zhai, Z. W., Weng, J. Q., Tan, C. X., Liu, X. H., Li, B. J., & Zhang, Y. G., (2016). *Lett. Drug Des. Discov.*, *13*, 324. (f) Duan, H., Ning, M., Chen, X., Zou, Q., Zhang, L., Feng, Y., Zhang, L., Leng, Y., & Shen, J., (2012). *J. Med. Chem.*, *55*, 10475. (g) Ali, A., Bansal, D., Kaushik, N. K., Kaushik, N., Choi, E. H., & Gupta, R., (2014). *J. Chem. Sci.*, *126*, 1091. (h) Wai, J. S., Williams, T. M., Bamberger, D. L., Fisher, T. E., Hoffman, J. M., Hudcosky, R. J., et al., (1993). *J. Med. Chem.*, *36*, 249.
10. Goetz, A. E., Shah, T. K., & Garg, N. K., (2015). *Chem. Commun.*, *51*, 34.
11. Timmins, G. S., Master, S., Rusnak, F., & Deretic, V., (2004). *Antimicrob. Agents Chemother.*, *48*, 3006.
12. Vannelli, T. A., Dykman, A., & Ortiz, D. M. P. R., (2002). *J. Biol. Chem.*, *277*, 12824.

13. (a) Dai, H., Yu, H. B., Liu, J. B., Li, Y. Q., Qin, X., Zhang, X., Qin, Z. F., Wang, T. T., & Fang, J. X., (2009). *ARKIVOC, VII*, 126. (b) Moradi, A., Navidpour, L., Amini, M., Sadeghian, H., Shadnia, H., Firouzi, O., Miri, R., Ebrahimi, S. E. S., Abdollahi, M., Zahmatkesh, M. H., & Shafiee, A., (2010). *Arch. Pharm. Chem. Life Sci., 9*, 509.
14. (a) Haval, K. P., & Argade, N. P., (2008). *J. Org. Chem., 73*, 6936. (b) Haval, K. P., & Argade, N. P., (2007). *Synthesis*, 2198. (c) Haval, K. P., Mhaske, S. B., & Argade, N. P., (2006). *Tetrahedron, 62*, 937. (d) Haval, K. P., & Argade, N. P., (2006). *Tetrahedron, 62*, 3557. (e) Haval, K. P., Kulkarni, R. S., Phatak, P. S., & Tigote, R. M., (2017). *Int. J. Sci. Res. Sci. Technol., 3*, 24. (f) Sathe, B. P., Phatak, P. S., Kadam, A. Y., Gulmire, A. V., Narvade, P. R., & Haval, K. P., (2018). *Int. Res. J. Sci. and Engin.,* A5, 99. (g) Haval, K. P., Sathe, B. P., Phatak, P. S., & Tigote, R. M., (2017). *Int. J. Sci. Res. Sci. Technol., 9*, 53.
15. (a) Sun, G. X., Yang, M. Y., Shi, Y. X., Sun, Z. H., Liu, X. H., Wu, H. K., Li, B. J., & Zhang, Y. G., (2014). *Int. J. Mol. Sci., 15*, 8075. (b) Salahuddin, M. A., & Shaharyar, M., (2014). *Bio. Med. Res. Int.*, 1–14. (c) Wang, X., Zhi, B., Baum, J., Chen, Y., Crockett, R., Huang, L., Eisenberg, S., Ng, J., Larsen, R., Martinelli, M., & Reider, P., (2006). *J. Org. Chem., 71*, 4021. (d) Zen, Y. M., Chen, F., & Liu, F. M., (2012). *Phosphorus Sulfur Silicon Relat. Elem., 187*, 421. (e) Sangani, C. B., Shah, N. M., Patel, M. P., & Patel, R. G., (2013). *Med. Chem. Res., 22*, 3831. (f) Ahn, S. H., Jang, S. S., Han, E. G., & Lee, K. J., (2011). *Synthesis*, 377. (g) Iino, T., Sasaki, Y., Bamba, M., Mitsuya, M., Ohno, A., Kamata, K., et al., (2009). *Biorg. Med. Chem. Lett., 19*, 5531.
16. Kulkarni, J. A., Kothari, M. N., & Baig, M. M. V., (2013). *Int. J. Adv. Biotechnol. Res., 4*, 324.

CHAPTER 9

SEPARATION OF COFFEE PULP BIOACTIVE PHENOLIC COMPOUNDS BY MPLC FRACTIONATION AND IDENTIFICATION BY HPLC-ESI-MS

JORGE E. WONG-PAZ,[1] SYLVAIN GUYOT,[2]
JUAN C. CONTRERAS-ESQUIVEL,[1] PEDRO AGUILAR-ZÁRATE,[1]
RAÚL RODRÍGUEZ-HERRERA,[1] and CRISTÓBAL N. AGUILAR[1*]

[1]*Bioprocesses and Bioproducts Group, Department of Food Research, School of Chemistry, Autonomous University of Coahuila, Saltillo, Coahuila, México*

[2]*INRA, UR1268 BIA, Team Polyphenol, Reactivity and Processing (PRP), BP–35327, 35653 Le Rheu, France*

Corresponding author. E-mail: cristobal.aguilar@uadec.edu.mx

ABSTRACT

Coffee pulp is the major by-product of the coffee industry, and its generation and accumulation is a big problem of contamination. Some strategies have been studied in order to reduce it. One of the most common strategies is turning waste into value-added products. In this study, the MPLC technique was successfully applied to the fractionation of the aqueous acetone extracts (AAE) from the coffee pulp. Seven fractions were obtained using MPLC. The fractions were characterized by reversed-phase HPLC-UV and ESI-MS. Four fractions were obtained as pure compounds according to the HPLC chromatogram. The ESI-MS showed that the main compound present in the acetone extract was caffeine. Additionally, some new masses observed (MW: 232, 357, and 532) had not been reported in the coffee pulp. The MS2 analysis allowed obtaining the main fragments of these new masses. Finally, these results provide new information about the characterization of some new compounds present in the coffee pulp.

9.1 INTRODUCTION

Nowadays, coffee is the most consumed drink in the world and is the second-largest traded commodity after crude oil [1]. World production of coffee in 2011 was almost 8.2 million tons [2]. As a consequence, to the great demand for coffee, enormous amounts of residues are produced by the coffee industry. Some of them may be toxic and represent serious environmental problems. Coffee pulp is the major by-product of the coffee industry representing around 29% dry-weight of the whole berry [3, 4]. Several attempts have been made in order to reduce this problem of contamination. One of the most common strategies is turning waste into value-added products [4].

Phenolic compounds have attracted a lot of interest for their potential positive impacts on human health related to their antioxidant properties and cell signaling action [5–7]. The recovery of such value-added compounds from processing by-products such as coffee pulp has become an interesting alternative. Until now, information about phenolic composition in the coffee pulp, unlike hydroxycinnamic acids (chlorogenic acid), is nonspecific and only generalized to the class of compounds present. In fact, an investigation on the characterization of the phenolic composition in coffee pulp was described by Ramirez-Coronel et al. [8]. This study pointed out the presence of four main classes of phenolic compounds, namely: hydroxycinnamic acids, flavonols, anthocyanidins, and flavan-3-ol (monomer and procyanidins, the later also called condensed tannins). Regarding procyanidins, the authors reported the presence of oligomers from dimer to hexamer by the use of normal-phase HPLC fractionation and MALDI-TOF analysis in an aqueous acetone extract (AAE) (purified on C18 Sep-Pak cartridges) from the coffee pulp (fresh and 3-day-old). However, the other phenolic acids are not well defined until now.

Several methods have been successfully proposed to fractionate and isolate phenolic compounds from natural products by TLC [9], liquid chromatography on Toyopearl TSK HW-40F [10], and Sephadex LH-20 [11], preparative HPLC [12] and, centrifugal partition chromatography [13].

Chromatographic methods using solid supports are preferred over a two-phase solvent system because the high resolution in the separations is obtained. Noticeably, these methods are complicated due to the use of solid supports that may absorb a part of the sample irreversibly. In addition, the equipment is relatively costly. However, both systems using solid supports and a two-phase solvent can be successfully applied and scaled up to isolate and purify phenolic compounds [14, 15]. Medium pressure liquid chromatography (MPLC) is an attractive alternative to troubleshooting above mentioned and additionally exhibits a higher handling capacity for industrial-scale production of natural products [16].

To continue and improve the current *in vitro* and to allow the *in vivo* assays, it is necessary to dispose of large amounts of pure bioactive compounds [13]. The recovery of nutritionally valuable phenolic compounds appears to be a promising strategy for the utilization of coffee pulp. However, adequate characterization and a feasible recovery process are needed. The aim of the present study was to fractionate and characterize an AAE from the coffee pulp by MPLC.

9.2 MATERIALS AND METHODS

9.2.1 RAW MATERIAL

The coffee pulp (*Coffea arabica*) was collected in Xilitla, San Luis Potosi, Mexico, in January 2013, directly from the waste. The sample was sun-dried for 72 h and immediately transported to Saltillo, Coahuila, Mexico to be finally dried at 60°C for 24 h in an oven (LABNET international, Inc.). The dried sample was ground to a fine powder and kept dry and darkness until use.

9.2.2 EXTRACTION PROCEDURE

The extraction of the phenolic compounds was carried out according to Ramirez et al. [8] with some modifications. Lipophilic compounds, sugars, and other phenolic compounds were first removed from the coffee pulp as follows: 500 grams of dried material was extracted with 2×2 L of hexane to remove lipophilic compounds. Then the residual solids were subjected to two successive extractions with ethanol (2×2 L). Then, phenolic compounds of interest were extracted using 2×2 L of aqueous acetone (70%, v/v). All extractions were carried out at 60°C for 30 min. The hexane and ethanol filtrates were discarded. AAE was first filtered through Whatman No. 1 and then on a nylon membrane (0.45 μm, Millipore). The AAE filtrates were combined, concentrated by evaporation under vacuum at 50°C, freeze-dried, and stored prior to purification. A sample of the freeze-dried AAE was analyzed by analytical RP-HPLC.

9.2.3 MPLC FRACTIONATION

Fractionation of the AAE from the coffee pulp was achieved by MPLC, including a ternary pump (Varian ProStar 230I, USA) and a PDA detector (Varian ProStar 330, USA) set at 280 nm and coupled to Workstation Multi-Instrument (V. 6.2) for data acquisition. For developing the proper fractionation conditions, a packed C18 column was used (250 × 21.4 mm, 10 μm, Microsorb 300, Dynamax). The filtrated sample (100 mg/123 mL of aqueous-ethanol, 12%, v/v) was injected through one of the pumping lines with a flow rate of 8 mL/min. Run was conducted at room temperature. The eluent was a gradient of aqueous acetic acid (3%, v/v; solvent A) and acetonitrile (solvent B). The following gradient was applied: initial, 0% B; 0–7 min, 20% B linear; 7–10 min, isocratic; 10–20 min, 30% B linear; 20–25 min, isocratic; 25–45 min, 40% B linear; 45–50 min, isocratic; 50–60 min, 50% B linear; 60–70 min, 60% B linear. The column was then washed and reconditioned. The collected polyphenolic fractions were concentrated 50°C during 24 h, filtered (0.45 μm, nylon), and injected directly into the HPLC and ESI-MS.

9.2.4 HPLC-ESI-MS

Analysis of the crude AAE before MPLC and fractions purified using MPLC were performed by Reversed-Phase High-Performance Liquid Chromatography, including an autosampler (Varian ProStar 410, USA), a ternary pump (Varian ProStar 230I, USA) and a UV-visible PDA detector (Varian ProStar 330, USA). Samples (10 μL) were injected onto a Denali C18 column (240 mm × 4.6 mm, 5μm, Grace, USA). The oven temperature was maintained at 30°C. The eluent was a gradient of aqueous acetic acid (3%, v/v; solvent A) and acetonitrile (solvent B). The flow rate was maintained at 1.2 mL/min, and elution of phenolic compounds was monitored at 245, 280, and 320 nm. Data processing was done by Workstation Multi-Instrument (V. 6.2). The following gradient was applied: initial, 3% B; 0–5 min, 9% B linear; 5–15 min, 16% B linear; 15–45 min, 50% B linear. The column was then washed and reconditioned. An ion trap mass spectrometer (Varian 500-MS IT Mass Spectrometer, USA) equipped with an electrospray ion source was used. Manual injection at an infusion flow rate of 50µL/min was load into the mass spectrometer source All MS experiments were carried out in the negative mode [M-H]-1. Nitrogen was used as nebulizing gas and helium as damping gas. The ion source parameters were: spray voltage 5.0 kV, and capillary voltage and temperature were 90.0 V and 350°C, respectively. Data were collected and processed using MS Workstation software (V 6.9). Full scan spectra were acquired in the m/z range 50–2000. Samples were firstly analyzed in full scan mode. MS/MS analyses were performed on a series of selected precursor ions.

9.3   RESULTS AND DISCUSSION

Figure 9.1 shows the typical chromatogram of the AAE from coffee pulp using analytical RP-HPLC. The peaks eluting before 5 minutes in the chromatogram are characterized and well known as highly polar compounds, and residual phenols and phenolic acids present in the acetone extract. The presence of chlorogenic acid (RT: 13.5 min) was also unambiguously confirmed according to its retention time and its UV spectrum by comparison to the commercial standard compound. It is also possible to observe a major peak in the AAE with a retention time of 14.6 min. Individual commercial standards of caffeine and caffeic acid have the same retention time of 14.6 min as the major peak observed in the AAE. The corresponding peak was marked with an "*" in Figure 9.1. Then the AAE sample was fractionated using the MPLC system.

The fractionation of the AAE from coffee pulp using MPLC led to the purification of eight fractions, which are numbered (I-VIII) in Figure 9.2. These fractions were directly analyzed by injection in RP-HPLC-UV-visible and by infusion in electrospray mass spectrometry (ESI-MS). The results are shown in Table 9.1. Only fraction VIII do not reveal any peak on the analytical RP-HPLC chromatogram (data not shown); therefore, this sample was discarded. In the other fractions (I-VII), one or several peaks were observed in the analytical RP-HPLC (Table 9.1).

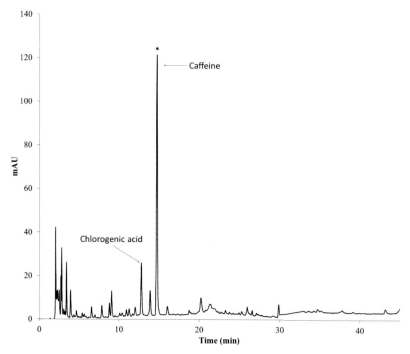

FIGURE 9.1 UV 280 nm HPLC chromatogram of the aqueous acetone extract using analytical RP-HPLC.

Interestingly, the fractions I, IV, V, and VII resulted in a clear chromatogram containing a major peak (Figure 9.3). It is important to mention that polar compounds as sugars and some phenolic acids and, other as fatty acids, well-characterized in coffee were removed in the MPLC isolation before eluting the first peak. This could be explained by the fact of the presence of ethanol when the sample of AAE was re-suspended played a role as mobile phase in the MPLC, limiting the retention of the polar compounds, including the chlorogenic acid. This is useful when it is required to remove highly polar compounds, and then prepare the sample in a solvent as ethanol to help remove these compounds when they are subjected to chromatography. The peak present in the fraction I (Figure 9.3) was clearly identified as the major peak observed in the typical chromatogram of AAE (Figure 9.1) with a retention time of 14.6 min. The other fractions (i.e., IV, V, and VII) revealed peaks for which no available standards having the same retention time were observed. Figure 9.3 also shows the Uv-visible spectrum for the major peak for each HPLC chromatogram. It is possible to note that fractions I, V, and VII have no absorbance at 320 nm, which is a typical wavelength of the hydroxycinnamic acids. Only the peak obtained in the fraction IV has a slight absorbance at 320 nm. Generally, all fractions also showed absorbance at or near 280 nm, which is a wavelength used to monitor the polyphenolic compounds due to the presence of aromatic rings in their structure.

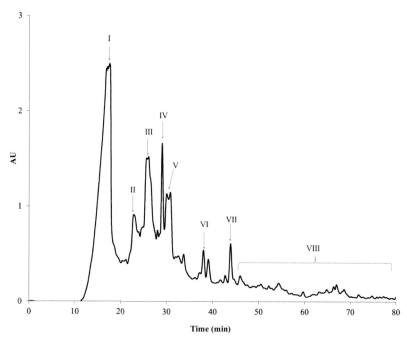

FIGURE 9.2   MPLC chromatogram (280 nm) of the acetone extract from coffee pulp marking the peak fraction manually collected.

Finally, the MS analysis was carried out to increase the information about these compounds isolated from the coffee pulp by MPLC. Amorim et al. [17] conducted a complete ESI-MS analysis of green and roasted coffees, which contains useful information to compare the typical compounds present. Table 9.1 shows the main molecular ions and the main productions on the MS2 spectrum that were detected by ESI-MS in each fraction in our study. As it was expected, the fraction I had the m/z corresponding to caffeine, which was confirmed with the MS/MS fragmentation pattern.

In the fraction II, III, and VI, several predominant m/z were obtained; however, it is difficult to establish a direct relation with HPLC chromatograms. Fraction II presented a predominant m/z of 365 in positive mode and fragments ions of 277 and 129. Similar m/z of 365 was clearly observed in green and roasted coffees in the work of Nunes et al. [18], concluding that corresponded to a di-hexose adduct [M+Na]$^+$ ion; though, the MS/MS analysis was different from the obtained in our work.

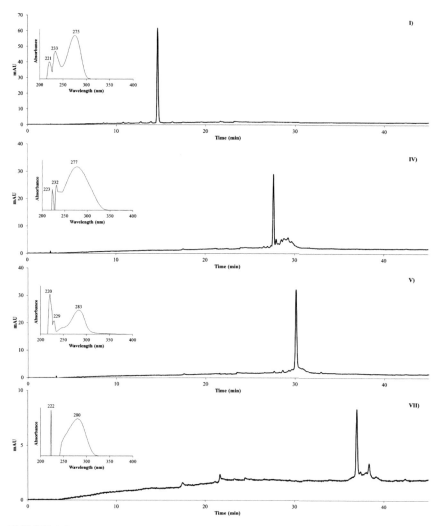

FIGURE 9.3   UV 280 nm HPLC chromatograms and the UV-Visible spectrum of the peak fraction obtained with a unique compound.

TABLE 9.1 Characterization of the Fractions Obtained by MPLC

Fraction	RT	Max Wavelength (nm)	Ionization Mode	Main m/z Observed in the Fraction	Main Product Ions in the MS/MS Spectrum
I	14.6	275	+	195 (100)	163, 135, 110
II	22.8	269	+	365 (100), 396 (30)	277, 129
	23.5	284			
	23.9	284			
	24.5	330			
	25.1	332			
III	26.1	283	-	319 (90), 374 (60), 515 (100)	353
	26.5	332			
IV	27.6	277	-	231 (100), 361 (80), 399 (63)	97
V	30.5	283	+	365 (100)	348, 333, 278, 277, 129
VI	33.4	275	-	356 (100), 397 (27)	338,310
	33.9	270			
VII	36.9	280	-	343 (30), 383 (80), 397 (90), 531 (100)	455, 437, 413, 409, 331

Footnote: MS/MS analyses were carried out for the mass with 100 of intensity.

(): relative abundance of the production in the MS/MS spectrum of [M-H]⁻

More information is necessary to conclude if this m/z corresponds to the oligosaccharide or another molecule. In fraction III, a common hydroxycinnamic acid in coffee pulp was clearly identified with m/z of 515, namely dicaffeoylquinic acid [19] and with a fragment ion of 353 [20]. Fraction IV, a predominant m/z of 231 in negative mode, was clearly observed. The MS/MS fragmentation shows a unique m/z of 97, indicating the loss of a fragment with 134 Da. Additional, the HPLC chromatogram showed a peak that could be linked with this mass. Interestingly the mass spectrum of the fraction V showed a single m/z of 365 in the positive mode as above was discussed for fraction II. An m/z of 356 was predominant in fraction VI with a fragment ion of 338 and 310, indicating a loss of 18 and 46 Da, respectively. Finally, the fraction VII had an m/z of 531 with a fragment pattern of 455 and 437 m/z. To best of our knowledge, the m/z of 231, 356, and 531 had never been reported in the coffee pulp. Further studies are needed to obtain a final characterization which to allow the complete elucidation of them.

9.4 CONCLUSION

MPLC was successfully used to the isolation of compounds from the coffee pulp, specially to obtain caffeine and phenols caffeine-free. New relevant information about the characterization of some new molecules present in coffee pulp was generated. Further studies are necessary to characterize these molecules and to evaluate their presence in coffee beans and the infusion of coffee beans.

ACKNOWLEDGMENT(S)

The authors wish to thank the Mexican Council for Science and Technology (CONACYT) for the financial support of students via a graduate scholarship.

KEYWORDS

- aqueous acetone extract
- bioactive compounds
- mass spectrometer
- medium pressure liquid chromatography (MPLC)
- polar compounds
- polyphenolic fractions

REFERENCES

1. Esquivel, P., & Jiménez, V. M., (2012). Functional properties of coffee and coffee by-products. *Food Research International*, *46*, 488–495. doi: 10.1016/j.foodres.2011.05.028.
2. FAOSTAT, (2013). Available at: http://faostat3.fao.org/home/index.html (Accessed on 13 November 2019).
3. Mussatto, S. I., Machado, E. M. S., Martins, S., & Teixeira, J. A., (2011). Production, composition, and application of coffee and its industrial residues. *Food Bioprocess Technology*, *4*, 661–672. doi: 10.1007/s11947–011–0565-z.

4. Murthy, P. S., & Madhava, N. M., (2012). Sustainable management of coffee industry by-products and value addition: A review. *Resources, Conservation and Recycling, 66*, 45–58. doi: 10.1016/j.resconrec.2012.06.005.
5. Valls, J., Millána, S., Martía, M. P., Borràsa, E., & Arola, L., (2009). Advanced separation methods of food anthocyanins, isoflavones and flavanols. *Journal of Chromatography A, 1216*, 7143–7172. doi: 10.1016/j.chroma.2009.07.030.
6. Fraga, C. G., & Oteiza, P. I., (2011). Dietary flavonoids: Role of (−)-epicatechin and related procyanidins in cell signaling. *Free Radical Biology and Medicine, 51*, 813–823. doi: 10.1016/j.freeradbiomed.2011.06.002.
7. Byun, E. B., Ishikawa, T., Suyama, A., Kono, M., Nakashima, S., Kanda, T., Miyamoto, T., & Matsui, T., (2012). A procyanidintrimer, C1, promotes NO production in rat aortic endothelial cells via both hyperpolarization and PI3K/Akt pathways. *European Journal of Pharmacology, 692*, 52–60. doi: 10.1016/j.ejphar.2012.07.011.
8. Ramírez, M. A., Marnet, N., Kolli, V. S. K., Roussos, S., Guyot, S., & Augur, C., (2004). Characterization and estimation of proanthocyanidins and other phenolics in coffee pulp (Coffea Arabica) by thiolysis-high performance liquid chormatography. *Journal of Agricultural and Food Chemistry, 52*, 1344–1349. doi: 10.1021/jf035208t.
9. Sathishkumar, T., & Baskar, R., (2014). Renoprotective effect of Tabernaemontana heyneana Wall. leaves against paracetamol-induced renotoxicity in rats and detection of polyphenols by high-performance liquid chromatography-diode array detector-mass spectrometry analysis. *Journal of Acute Medicine.* doi: 10.1016/j.jacme.2014.02.002.
10. Yanagida, A., Kanda, T., Shoji, T., Ohnishi-Kameyamab, M., & Nagata, T., (1999). Fractionation of apple procyanidins by size-exclusion chromatography. *Journal of Chromatography A, 855*, 181–190. doi: 10.1016/S0021–9673(99)00684–6.
11. Jerez, M., Touriño, S., Sineiro, J., Torres, J. L., & Núñez, M. J., (2007). Procyanidins from pine bark: Relationships between structure, composition and antiradical activity. *Food Chemistry, 104*, 518–527. doi: 10.1016/j.foodchem.2006.11.071.
12. Shoji, T., Masumoto, S., Moriichi, N., Kanda, T., & Ohtake, Y., (2006). Apple (Malus pumila) procyanidins fractionated according to the degree of polymerization using normal-phase chromatography and characterized by HPLC-ESI/MS and MALDI-TOF/MS. *Journal of Chromatography A, 1102*, 206–213. doi: 10.1016/j.chroma.2005.10.065.
13. Delaunay, J. C., Castagnino, C., Chèze, C., & Vercauteren, J., (2002). Preparative isolation of polyphenolic compounds from *Vitis vinifera* by centrifugal partition chromatography. *Journal of Chromatography A, 964*, 123–128. doi: 10.1016/S0021–9673(02)00355–2.
14. Sutherland, I. A., (2007). Recent progress on the industrial scale-up of counter-current chromatography. *Journal of Chromatography A, 1151*, 6–13. doi: 10.1016/j.chroma.2007.01.143.
15. Hopmann, E., Frey, A., & Minceva, M., (2012). A priori selection of the mobile and stationary phase in centrifugal partition chromatography and counter-current chromatography. *Journal of Chromatography A, 1238*, 68–76. doi: 10.1016/j.chroma.2012.03.035.
16. Wang, Y., Zhang, H., Liang, H., & Yuan, Q. (2013). Purification, antioxidant activity and protein-precipitating capacity of punicalin from pomegranate husk. *Food Chemistry, 138*(1), 437–443.

17. Amorim, A. C. L., Hovell, A. M. C., Pinto, A. C., Eberlin, M. N., Arruda, N. P., Pereira, E. J., Bizzo, H. R., Catharino, R. R., Filho, Z. B. M., & Rezende, C. M., (2009). Green and roasted arabica coffees differentiated by ripeness, process and cup quality via electrospray ionization mass spectrometry fingerprinting. *Journal of the Brazilian Chemical Society, 20*, 313–321. doi: 10.1590/S0103–50532009000200017.
18. Nunes, F. M., Domingues, M. R. R., & Coimbra, M. A., (2005). Arabinosyl and glucosyl residues as structural features of acetylated galactomannans from green and roasted coffee infusions. *Carbohydrate Research, 340*, 1689–1698. doi: 10.1016/j.carres.2005.05.002.
19. Ramírez-Martínez, J. R., (1988). Phenolic compounds in coffee pulp: Quantitative determination by HPLC. *Journal of the Science of Food and Agriculture, 43*, 135–144. doi: 10.1002/jsfa.2740430204.
20. Gouveia, S. C., & Castilho, P. C., (2013). *Artemisia annua* L.: Essential oil and acetone extract composition and antioxidant capacity. *Industrial Crops and Products, 45*, 170–181. doi: 10.1016/j.indcrop.2012.12.022.

CHAPTER 10

TRICHODERMA ASPERELLUM AS BIOLOGICAL CONTROL AGENT: FUNGAL CELLULASE AND SPORE PRODUCTION BY SOLID-STATE FERMENTATION

REYNALDO DE LA CRUZ-QUIROZ,[1] SEVASTIANOS ROUSSOS,[2] RAÚL RODRÍGUEZ-HERRERA,[1] DANIEL HERNANDEZ-CASTILLO,[3] and CRISTÓBAL N. AGUILAR[1*]

[1]*Bioprocesses and Bioproducts Research Group, Food Research Department, Autonomous University of Coahuila, 25280, Saltillo, México.*

[2]*Mediterranean Institute of marine and terrestrial Biodiversity and Ecology, Marseille, France*

[3]*Agricultural Parasitology Department, Antonio Narro Agrarian Autonomous University, Buenavista, Saltillo, Coahuila, México*

Corresponding author. E-mail: cristobal.aguilar@uadec.edu.mx

ABSTRACT

Around the world, agro-industrial companies generate significant quantities of wastes, including husks, peels, leaves, etc. They are cheap and available sources with the potential to produce a great variety of added-value products. Agroindustrial biomasses can be used as support and substrate for the growth of microorganisms in solid-state fermentation (SSF) process. In the present work, corncob, sugarcane bagasse (SCB), and coconut husk were substrates evaluated for spore and cellulase production by *Trichoderma asperellum* under SSF culture conditions. The best results were showed using corncob as a substrate. The sporulation reached on corncob was 9.98×10^8 spores/g CS, and the values of enzyme activities were 2.08 and 2.28 U/g CS for endoglucanase and exoglucanase, respectively. According to the results obtained in this study, SCB and corncob without pretreatment are suitable materials for the production of cellulases and spores by *T. asperellum* T2–10 under SSF.

10.1　INTRODUCTION

Biorefineries and traditional bioprocesses have generated high interest, especially in countries with abundant agro-industrial wastes, because it is an attractive biotechnological alternative to make easy the biotransformation of those wastes to value-added compounds. The disposition and management of solid organic wastes are a big issue worldwide. The high generation of wastes by the food, agricultural, and forestry industries are not well disposed of, and the main problem is the fast susceptibility to microbial contamination [1, 2]. In Mexico, the generation of agro-industrial wastes reached 5 million tons per year [3]. These kinds of materials are an important source of carbohydrates, proteins, cellulose, and hemicelluloses, and therefore, the potential to be used as nutrients and energy sources for several microorganisms to synthesize different types of value-added compounds [4, 5].

The solid-state fermentation (SSF) systems have generated high interest, especially in countries with abundant agro-industrial wastes, because it is an attractive biotechnological alternative to make easy biotechnological transformations of those wastes to value-added compounds [6]. Organic acids, flavors, polysaccharides, biodegradable plastics, biomass, dietary fiber, pharmaceuticals, acetone, ethanol, hydrogen, and enzymes are the main products obtained from SSF [7, 8]. SSF has several advantages, such as low energy requirements, the simplicity of the process, cheap aeration, no rigorous control of the fermentation process, and low generation of liquid residues [9]. In this way, filamentous fungi seem to be the organisms most adaptable to SSF conditions [10, 11].

Biological control agents (BCA) are one of the most required products in modern agriculture, and they are traditionally produced in submerged fermentation systems, with low yield, effectivity, and stability. Particularly, the genus *Trichoderma* is an important producer of cellulolytic enzymes used at the industry level, and its spores are used commonly as a biocontrol agent (BCA) against pest in food crops. In that way, it is possible to produce both products mentioned above under SSF culture conditions and several agroindustrial wastes [12]. Cellulases and spores have been produced under SSF conditions using substrates, such as wheat bran, oat straw, cotton husks, rice straw, corncob, corn stover, SCB, wet corn grains, among others [13–15].

The present study provides quantitative data relating to the use of agroindustrial wastes for high yields of cellulolytic enzymes and spores from *T. asperellum* under SSF. As such, it helps to design BCA. The main goal of the present work was to explore agroindustrial wastes suitable for high yields of cellulase and spores from *T. asperellum* under SSF. The results will establish the unitary operations required to develop a cheap and efficient bioprocess to generate value-added products of *Trichoderma* fungus.

10.2 MATERIALS AND METHODS

10.2.1 MICROORGANISM AND CULTURE CONDITIONS

*Trichoderma asperellum*T2–10 was kindly proportioned by the Agricultural Parasitology Department-Universidad Autónoma Agraria Antonio Narro (UAAAN), Saltillo, México. The commercial strain *Trichoderma harzianum* (THR) was used as a control. The fungal strains were cultivated and conserved in a milk-glycerol 8.5% solution. Potato dextrose agar (PDA) medium was used to reactivate fungal strains. PDA (5 mL) was placed into HACH® tubes, and then they were closed and sterilized at 121° C for 15 min. Tubes on slant were inoculated with the fungal strains and incubated at 30° C for 5 days. After that, the tubes were conserved at ± 4°C.

10.2.2 SUBSTRATES

SCB was proportioned by the Food Research Department-Universidad Autonoma de Coahuila (UAdeC), corncob (CC) donated by the Mexican Institute of Maize-UAAAN and coconut fiber (CF) proportioned by COPEMASA Colima, México. Vegetal materials were dried, ground, fractioned (300–1680 μm), and stored under low moisture conditions until further evaluations. These materials were used as substrates during SSF without pretreatment. In addition, agro-industrial wastes were characterized to determine the percentage of cellulose, hemicellulose, and lignin, according to Van Soest et al. [16].

10.2.3 SOLID STATE FERMENTATION

The capacity of *Trichoderma* to growth over the surface of the substrate, sporulation index, and cellulase activities were evaluated. Petri plates were packed with the substrates (Moisture at 70%) at the height of 5 mm. Inoculation was done by placing a plug of PDA-*Trichoderma* on the center of the plate and incubated at 29 °C for 96 h. The surface growth rate was evaluated by measuring the colony size in relation to time. The determination was performed from the center of the Petri plate to the four cardinal points using a Vernier caliper. Spore counting was done at the end of SSF by mixing 1 g of fermented material and 100 mL of distilled water in an Erlenmeyer flask; after that, the suspension of spores was counted using a hemocytometer. The fermented material was placed in Falcon® tubes with 10 mL of distilled water. The enzymatic extract was homogenized on a vortex (1 min) for further determination of cellulases.

10.2.4 CELLULASE ACTIVITY DETERMINATION

Endoglucanase activity was assayed using 1% carboxymethylcellulose in sodium citrate buffer (50 mM, pH 4.8) at 50°C for 30 min [12]. Exoglucanase activity was measured using filter paper Whatman No.1 (1 cm x 5 cm) in sodium citrate buffer (50 mM, pH 4.8) at 50°C for 60 min in according to with Nava-Cruz et al. [12]. After the end of both reactions, the concentration of sugars released was determined by the colorimetric method described by Miller [17]. An enzyme activity (U) was defined as the amount of enzyme that catalyzes the release of 1 µmol of glucose per minute.

10.2.5 DESIGN AND STATISTICAL ANALYSIS

In this study, a bifactorial re-arrangement (3 x 2) was used. The factors were substrates (three levels) and fungal strains (two levels). Spore production, surface growth rate, and cellulase production were the response variables. Data were analyzed by ANOVA using STATISTICA 7.0 software, and mean comparisons were compared using Tukey's multiple range test. A p-value of less than 0.05 was used to define significant differences.

10.3 RESULTS AND DISCUSSION

T. asperellum T2–10 strain showed a surface growth rate of 0.594 and 0.409 mm/h on CC and SCB, respectively. The commercial strain THR showed values of 0.474 and 0.318 mm/hon CC and SCB, respectively. The higher values of superficial growth rates were obtained using corn cob (CC) as a substrate by both strains. Any strain showed growth over CF. Sporulation index on CC was 1.74×10^9 and 9.98×10^8 spores/g CS for THR and *T. asperellum*T2–10, respectively. In the case of SCB, the values obtained were 2.51×10^8 and 5.47×10^7 spores/ g CS for THR and *T. asperellum*T2–10, respectively (Table 10.1). The values of sporulation on CC were higher four to seven times over than on SCB.

The values of endoglucanase and exoglucanase activities were not significantly different between THR and *T. asperellum*T2–10. The same behavior of activities was observed between CC and SCB. All enzyme activities were within the range of 2.07 to 2.69 U/g CS (Table 10.1). The main components, cellulose, hemicellulose, and lignin of each substrate, were evaluated (Table 10.2). The high concentration of cellulose was determined on CF (51.90%), followed by SCB and CC. Hemicellulose was present at 39.86% in CC, followed by SC and CF. In the case of lignin, a high value was observed in CF (22.89%), followed by low quantities on SCB and CC.

TABLE 10.1 Cellulase and Spore Production by *Trichoderma* Using Corn Cob and Sugarcane Bagasse on SSF

Strains	Endoglucanase (U/g)		Exoglucanase (U/g)		Sporulation (Spores/g)	
	CC	SCB	CC	SCB	CC	SCB
T. asperellum T2–10	2.08 a	2.11 a	2.28 a	2.10 a	9.98×10^8b	5.47×10^7d
THR Commercial	2.07 a	2.36 a	2.69 a	2.39 a	1.74×10^9a	2.51×10^8c

*Different words indicate significant differences between the same response variable. Corn cob (CC), Sugarcane Bagasse (SCB).

The success of the SSF process depends on an appropriate selection of substrate, which should be an effective source of nutrients to be used by a specific microorganism [18]. However, the use of substrates on

SSF is closely related to factors such as availability, the cost of material, particle size, porosity, and chemical composition [19]. On the present research, surface growth rate, sporulation index, and cellulase activities were the parameters evaluated to explore the feasibility of substrates to be used on SSF.

TABLE 10.2 Main Components in the Fibrous Wastes

Fibrous Waste	Main Components% w/w		
	Cellulose	Hemicellulose	Lignin
Corn cob	32.29	39.86	4.60
Sugarcane bagasse	39.32	29.16	8.27
Coconut fiber	51.90	6.88	22.89

Commercial THR and *T. asperellum* T2–10 were unable to growth over CF as a substrate, which could be mainly related to the chemical composition. CF has a high concentration of cellulose and a few quantities of hemicellulose to be used as a carbon source [20]. However, CF also has a high concentration of lignin, which is the main protector of polysaccharides presents in the cell wall of a plant [21, 22]. It is known that lignin is a limiting factor to the hydrolysis of cellulose and hemicellulose to release monosaccharides, but in addition, FC is reported as a container of some secondary metabolites, which act like antimicrobial agents inhibiting the development of microorganisms [23]. Similar results were reported by Hong et al. [18], where they evaluated the production of cellulases, hemicellulases, and fermentable sugars released on the process by strains of *Aspergillus* and *Trichoderma.* Several substrates also were evaluated; however, all strains were unable to grow on CF as a substrate.

On the other hand, both *Trichoderma* strains (THR and T2–10) showed important growth and sporulation over SCB and CC. Some experiments about sporulation from the genus of *Trichoderma* are reported showing values of 1.0×10^8, 7.5×10^8, and 7.7×10^9 spores/g by *T. martinale, T. reesei,* and *T. asperellum*, respectively [13, 24, 25]. In the present case, both substrates SCB and CC showed a similar percentage of cellulose 39.32 and 32.29%, respectively. In addition, they had a high concentration of hemicellulose but a few quantities of lignin, as mentioned for forestry residues by Lah et al. [26]. The high growth development and spore production on these substrates are closely related to the low concentration of lignin, which confirms its protection role.

To develop fungal biomass during SSF is necessary, a saccharification process of the substrate using lytic enzymes such as cellulases. In this process, monosaccharides are released to serve as carbon and energy source. In the present study, the enzyme activities obtained in all experiments have not a significant difference among every treatment (strains and substrates). Low enzyme activities were observed by other researchers, such as Lah et al. [26], who evaluated palm kernel cake (PKC) and defatted PKC as substrates under SSF conditions by *Trichoderma* spp., reporting an exoglucanase activity of 6.9 and 16.1 U/g, respectively. An experiment using a combination of substrates including CC, rice straw, wheat bran, soybean cake powder, corn steep liquor under SSF conditions by *T. longibranchiatum* was reported by Xie et al. [27]. They reported values of 40.9 and 99.7 U/g of exoglucanase and endoglucanase activities, respectively. Rahnama et al. [28] evaluated *T. harzianum* on rice straw as substrate obtaining 6.25 and 111.35 U/g for exoglucanase and endoglucanase.

Ingredients such as liquors and nutrients solutions have been added to enhance the SSF and producing high enzyme activities. However, less information is generated on the use or improvement of material without the addition of supplements to influence the SSF process more feasible and economical to the industry. In addition, it is necessary to find fibrous substrates with low lignin concentration or apply physical or chemical pretreatments that allow releasing the polysaccharides as carbon and energy source [29].

10.4 CONCLUSION

Under the conditions used in the present study, SCB and CC were the substrates that favor cellulases and spores production by *Trichoderma asperellum* T2–10 under SSF. CC without pretreatment was the best substrate to produce spores from *T. asperellum* T2–10 under SSF. Results showed that CF was not suitable for cellulase and spore production by *Trichoderma* strains. As a perspective, the process of cellulases and spore production needs optimization of the culture conditions to enhance the yields of both products.

ACKNOWLEDGMENTS

Authors thank Autonomous University of Coahuila and the National Council of Science and Technology (CONACYT-Mexico) for financial support through the project No. 373326.

KEYWORDS

- **biocontrol agent**
- **biomass**
- **biopesticide**
- **lytic enzyme**
- **solid waste**
- **solid-state fermentation**

REFERENCES

1. Lai, W. T., Khong, N. M. H., Lim, S. S., Hee, Y. Y., Sim, B. I., Lau, K. Y., & Lai, O. M., (2017). A review: Modified agricultural by-products for the development and fortification of food products and nutraceuticals, *Trends Food Sci. Tech., 59,* 148–160.
2. Salgado, J. M., Max, B., Rodríguez-Solana, R., & Domínguez, J. M., (2012). Purification of ferulic acid solubilized from agroindustrial wastes and further conversion into 4-vinyl guaiacol by *Streptomyces setonii* using solid state fermentation, *Ind. Crop Prod., 39,* 52–61.
3. Robledo-Narváez, P. N., Muñoz-Páez, K. M., Poggi-Varaldo, H. M., Ríos-Leal, E., Calva-Calva, G., Ortega-Clemente, L. A., Rinderknecht-Seijas, N., Estrada-Vázquez, C., Ponce-Noyola, M. T., & Salazar-Montoya, J. A., (2013). The influence of total solids content and initial pH on batch biohydrogen production by solid substrate fermentation of agroindustrial wastes, *J. Environ. Manag., 128,* 126–137.
4. Ashok, A., Doriya, K., Rao, D. R. M., & Kumar, D. S., (2017). Design of solid state bioreactor for industrial applications: An overview to conventional bioreactors, *Biocatal. Agric. Biotechnol., 9,* 11–18.
5. Stabnikova, O., Wang J. Y., & Ivanov, V., (2010). Value-added biotechnological products from organic wastes. In: Wang, L. K., Ivanov, V., & Tay, J. H., (eds.), *Environmental Biotechnology* (pp. 343–394). Humana Press, Totowa, NJ.

6. Buenrostro-Figueroa, J., Ascacio-Valdés, A., Sepúlveda, L., De La Cruz, R., Prado-Barragán, A., Aguilar-González, M. A., Rodríguez, R., & Aguilar, C. N., (2014). Potential use of different agroindustrial by-products as supports for fungal ellagitannase production under solid-state fermentation. *Food Bioprod. Process, 92*(4), 376–382.

7. López-Pérez, M, & Viniegra-González, G., (2016). Production of protein and metabolites by yeast grown in solid state fermentation: Present status and perspectives. *J. Chemical. Technol. Biot., 91*(5), 1224–1231.

8. Thomas, L., Larroche, C., & Pandey, A., (2013). Current developments in solid-state fermentation. *Biochem. Eng. J., 81*, 146–161.

9. Roussos, S., Olmos, A., Raimbault, M., Saucedo-Castañeda, G., & Lonsane, B. K., (1991). Strategies for large scale inoculum development for solid state fermentation system: Conidiospores of *Trichoderma harzianum*. *Biotechnol. Tech., 5*(6) 415–420.

10. Carrillo-Sancen, G., Carrasco-Navarro, U., Tomasini-Campocosio, A., Corzo, G., Pedraza-Escalona, M. M., & Favela-Torres, E., (2016). Effect of glucose as a carbon repressor on the extracellular proteome of *Aspergillus niger* during the production of amylases by solid state cultivation. *Process Biochem., 51*(12) 2001–2010.

11. Mata-Gómez, M., Mussatto, S. I., Rodríguez, R., Teixeira, J. A., Martinez, J. L., Hernandez, A., & Aguilar, C. N., (2015). Gallic acid production with moldy polyurethane particles obtained from solid state culture of *Aspergillus niger* GH1. *Appl. Biochem. Biotechn., 176*(4) 1131–1140.

12. Nava-Cruz, N. Y., Contreras-Esquivel, J. C., Aguilar-González, M. A., Nuncio, A., Rodríguez-Herrera, R., & Aguilar, C. N., (2016). Agave atrovirens fibers as substrate and support for solid-state fermentation for cellulase production by *Trichoderma asperellum*. *3 Biotech., 6*(1) 1–12.

13. Flodman, H. R., & Noureddini, H., (2013). Effects of intermittent mechanical mixing on solid-state fermentation of wet corn distillers grain with *Trichoderma reesei*. *Biochem. Eng. J., 81*, 24–28.

14. Ortiz, G. E., Guitart, M. E., Cavalitto, S. F., Albertó, E. O., Fernández-Lahore, M., & Blasco, M., (2015). Characterization, optimization, and scale-up of cellulases production by *Trichoderma reesei* cbs 836.91 in solid-state fermentation using agro-industrial products. *Bioprocess Biosys. Eng., 38*(11), 2117–2128.

15. Raghuwanshi, S., Deswal, D., Karp, M., & Kuhad, R. C., (2014). Bioprocessing of enhanced cellulase production from a mutant of *Trichoderma asperellum* RCK2011 and its application in hydrolysis of cellulose. *Fuel, 124*, 183–189.

16. Van Soest, P. J., Robertson, J. B., & Lewis, B. A., (1991). Methods for dietary fiber, neutral detergent fiber, and nonstarch polysaccharides in relation to animal nutrition, *J. Dairy Sci., 74*(10), 3583–3597.

17. Miller, G. L., (1959). Use of dinitrosalicylic acid reagent for determination of reducing sugar. *Anal. Chem., 31*(3), 426–428.

18. Hong, L. S., Ibrahim, D., & Omar, I. C., (2011). Lignocellulolytic materials-as a raw material for the production of fermentable sugars via solid state fermentation. *Asian J. Sci. Res., 4*, 53–61.

19. Couto, S. R., & Sanromán, M. Á., (2005). Coconut flesh: a novel raw material for laccase production by *Trametes hirsuta* under solid-state conditions: Application to Lissamine green B decolorization. *J. Food Eng., 71*(2), 208–213.

20. Rencoret, J., Ralph, J., Marques, G., Gutiérrez, A., Martínez, Á. T., & Del Río, J. C., (2013). Structural characterization of lignin isolated from coconut (*Cocos nucifera*) coir fibers. *J. Agr. Food Chem., 61*(10), 2434–2445.
21. Neutelings, G., (2011). Lignin variability in plant cell walls: Contribution of new models. *Plant Sci., 181*(4), 379–386.
22. Ojumu, T. V., Solomon, B. O., Betiku, E., Layokun, S. K., & Amigun, B., (2003). Cellulase production by *Aspergillus flavus* Linn isolate NSPR 101 fermented in sawdust, bagasse and corncob. *Afr. J. Biotechnol., 2*(6), 150–152.
23. Kang, S. W., Park, Y. S., Lee, J. S., Hong, S. I., & Kim, S. W., (2004). Production of cellulases and hemicellulases by *Aspergillus niger* KK2 from lignocellulosic biomass. *Bioresource Technol., 91*(2), 153–156.
24. De Los Santos-Villalobos, S., Hernández-Rodríguez, L. E., Villaseñor-Ortega, F., & Peña-Cabriales, J. J., (2012). Production of *Trichoderma asperellum* T8a spores by a "home-made" solid-state fermentation of mango industrial wastes. *BioResources, 7*(4), 4938–4951.
25. Hanada, R. E., Pomella, A. W. V., Soberanis, W., Loguercio, L. L., & Pereira, J. O., (2009). Biocontrol potential of *Trichoderma martiale* against the black-pod disease (*Phytophthora palmivora*) of cacao. *Biol. Control., 50*(2), 143–149.
26. Lah, T. N. T., Norulaini, N. A. R. N., Shahadat, M., Nagao, H., Hossain, M. S., & Omar, A. K. M., (2016). Utilization of industrial waste for the production of cellulase by the cultivation of *Trichoderma* via solid state fermentation. *Environ. Process, 3*(4), 803–814.
27. Xie, L., Zhao, J., Wu, J., Gao, M., Zhao, Z., Lei, X., Zhao, Y., Yang, W., Gao, X., Ma, C., Liu, H., Wu, F., Wang, X., Zhang, F., Guo, P., & Dai, G., (2015). Efficient hydrolysis of corncob residue through cellulolytic enzymes from *Trichoderma* strain G26 and l-lactic acid preparation with the hydrolysate. *Bioresource Tech., 193*, 331–336.
28. Rahnama, N., Shah, U. K. M., Foo, H. L., Rahman, N. A. A., & Ariff, A. B., (2016). Production and characterization of cellulase from solid state fermentation of rice straw by *Trichoderma harzianum* SNRS3. *Pertanika J. Trop. Agr. Sci., 34*(4), 507–531.
29. Zeng, Y., Zhao, S., Yang, S., & Ding, S. Y., (2014). Lignin plays a negative role in the biochemical process for producing lignocellulosic biofuels. *Curr. Opin. Biotech., 27*, 38–45.

CHAPTER 11

KNOWLEDGE DEMOCRATIZATION AND THE HIDDEN FACE OF PALM OIL BIODIESEL

FRANCISCO TORRENS[1*] and GLORIA CASTELLANO[2]

[1]Institute for Molecular Science, University of Valencia, PO Box 22085, E-46071 Valencia, Spain

[2]Department of Experimental Sciences and Mathematics, Faculty of Veterinary and Experimental Sciences, Valencia Catholic University Saint Vincent Martyr, Guillem de Castro-94, E-46001 Valencia, Spain

*Corresponding author. E-mail: torrens@uv.es

ABSTRACT

The individual, open, off the record certain and idiomatic quality that at the moment and another time Fuster's school conversation scholarships engrosses a stylistic novelty that, in addition to stamping him a stout private trademark, commencing to utilize roads aggravating and, regularly, original in the conducts of sharing facts: A quantity of paths of inestimable importance for the defy of knowledge dispersal and facts democratization. The deliberation amounts to the initial end signifying abstract and linguistic paths: the list and study of Fusterian communication akin to and antiseptic in opposition to the refinement and murkiness of specific varieties of school words, an remedy in opposition to stoppage in knowing original data, an antitoxic that, perfectly, sanctions agreeable, vigorous and efficient information for knowledge popularization. Fuster's suggestions denote, as a minimum, an attempt to add, with the missiles of good sense, to one of the reasons of extremely significant present subject in current civilization: that of conquering nervousness, technocracy, stubbornness, despotism or unawareness ghosts, defending, consequently, civilization entitlement to fantasize about an improved prospect with the progressing information take-over. It results, there is no necessity to tell it, a confront against which Fuster, in the van places, did not desire to exclude: that of discipline dialogues for an effective and real information democratization. This work is finished with a unpaid employees' point of view on the concealed countenance of palm oil biodiesel and the extinction of the plants.

11.1 INTRODUCTION

Setting the scene: the discourses of science, Joan Fuster, the democratization of knowledge, the hidden face of palm oil biodiesel, and the extinction of the species. The subjective, free, informal confident and colloquial tone that now and again Fuster's academic discourse grants involves a stylistic originality that, besides imprinting him a strong personal hallmark, beginning to use roads provoking and, frequently, new in the ways of communicating knowledge; some roads of incalculable interest for the challenge (crucial in present technology and information society) of science spreading and knowledge democratization. Fuster's (ideological, stylistic) proposals mean, at least, an effort to contribute, with the weapons of reason, to one of the causes of highly important current issue in present society: that of overcoming uneasiness, technocracy, dogmatism, totalitarianism or ignorance phantoms, protecting, so, humanity right to dream about a better future with the progressive knowledge conquest. It is, no need exists to say it, a challenge in front of which Fuster, in the van positions, did not want to keep out: that of science discourses for an efficacious and true knowledge democratization.

It was reviewed fads and fallacies in the name of science, the curious theories of modern pseudoscientists, and the strange, amusing, and alarming cults that surround them as a study in human gullibility [1]. The scientific attitude was revised [2]. The following hypotheses (H) were proposed on biofuel economic and ethical risks.

- H1. (Fidel Castro, 2003). Biofuels generation from edible feed-stocks is in competition with food production.
- H2. (Fidel Castro, 2003). Generation of biofuels from edible feed-stocks increases food prices.
- H3. (Fidel Castro, 2007). The use of food to produce biofuel will affect region food security.

The trap of diversity was discussed as to how neoliberalism fragmented the identity of the *working class* [3]. The societies of the persons without value were analyzed as the Fourth Industrial Revolution, de-substantiation of capital, and generalized de-valorization [4]. Tarín Sanz and Rivas Otero reviewed the working class as a possible subject of change in the 21st century [5].

In earlier publications, it was reported the periodic table of the elements (PTE) [6–8], quantum simulators [9–17], science, ethics of developing sustainability *via* nanosystems, devices [18], *green nanotechnology* as an approach towards environment safety [19], molecular devices, machines as hybrid organic-inorganic structures [20], PTE, quantum biting its tail, sustainable chemistry [21], quantum molecular spintronics, nanoscience, and graphenes [22]. It was informed cancer, its hypotheses [23], precision personalized medicine from theory to practice, cancer [24], how human immunodeficiency virus/acquired immunodeficiency syndrome (HIV/AIDS) destroy immune defenses, hypothesis [25], 2014 emergence, spread, uncontrolled Ebola outbreak [26, 27], Ebola virus disease, questions, ideas, hypotheses, models [28], metaphors that made history, reflections on philosophy, science, and deoxyribonucleic acid (DNA) [29], scientific integrity, ethics, science communication, psychology [30], capital *vs.* nature contradiction, inclusive spreading of science [31], and past, present, and future of reflections on (palaeo)climate and global changes [32]. In the present report, it is reviewed some reflections on Joan Fuster's academic discourse, the discourses of science, Fuster, the democratization of knowledge, the hidden face of palm oil biodiesel, and the extinction of the species. The aim of this work is to compare two different discourses of science spreading: The first is Fuster's democratization of knowledge; the second is voluntary workers' speech on the hidden face of palm oil biodiesel and the extinction of the species. This study deals with initiating a debate by suggesting a number of questions, which can arise when addressing subjects of science spreading, etc., and their points of view from the democratization of knowledge and activism.

11.2   JOAN FUSTER'S ACADEMIC DISCOURSE

The personal, liberated, unofficial sure and informal tenor that at the present and once more Joan Fuster's educational dialogue funding engages a stylistic innovation that, as well printing him a robust individual seal, starting to employ roads inciting and, often, novel in the habits of conveying information: A number of ways of untold concern for the confront (vital in current expertise and information civilization) of discipline distribution and information democratization. The thought is the preliminary tip symptomatic of theoretical and linguistic ways: the register and examination of Fusterian discussion similar to and antiseptic against the sophistication and cloudiness of particular types of educational communication, a cure against breakdown in comprehending novel information, an antitoxic that, ultimately, legalizes enjoyable, energetic and effective education for discipline vulgarization.

11.3 DISCOURSES OF SCIENCE: JOAN FUSTER AND KNOWLEDGE DEMOCRATIZATION

The same *science* concept turned, nowadays, a high absolute: One of these untouchables that Fusterian rationalism would recommend disinfecting [33]. Among other things, because science categorical conception is frontally contradictory with the same method that defines it. Always, it results evident that the science concept includes broad ideas and activities heterogeneity: Heterogeneity directly proportional to that of scientific-discourses types (*cf.* Figure 11.1). In addition, in the midst of this ocean of possible discourse types, Fusterian academic discourse represents, in the particular Catalan-culture framework, a model that fills with enthusiasm (which fills with enthusiasm pragmatic philological research) by reason of the singularities in wide-supply spreading. Naturally, there should be still to take into account another aspect, in the just valuation of the discourse type and the interest that it presents in the case of a language as Catalan: the socio-linguistic perspective. Because in the present Catalan situation, in which to slow down the linguistic substitution process was not got, and normalizing appropriateness is hardly confirmed timidly, the social prestige of science and the language in that this is vehiculated cannot be, of course, a negligible factor. That Catalan-speaking persons look into their own language as a *science language* unquestionably contributes to lost-prestige return. In addition, the social prestige of a language, naturally, presents a specific weight somewhat contemptible in the possibilities of normalization or strict survival. On the contrary, people could not leave aside either, in consideration, the positive influence of language on science and its propagation possibilities. It is not now the moment of remembering the infinite fan of possibilities that a language as Catalan (with all the universe of affective connotations and exclusive mechanisms of knowledge representation) can offer for science-communication yield. In addition, it is that (to say it fast) communicating science in Catalan, inside the Catalan-speaking community, brings some immeasurable advantages in relation to the sole and exclusive use of Castilian for such a purpose: some advantages that no education or communication specialist would dare to question. In spite of a global and generic consideration (independent of the particular instance of a socio-linguistic context as that of each of the territories that integrate the Catalan domain), one should put the emphasis on the social dimension of science popularization discourses. On scientific knowledge spreading depends, in all developed world and, maybe still more, in depressed countries, success in the use of the resources and applications that progress brings. On science, democratization can depend, as Fuster observed, that the model society that people construct be that of either an intelligently industrious leisure or technocratic despotism. Closing the circle: On the ability that people be able to show on science words depends, definitively, the probability of the possible utopia (comforts, rights, and possibilities equality, services, personal autonomy, efficacious medical care, cultural enjoyment, etc.). Told and debated: On they depend not on few happiness aspirations. Joan Fuster's (ideological, stylistic) proposals mean, at least, an effort to contribute, with the weapons of reason, to one of the causes of highly important current issue in present society: that of overcoming uneasiness, technocracy, dogmatism, totalitarianism or ignorance phantoms, protecting, so, humanity right to dream about a better future with the progressive knowledge conquest. It is, no need exists to say it, a challenge in front of which Fuster, in the van positions, did not want to keep out: that of science discourses for an efficacious and true knowledge democratization.

11.4   HIDDEN FACE OF THE BIODIESEL OF PALM OIL: THE EXTINCTION OF SPECIES

A necessity exists for giving up using palm oil mixed with diesel (*cf.* Figure 11.2) [34]. On February 1, 2019, European Commission in Madrid (Spain) presented a document (delegated act) that explained how to distinguish the biodiesels with high CO_2 emissions from the rest, and exclude the formers from renewable-energy consideration, which would mean that palm and soya oils would give up utilized to produce biodiesel. Till 7% of the diesel that one puts in his vehicle or the bus that moves you put is biodiesel. In Spain, the largest part is made with palm oil. Although unknown, biodiesel consumption in the EU supposes 51% of production above food and cosmetics together. People have an opportunity for reverting this. Palm oil plantations devastate Indonesia and Malaysia rainforests, as well as in a number of Central-America and tropical-Africa countries. They destroy rainforests and biodiversity. In addition, they suppose enormous amounts of emissions of *greenhouse effect* (GHE) gases and are bound to infringements of the human rights of the local communities where they settle. That said above is of special interest in the areas of transport, energy, conservation, anti-globalization, and agroecology.

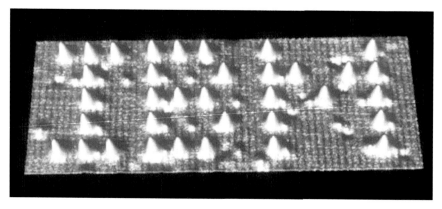

FIGURE 11.1   Science spreading in the science nanotechnology community.

11.5   FINAL REMARKS

From the present results and discussion, the following final remarks can be drawn.

1. The trap of diversity is how neoliberalism fragmented the identity of the *working class*. Biofuel has economic and ethical risks increasing food prices and decreasing regional food security. At the beginning of 21st century, together with *the fundamental contradiction* described by Marx at least two others exist, crossed, and non-assimilable, without which the *political subjects* question

cannot be tackled: the one that faces capital *vs.* nature and the other that opposes, in the political and geographic plane, actions *vs.* representations. To take the capital/nature contradiction seriously forces to accept, *vs.* classical Marxism, that *the productive forces are at the same time destructive forces* and their development, far from securing without brake emancipation, should be controlled and stopped/reverted. The universal *consumer middle class*, cracked today, is inseparable from the two other contradictions above.

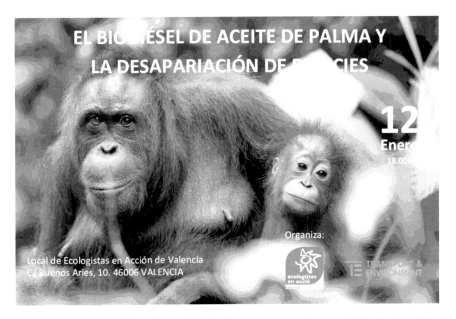

FIGURE 11.2   The hidden face of the biodiesel of palm oil: palm oil biodiesel and the extinction of species.

2.   Joan Fuster's (ideological, stylistic) proposals mean, at least, an effort to contribute, with the weapons of reason, to one of the causes of highly important current issue in present society: that of overcoming uneasiness, technocracy, dogmatism, totalitarianism or ignorance phantoms, protecting, so, humanity right to dream about a better future with the progressive knowledge conquest. It is, no need exists to say it, a challenge in front of which Fuster, in the van positions, did not want to keep out: that of science discourses for an efficacious and true knowledge democratization.

3. During the next decades, humankind must face severe restrictions on energy production. Worldly, most part of the energy is produced on the basis of hydrocarbons combustion, and the trend will be to the substitution of the use of fossil fuels with the so-called *renewable energies*. While other forms of energy production will not be feasible on a large scale, a man should be accustomed to optimize the existing processes and reduce the use of hydrocarbons. Governments must encourage the public financing of research on technologies of renewable energies that finally will cause the solution that the climatic change obliges.

ACKNOWLEDGMENTS

The authors thank the support from Generalitat Valenciana (Project No. PROMETEO/2016/094) and Universidad Católica de Valencia *San Vicente Mártir* (Project No. 2019-217-001).

KEYWORDS

- academic discourse
- activism
- agroecology
- anti-globalization
- biodiesel action
- Catalan culture
- Catalan language
- green chemistry
- Joan Fuster
- science discourse
- science spreading
- species extinction
- voluntary worker

REFERENCES

1. Gardner, M., (1957). *Fads and Fallacies in the Name of Science: The Curious Theories of Modern Pseudoscientists and the Strange, Amusing and Alarming Cults that Surround Them: A Study in Human Gullibility*, Dover: New York, NY.
2. Grinnell, F., (1992). *The Scientific Attitude*. Guilford: New York, NY.
3. Bernabé, D., (2018). *La Trampa de la Diversidad: Cómo el Neoliberalismo Fragmentó la Identidad de la Clase Trabajadora*. Akal: Tres Cantos, Madrid, Spain.
4. Piqueras, A., (2018). *Las Sociedades de las Personas sin Valor: Cuarta Revolución Industrial, Des-Substanciación del Capital, Desvalorización Generalizada*. El Viejo Topo: Vilassar de Dalt, Barcelona, Spain.
5. Tarín, S. A., & Rivas, O. J. M., (2018). *La Clase Trabajadora: ¿Sujeto de Cambio en el Siglo XXI?*. Siglo XXI: Tres Cantos, Madrid, Spain.
6. Torrens, F., & Castellano, G., (2015). Reflections on the nature of the periodic table of the elements: Implications in chemical education. In: Seijas, J. A., Vázquez, T. M. P., & Lin, S. K., (eds.), *Synthetic Organic Chemistry* (Vol. 18, pp. 1–15). MDPI: Basel, Switzerland.
7. Torrens, F., & Castellano, G., (2018). Nanoscience: From a two-dimensional to a three-dimensional periodic table of the elements. In: Haghi, A. K., Thomas, S., Palit, S., & Main, P., (eds.), *Methodologies and Applications for Analytical and Physical Chemistry* (pp. 3–26). Apple Academic–CRC Press: Waretown, NJ.
8. Torrens, F., & Castellano, G. Periodic table. In: Putz, M. V., (ed.), *New Frontiers in Nanochemistry: Concepts, Theories, and Trends*. Apple Academic–CRC: Waretown, NJ, (In Press).
9. Torrens, F., & Castellano, G., (2015). Ideas in the history of nano/miniaturization and (quantum) simulators: Feynman, education and research reorientation in translational science. In: Seijas, J. A., Vázquez, T. M. P., & Lin, S. K., (eds.), *Synthetic Organic Chemistry* (Vol. 19, pp. 1–16). MDPI: Basel, Switzerland.
10. Torrens, F., & Castellano, G., (2015). Reflections on the cultural history of nanominiaturization and quantum simulators (computers). In: Laguarda, M. N., Masot, P. R., & Brun, S. E., (eds.), *Sensors and Molecular Recognition* (Vol. 9, pp. 1–7). Universidad Politécnica de Valencia: València, Spain.
11. Torrens, F., & Castellano, G., (2016). Nanominiaturization and quantum computing. In: Costero, N. A. M., Parra, Á. M., Gaviña, C. P., & Gil, G. S., (eds.), *Sensors and Molecular Recognition* (Vol. 10, pp. 31–1–5). Universitat de València: València, Spain.
12. Torrens, F., & Castellano, G., (2018). Nanominiaturization, classical/quantum computers/simulators, superconductivity, and universe. In: Haghi, A. K., Thomas, S., Palit, S., & Main, P., (eds.), *Methodologies and Applications for Analytical and Physical Chemistry* (pp. 27–44). Apple Academic–CRC: Waretown, NJ.
13. Torrens, F., & Castellano, G., (2018). Superconductors, superconductivity, BCS theory and entangled photons for quantum computing. In: Haghi, A. K., Aguilar, C. N., Thomas, S., & Praveen, K. M., (eds.), *Physical Chemistry for Engineering and Applied Sciences: Theoretical and Methodological Implication* (pp. 379–387). Apple Academic–CRC: Waretown, NJ.
14. Torrens, F., & Castellano, G., (2018). EPR paradox, quantum decoherence, qubits, goals and opportunities in quantum simulation. In: Haghi, A. K., (ed.), *Theoretical*

Models and Experimental Approaches in Physical Chemistry: Research Methodology and Practical Methods (Vol. 5, pp. 317–334). Apple Academic–CRC: Waretown, NJ.

15. Torrens, F., & Castellano, G. (2019). Nanomaterials, molecular ion magnets, ultrastrong and spin-orbit couplings in quantum materials. In: Vakhrushev, A. V., Haghi, R., De Julián-Ortiz, J. V., & Allahyari, E., (eds.), *Physical Chemistry for Chemists and Chemical Engineers: Multidisciplinary Research Perspectives* (pp. 181–190). Apple Academic–CRC: Waretown, NJ.

16. Torrens, F., & Castellano, G. (2019). Nanodevices and organization of single ion magnets and spin qubits. In: Balköse, D., Ribeiro, A. C. F., Haghi, A. K., Ameta, S. C., & Chakraborty, T., (eds.), *Chemical Science and Engineering Technology: Perspectives on Interdisciplinary Research* (pp. 181–190). Apple Academic–CRC: Waretown, NJ, (In Press).

17. Torrens, F., & Castellano, G. Superconductivity and quantum computing via magnetic molecules. In: Haghi, A. K., (ed.), *New Insights in Chemical Engineering and Computational Chemistry*. Apple Academic–CRC: Waretown, NJ, (In Press).

18. Torrens, F., & Castellano, G. Developing sustainability via nanosystems and devices: Science-ethics. In: Balköse, D., Ribeiro, A. C. F., Haghi, A. K., Ameta, S. C., & Chakraborty, T., (eds.), *Chemical Science and Engineering Technology: Perspectives on Interdisciplinary Research*. Apple Academic–CRC: Waretown, NJ, (In Press).

19. Torrens, F., & Castellano, G. Green nanotechnology: An approach towards environment safety. In: Vakhrushev, A. V., Ameta, S. C., Susanto, H., & Haghi, A. K., (eds.), *Advances in Nanotechnology and the Environmental Sciences: Applications, Innovations, and Visions for the Future*. Apple Academic–CRC: Waretown, NJ, (In Press).

20. Torrens, F., & Castellano, G. Molecular devices/machines: Hybrid organic-inorganic structures. In: Pourhashemi, A., Deka, S. C., & Haghi, A. K., (eds.), *Research Methods and Applications in Chemical and Biological Engineering*. Apple Academic–CRC: Waretown, NJ, (In Press).

21. Torrens, F., & Castellano, G. The periodic table, quantum biting its tail, and sustainable chemistry. In: Torrens, F., Haghi, A. K., & Chakraborty, T., (eds.), *Chemical Nanoscience and Nanotechnology: New Materials and Modern Techniques*. Apple Academic–CRC: Waretown, NJ, (In Press).

22. Torrens, F., & Castellano, G. Quantum molecular spintronics, nanoscience and graphenes. In: Haghi, A. K., (ed.), *Molecular Physical Chemistry*. Apple Academic–CRC: Waretown, NJ, (In Press).

23. Torrens, F., & Castellano, G. Cancer and hypotheses on cancer. In: Pogliani, L., Torrens, F., & Haghi, A. K., (eds.), *Molecular Chemistry and Biomolecular Engineering: Integrating Theory and Research with Practice*. Apple Academic–CRC: Waretown, NJ, (In Press).

24. Torrens, F., & Castellano, G. Precision personalized medicine from theory to practice: Cancer. In: Haghi, A. K., (ed.), *Molecular Physical Chemistry*. Apple Academic–CRC: Waretown, NJ, (In Press).

25. Torrens, F., & Castellano, G., (2014). AIDS destroys immune defenses: Hypothesis. *New Front. Chem., 23*, 11–20.

26. Torrens-Zaragozá, F., & Castellano-Estornell, G., (2015). Emergence, spread and uncontrolled Ebola outbreak. *Basic Clin. Pharmacol. Toxicol., 117*(2), 38–38.

27. Torrens, F., & Castellano, G., (2014). Spread/uncontrolled Ebola outbreak. *New Front. Chem.*, *24*, 81–91.

28. Torrens, F., & Castellano, G., (2016). Ebola virus disease: Questions, ideas, hypotheses and models. *Pharmaceuticals*, *9*, 14–6–6.

29. Torrens, F., & Castellano, G. Metaphors that made history: Reflections on philosophy/science/DNA. In: Haghi, A. K., (ed.), *Molecular Physical Chemistry*. Apple Academic-CRC: Waretown, NJ, (In Press).

30. Torrens, F., & Castellano, G. Scientific integrity/ethics: Science communication and psychology. In: Haghi, A. K., (ed.), *Molecular Physical Chemistry*. Apple Academic–CRC: Waretown, NJ, (In Press).

31. Torrens, F., & Castellano, G. Capital vs. nature contradiction and inclusive spreading of science. In: Haghi, A. K., (ed.), *Concepts, Theories, and Trends in Physical Chemistry*. Apple Academic–CRC: Waretown, NJ, (In Press).

32. Torrens, F., & Castellano, G. Reflections on (Palaeo)climate/global changes: Past/present/future. In: Haghi, A. K., (ed.), *Physical Chemistry for the Life Sciences*. Apple Academic – CRC, Waretown, NJ, (In Press).

33. Borja, I., & Sanz, J., (2013). *Els Discursos de la Ciència: Joan Fuster i la Democratització del Coneixement*. Càtedra Joan Fuster No. 16, Universitat de València: València, Spain.

34. Ecologistes en Acció València, personal communication.

CHAPTER 12

NANOBIOCOMPOSITES, BIOMIMETIC NANOCOMPOSITES, AND BIOLOGICALLY INSPIRED NANOCOMPOSITES

SHRIKAANT KULKARNI

Assistant Professor, Vishwakarma Institute of Technology, Department of Chemical Engineering, 666, Upper Indira Nagar, Bibwewadi, Pune – 411037, India. Mobile: +91-9970663353

*Corresponding author. E-mail: shrikaant.kulkarni@vit.edu

ABSTRACT

Natural nanobiocomposites as the name itself implies, are the composite materials having natural origin with structure on the nanoscale; biomimetic nanocomposites are synthetically derived nanocomposite materials by the processes that mimic the biology of their naturally occurring counterparts in terms of their function, biocompatibility, and biodegradability; and biologically inspired nanocomposites are the ones which are created through processes that are inspired by either a biological process or a biological material, but neither by attempting to mimic their naturally occurring counterparts, or directly copying the mechanism by virtue of which biological material is formed. This chapter takes an overview of natural nanobiocomposites, biomimetic nanocomposites, and biologically inspired synthetic nanocomposites.

12.1 INTRODUCTION

Nanostructured and nanocomposite materials commonly encountered in biology are created by self-organization and directed assembly of naturally occurring macromolecules and inorganic materials. Over the last decade, materials scientists and chemists have undertaken considerable research initiatives to design and develop synthetic analogs by trying to mimic biology of their natural counterparts and, more importantly, to ascertain the design protocols of the systems having biological origin. Efforts have also been made to create innovative materials on learning from the way biological materials form, with properties distinct from the incumbent biological systems. Natural materials no doubt possess exquisite properties not observed in synthetic materials and therefore all the efforts are directed towards designing and developing application driven synthetic materials. Biological systems are amenable to produce exquisite materials at or near ambient temperature in aqueous environments, as against most of the synthetic ones which produce often inferior materials to natural analogs demand drastic temperature and pressure conditions as well as and hazardous chemicals [1–3].

Biological nanocomposite materials can be either inorganic, organic in entirety, or a combination of both organic and inorganic ones. The final material derived by one or the other synthetic processes may not have a structure necessarily belonging to a particular class or family of organic materials. E.g. a biological nanocomposite in which the organic material loses its character in the ultimate product is the enamel of the mature human tooth, which is hydroxyapatite (95% by wt). During tooth formation, enamel does consist of a composite of proteins (primarily amelogenin and enamelin) and hydroxyapatite; however, as the tooth develops the proteins are found to be removed. The presence of the proteins, and the organized self-assembled structures formed by them with other biological macromolecules, however are instrumental in generating the final structure of the enamel, which imparts the observed toughness property. The best known example of a combination of inorganic and organic structural composite wherein both the phases remain intact in the final product is the aragonitic nacreous layer of the abalone shell, with outstanding strength attributed to its organic/inorganic layered nanocomposite structure, in which ceramic layers (crystalline) are interfaced with highly organic layers (elastic). However, exceptional properties of the abalone shell are not only due to its layered structure but according to many researchers there may many other factors yet be unraveled which are responsible for their characteristic behavior . Synthetic routes or pathways adopted over last about 10 years to create such a structure which resemble with the abalone shell, till now the developed material has properties quite inferior than its natural analog (abalone shell). Thus the synthetic structures have limited applications due to their poor characteristics profile. However, with the advent and advancement in many exciting scientific discoveries, technologies and tools made over the time, there is huge promise and potential for the design and development of innovative materials in the near future [4].

Many more attempts to mimic biology have not been fructified much in generating engineering materials as one would have expected. Biological materials are characterized by their formation over a span of days to years, consisting of limited set of elements, and are designed for use within a given temperature range. However synthetically derived engineering materials have to be made rapidly (hours or minutes) and generally should work over a broad range of temperature and other environmental conditions. The mismatch between the demands of engineering materials and of biological materials has led many scientists to rethink their strategy, that rather than going for directly copying biology, a much better philosophy would be understand from biology, the mechanism of how biological systems work and translate this knowledge to develop new synthetic materials. This may or may not involve the use of some biological molecules, but certainly not to 'copy' biological processes per se [5].

The development of solids possessing well defined nanometer-scale structures and properties is a huge challenge of immense interest in the synthesis of novel materials. The techniques ranging from scanning microscopy to molecular self-assembly have come up over the time for the creation of nanostructured materials [6–14]. Careful control and maneuvering of molecular architecture, self-assembly can yield many different configurations of nanostructured organics. There is an enormous potential in creating novel materials by mineralizing, polymerizing, or replicating these organized structures and is quite interesting too. E.g. mineral growth within and at the surface of lipid aggregates has led to the formation of unexpected morphologies, like mineralized tubules and disks [15, 16]. Coassembly of molecular species and mineral-phase precursors into mesoporous template structure is an another approach which can be adopted to control mineral growth through self-assembly. This methodology has been materialized in the widely investigated development of mesoporous oxides [17–23].

12.2 NATURALLY OCCURRING NANOCOMPOSITE MATERIALS

Biology has many examples possessing nanoscale structures, and the functionality shown by these materials is due to the nanoscale dimensions of the structure. Lipid cellular membranes, ion channels, proteins, DNA, actin, spider silk, etc. are few examples of nanoscale materials in Biology. All of these structures, possess 1D, and often 3D, nanoscale structures. The properties of many of the biological materials are having nanoscale structure and, as the matrix is composed of discrete nanoscale building blocks, these can be considered as nanocomposite materials. For example, proteins in their active form (folded) are composed of domains with varying degree of hydrophilic and hydrophilicity character, as well as alpha helixes, beta sheets, and turns as structural features (configurations). The assembly of proteins into these complex structures having nano-sized domains with different chemical properties gives proteins, and many other biomolecules, their intriguing properties. Because these chemically distinct domains by virtue of their acidic, basic, hydrogen-bonding, hydrophilic, or hydrophobic behavior, can interact in many different ways with different substrates (minerals). Host of the inorganic/organic composite materials are formed by these highly complex biomolecular structures.

12.3 ORGANIC NANOCOMPOSITE

Organic nanocomposite with outstanding properties, with best example as Dragline spider silk, makes up the spokes of a spider web, is tougher by five folds than steel by weight and can stretch 30%–40% without rupturing. However, the elastic modulus of silk is far less than that of steel. Applications which demand flexibility and toughness in preference, a synthetic pathway to synthesize a material with properties close to spider silk would be exceedingly important. The strong core of spider silk is constituted primarily by two protein components that self-assemble into regions of crystallinity and non-crystallinity. The crystalline regions (alternating alanine-rich blocks), impart hardness [24–26], while the amorphous or non-crystalline regions (glycine-rich blocks), impart elasticity [27]. An amorphous organic matrix is responsible for the exceptional properties of spider silk in the nanocomposite structure of organic nanocrystals.

Mere knowledge of the molecular structure of spider silk will not suffice the needs of creating a synthetic material with requisite properties.

Inside the spider, the silk precursor (lyotropic liquid crystal) exists as 50% silk. As the silk is excreted, the protein molecules that constitute silk fold are aligned as they interact followed by moving through the spinneret, resulting into a complex and insoluble nanostructured fiber. The spider silk made up of crystalline (highly or less oriented crystals) and amorphous regions [28, 29]. The less oriented crystalline regions may help to bridge the highly oriented crystalline regions with the amorphous ones mechanically. This three-phase morphological structure has properties superseding a similar kind of two-phase system because of better cohesion between the phases, ascribed to the small difference in mechanical properties leading to better interfacial adhesion between the various domains.

Recently, a synthetic spider silk-like material with properties approaching those of natural spider silk has been created. Because of their high complexity, the silk precursors could not be created by conventional organic synthesis but by expressing two of the dragline silk genes in mammalian cells [30]. The resulting soluble recombinant dragline silk proteins were wet-spun into fibers of diameters (10 to 40 μ). After a postspinning draw, fibers with mechanical properties close to natural spider silk were obtained. The fibers were highly birefringent, showing a high degree of chain orientation, but it is not yet known whether the internal nanostructure of the fibers resemble with that of natural spider silk or otherwise. Work is now underway to have a herd of goats (transgenic) that express spider silk proteins and excrete them in their milk, sufficient enough for silk protein manufacturing.

12.3.1   SELF ASSEMBLY

Natural organic/inorganic nanocomposites are also formed through self-assembly. The two extremes of the mechanism for formation of natural nanocomposites involve either the formation of organic matrix first, followed by mineralization, or the organic and inorganic materials assemble together into the nanostructured composite. However there is no example to show that the inorganic structure forms first, followed by organic structure as per first mechanism. Most biological composites appear to form through the first route; an organic structure forms first, followed by the nucleation directed biologically and the growth of a mineral phase subsequently. However, it is also observed that the organic matrix restructures and reorganizes continuously as the mineral deposits, which is similar to the second mechanism. Given both of these mechanisms, the organic material is normally composed of an host of diverse macromolecules, proteins and other biopolymers.

12.4   BIOLOGICAL NANOCOMPOSITES

Biological nanocomposites are the ones in which the mineral phase is simply deposited onto or interspersed within an organic matrix structure. Further higher level of complexity is shown by examples in which the structure of the mineral phase is clearly influenced by the organic matrix structure. The greatest complexity is where the mineral is associated with the organic phase intimately to a structure with distinct and superior properties to those of either the mineral or organic phase in isolation.

12.4.1   BIOLOGICALLY SYNTHESIZED NANOPARTICLES

The simplest example of a biological nanocomposite, is grasses. Many grass species precipitate silica (SiO_2) nanoparticles as a part of their cellular structures. These silica nanoparticles found within the cells have varying degrees of morphologies like sheet, globular, or rod-like, with characteristic nanoscale range which vary from few to tens of nm [31]. The cause of silica precipitation by the cells is yet to be ascertained, although it may simply be the way in which the plant sequesters silica nanoparticles, which it continuously absorbs in the form of some silica-containing soluble species. If the plant fails to sequester silica, it would accumulate which has a potential to limit growth. The plant may be unaccepted as food at very high concentrations of silica in them [32], e.g., the species horsetails contains (20%–25% wt.) of silica, magnetic bacteria, contain magnetite (Fe_3O_4) nanocrystals (40 nm in diameter) exhibit a net magnetic moment, when subjected to the earth's magnetic field align themselves in the direction of magnetic field. The direction of their locomotion is attributed to the presence of these magnetic (Fe_3O_4) nanocrystals. The behavior of an individual magnetic bacterium, points in a preferred direction, and continuously explores fresh territory as it moves on unlike a bacterium follows a random walk which is bereft of magnetic nanoparticles exhibit random walk, thus the latter lowers the probability of movement into fresh territory. Other bacteria precipitating mineral greigite (Fe_3S_4) within their cell structures behave in the similar fashion as to those containing magnetite (Fe_3O_4) nanocrystals.

12.4.2   *BIOLOGICALLY SYNTHESIZED NANOSTRUCTURES*

Nanostructures and nanocomposite materials synthesized by biological organisms are much complex than nanoparticles. These structures are found different forms, right from needles and plates to complex 3D nanostructures, and are characterized by many distinct and exciting chemical, mechanical, and optical properties. Biological nanostructure formation pathways are although difficult to describe in a single mechanism, as there may several routes followed for their formation. The order of preference may be first biological structure forms first, followed by inorganic phase. It means that the organic matrix forms first, limiting the growth of the inorganic filler material phase. However, that the organic matrix is polymeric which is prone to deformation in response to the growing inorganic phase.

Bacteria are amenable to form more complex nanostructures apart from nanoparticles. Bacteria in general are instrumental in a vast amount of mineral deposition and can contribute substantially to mineral deposits at the bottom of water bodies. Mineral formation, e.g., gypsum ($CaSO_4$) in the close neighborhood of bacteria is generally driven by a biologically induced change in the pH or ionic strength in the vicinity of individual bacteria due to their respiration. This localized change in the environment lowers the dissolution tendency of certain mineral compounds, effecting their precipitation. A layer of proteins (S-layer) on the bacteria surface are responsible for the alteration in the structure of minerals deposited, in the form of complex nanostructures by templating [33, 34]. The exact mechanism of the mineral templating is yet to be elicited, but preferred adsorption sites on the S-layer must be responsible for heterogeneous nucleation of mineral, rather than a regular structure. During the growth of the mineral nuclei, they agglomerate, resulting into a thin, but periodically structured film of gypsum. The complexity of this structure is attributed to the pores resulted in the inorganic layer which may permeate the bacterium to exchange nutrients with its surroundings subsequent to the mineral phase formation. Formation of a dense solid film of Gypsum, would inhibit the respiration of bacteria, thereby killing it. Inorganic nanostructures of these length scales are of immense importance for varied high technology applications. Genetically engineered bacteria which express proteins and form S-layers can form technologically significant nanostructures for advanced applications and there is huge potential in biosynthesizing materials.

Higher forms of organisms too create inorganic/organic composite structures. For example, the sea urchin spine is a single crystal containing calcite (inorganic material), with only about 0.02% glycoproteins (organic material) trapped within the crystal lattice of the spine [35]. However, this very small amount of organic matter (glycoproteins) imparts the extremely high toughness and distinct fracture properties of the spine. The spine is found to be much tougher against its synthetic counterpart containing either single-crystalline or polycrystalline calcite. Fracture mode of the spine is amazing and the fracturing is found to take place along a preferred crystallographic direction, in semblance with most single crystals, and has conchoidal cleavage (smooth rounded fracture surface), just like glassy materials quite unlike most of the crystalline ceramic materials. The toughening mechanism is still not fully known but is partially due to the dispersion of nanoscale protein molecules in the crystal lattice of spine (matrix).

Another sea creature named abalone that creates an organic/inorganic composite that is of tremendous importance from the point of view of creature's survival. The nacreous (mother-of pearl) layer of the abalone shell consists of alternating layers of aragonite platelets (500-nm-thick) and an organic matrix sheets (30-nm-thick). The thickness and strength of the composite structure is attributed to matrix. The composite structure shows a fracture toughness 3000 times more than inorganic aragonite [32]. The organic matrix defines not only crystallographic orientation of aragonite plates but also limit their size and shape.

Another excellent example of a biological nanocomposite with complex structure and function is bone. Bone must exhibit multifaceted role. It must be characterized by high strength, yet low weight; it must respond to applied stresses, in such a way that it doesn't deform under the applied stress; it must adequately porous to allow oxygen and nutrients to diffuse to the cells within the bone, The pores can't lead to fractures; finally, it must work as a storage for minerals, but simultaneously should not allow itself to demineralize and thereby weaken. Bone exists in several forms; lamellar bone provides the structural properties of long bones in mammals and other species and is the subject of the following discussion, adapted from [36, 37]. The basic structure of bone is a mineralized collagen fibril ($\approx$65% mineral), and the remainder is organic material and water. The collagen phase of bone consists of individual fibrils ($\approx$ 80–100 nm diameter). These fibrils further are in turn consists of triple helix of polypeptide chains assemblies (diameter 1.5 nm and length 300 nm). The mineral phase of the bone is carbonated apatite $(Ca_5(PO_4,CO_3)_3(OH))$, which develops as platelets (50-nm-long, 25-nm-wide, 1.5–4 nm thick). These platelets lie within the collagen fibrils, with only a small number of polypeptide chains between each platelet responsible for maximizing the compressive strength of the bone.

Bone is an excellent example of a self-healing biological nanocomposite in which an organic host phase is formed, followed by highly regulated mineralization processes. The exact mechanism for this whole process is not known clearly, but substantial progress is being made in understanding it. Clearly, biological systems can create a host of diverse inorganic materials; however, although they are limited in terms of material selection. Metals, polymers, semiconductors, and ceramics cannot be synthesized by biological processes, because of non-availability of the suitable precursors in the natural environment, the precursors are hazardous, and/or the product is unstable in the presence of water and/or oxygen. All this has triggered a serious interest in mimicking the biological systems to develop synthetic nanocomposites from materials other than those found in biology, thus fulfilling the demands of both the biological and synthetic worlds.

12.4.3 BIOLOGICALLY DERIVED SYNTHETIC NANOCOMPOSITES

There is an immense interest in exploring the sophisticated mechanisms adopted by biological systems in order to design the synthetic procedures to create innovative and novel materials nanostructures with potentially, unique properties which otherwise would be difficult to obtain. Purely biological routes have been followed only a limited types of materials. It is difficult or impossible to synthesize the unique building blocks in the laboratory like proteins, DNA, RNA, and many other small but highly functional molecules which are offered by Biology.

12.4.4 PROTEIN-BASED NANOSTRUCTURES

Protein S-layers on the surface of bacteria are responsible for creating complex synthetic nanostructures. The variety in S-layer structures, with their chemical functionalization potential, make them ideal candidates for the synthesis of nanostructures. S-layers are 2D protein crystals that have oblique, square, or hexagonal lattice symmetry with lattice constants between 3 and 30 nm. An amenable to potential nanostructure formation, and thereby to enable bacterial respiration, S-layers possess characteristic but identical surface chemistry and pore size – properties that cater to the needs of nanostructure and nanocomposite fabrication. S-layer was used to template a periodic structure into a thin metal film (1-nm-thick metal (Ta/W)) having 15-nm holes periodically arranged in a triangular lattice with a lattice constant of 22 nm, by first adsorbing S-layer fragments onto an amorphous carbon support film followed by evaporation of a 1.2-nm thick film of Ta/W onto the S-layer at 408° angle to substrate surface. The transmission electron microscope (TEM), confirms that a metal film contained a periodic array of holes in the S-layer template [38, 39]. Creating such a nanostructure today in itself would still be a great challenge, even with a modern tools e-beam lithography system, an S-layer was used to create nanostructured semiconductor films of the semiconductor CdS [13] again confirmed by TEM [32].

12.4.5   DNA-TEMPLATED NANOSTRUCTURES

DNA holds a great promise and potential as a building block for nano-composite materials. It can be linked to a wide range of substrates, with specificities that supersede any of the synthetic molecule, is robust, can be synthesized on mass scale relatively, and can be functionalized by attaching fluorescent molecules for the rapid detection of binding moieties. The use of DNA to assemble and develop nanocomposites and nanostructures is only in its infancy, and the preliminary work done so far however indicates the huge potential of DNA-based assembly techniques hold.

A few of the approaches that have been investigated so far include:

- the mineralization of DNA,
- the ususe of DNA to assemble nanoparticles, and
- the uuse of DNA to assemble much larger colloidal particles.

However, the number of possibilities is very large, and substantial work on DNA-mediated assembly of nanostructures is currently underway. The use of plasmid DNA as a template for mineralization was first explored in 1996 [40]. The best example of DNA-mediated nanostructure can be seen in the nanoparticle assembly [41], which could be examined by UV/visible spectroscopy, because the absorption characteristics of gold nanoparticles change greatly when they aggregate, due to changes in the surface plasmon.

This is similar to the approach used to make DNA-linked aggregates; however, because each nanoparticle contains only one DNA strand, hybridization doesn't form an aggregated structure, but rather, dimmers, Trimers of gold nanoparticles were also developed with the help of a similar approach, except that nanoparticles with one strand of DNA of three different sequences was mixed with a strand of DNA complimentary to all three of the DNA strands on the surface of the nanoparticles [42, 43]. Recently, it was observed that DNA can assemble much larger colloidal particles into 3D assemblies with shapes controlled. The approach is very similar to the nanoparticles assembly; however, here the findings after hybridization are assemblies of colloidal particles with controlled connectivity [44].

12.4.5.1   PROTEIN ASSEMBLY

To achieve a same level of complexity to that which can be obtained by DNA-based assembly, one can genetically engineer or identify biological organisms that recognize and bind with a great degree of specificity to selective minerals, semiconductors, and metals. For example, *Escherichia coli* containing genetic sequences specific for recognizing and binding iron oxide but not other metal surfaces was identified and multiplied. Bacteria that would specifically adhere to iron oxide were identified via serial enrichment from a population of bacteria [45].

The experimental procedure was as follows: A population of genetically engineered *E. coli* was exposed to iron oxide (Fe_2O_3) particles. The bacteria that adhered to the iron oxide were collected, and the leftover were discarded. After repeating this procedure several times, bacteria with high degree of specificity for iron oxide were obtained. Only a selective bacterial bind to iron oxide particles which have the unique genetic disposition express proteins on their outer surface whose sequences are a function of their genetic makeup.

It is also possible to identify protein sequences that preferentially attach to specific metal surfaces, and also to metal nanoparticles., A library of 107 different polypeptides 14 or 28 amino acids long was developed on undertaking various biological experiments. Then, the polypeptides that bind selectively to the metal surface were isolated, and their sequences were determined [46]. This approach is very powerful because of the large number of molecular sequences that can be examined simultaneously in a single experiment. From a technological point of view, it is exciting to explore the possibility of identifying semiconductor surfaces and semiconductor nanoparticles with the help of this procedure [47]. The fallout of mixing a nanoparticle-binding phage with nanoparticles is 'decoration' of the phage with nanoparticles, with the phage that contains the polypeptide with specific binding sites [48]. Depending on the experimental conditions and phage design, it may even be possible to bind single nanoparticles to an individual phage or assemble the nanoparticles into defined architectures, although these days multiple nanoparticles are artistically are decorated in a random fashion on a phage.

12.5   BIOLOGICALLY INSPIRED NANOCOMPOSITES

The characteristic properties of biocomposites and synthetic routes adopted for their design and development are the driving forces for conduction wide spread research in this area. However, there was a misconception earlier that it is not always necessary or even desirable to use biologically derived materials for host of applications and that it may be possible simply to use biology as a cue for synthetically derived nanocomposites. It is, however, quite interesting to regard biological systems as an inspiration for nanocomposites by virtue of their unique characteristics that would be most sought after in synthetic materials. However, direct mimicking of biology will be confined to a handful of specific materials and nanostructures. However, thoroughly studying the mechanisms followed by biological systems will help go a long way in learning how to form complicated nanostructures and the potential property profile of these synthetic derived nanostructures, should provide a roadmap in successfully synthesizing them. Of course, just a semblance between the synthetic material and a natural process or the process of forming that material and a natural synthesis does not necessarily mean that the scientists and engineers were inspired by biological mechanisms.

Much can be learned from biological systems to further the development of synthetic approaches to the formation of complex inorganic structures through routes to nanostructure formation like:

- liquid crystal templating;
- colloidal particle templating;
- block copolymer templating;
- surfactant-inorganic self-assembly (mesoporous silica being the most famous of this approach to nanostructure formation) invokes many of the tenets of biologically directed mineral growth.

As discussed earlier, biological systems rely on self-assembly and mineralization in the synthesis of hard inorganic structures such as shells, teeth, and bone [11], and their approaches to materials fabrication can give rise to synthetic systems. Often, the term 'biomimetic' has been applied to any approach using biological mechanisms for the self-assembly in the synthesis of nanocomposite materials.

Biological systems use both self-assembling molecules, and great levels of molecular organization as a very vital part of an organism's inorganic structure development. However, it would be difficult to simulate this process but at the infancy stage in the laboratory. Biological processes are greatly dynamic, with very specific proteins and other molecules being created and transported in huge numbers to very specific locations, with control of high order. The well known synthetic systems are nothing but simple approximations of life and generally are too primitive to be considered as those which are mimicking biology in true sense. Although the synthetic systems are simple approximations of biological systems, still lot much can be learnt by trying for mimicking the living systems [8]. For example, the synthesis of mineral phases in a self-organized matrix have truely mimicked many biological systems as far as the mineralization processes of them is concerned. Many examples of matrix-mediated biological mineralization processes can be cited like the reliance of bacteria, plants, shells, and even mammals on organically driven growth of mineral phases to remediate byproducts (bacteria and plants) [31, 33, 34], create exoskeletons (shells) [49], and grow teeth (mammals) [35]. If during the synthetic process, organic molecules are introduced into the mineral phase, the material resulting may have a semblance with the spicule of a sea urchin, which possess (<1%) protein distributed into the crystal lattice [35].

Although synthetic systems have low degree of sophistication, still they do have comparative advantages over their biological counterparts. Biological systems operate with the use of small number of elements and compounds, unlike synthetic systems which can be designed to use a broad range of elements and compounds, many of which would be hazardous to the health of most of biological organisms. The comparative account between biological and synthetic systems based on various parameters is given in Table 12.1.

TABLE 12.1 Comparison Between Biological Synthetic Systems

Property	Biological Systems	Synthetic Systems
Temperature	Form and operate near ambient temperature in presence water and oxygen	Form and operate under a wide range temperature and at harsher conditions
Reaction time	More (days to months)	Less
Response to external stimuli	Positively responds in time, e.g., bone	May not respond positively like biological ones
Time scales and applications	Long time scales for formation, limited applications	Short time scales for formation, wider applications
Self assembly	Wide range of composites and inorganic nanostructures synthesized	Narrow range of composites and inorganic nanostructures synthesized

Biological systems have large amounts of lipids (soap-like molecules), many biological macromolecules, including proteins which self-assemble to form the cell membranes, and smaller vesicles within the cell. These membranes provide the protection to the cell contents, and to provide synthetic microreactors for biological processes. The syntheses in self-assembled microreactors is biologically inspired in that sense, has been used to the advantage by many investigators to synthesize nanoparticles and nanocomposites.

Zero-dimensional nanomaterials are, called as nanoparticles. The study of semiconductor nanoparticles in general is of great interest, because the electronic and optical properties of them change substantially as the particles reduced to the nanoscale regime, which is attributed to the quantum confinement of electrons within the particle, although surface-area to volume ratio also play a vital role [50–52]. The most sought after nanoparticles for fundamental studies belonged to semiconductor particles (II–VI group), due to their scientifically and technologically exciting properties. Synthetic methodologies for the creation of metal sulfide and selenide quantum dots and their assembly into higher-order architectures have been studied widely [53–57]. Metal sulfides and other semiconductors, to be obtained in nanostructures one of the characteristic dimension should at least be <10 nm [58].

Semiconducting nanoparticles are generally synthesized through following routes:

- Grinding of coarse chunks, generally generates a very polydisperse particles, and introduces too many contaminates for most applications.
- Gas-phase synthesis is essentially a vaporization and condensation process – a crucible containing the desired semiconductor (or other material) is heated until it starts to sublime, and then an inert carrier gas is flown over the material. The carrier gas then is then made to pass through a cool region where the gaseous semiconductor atoms or molecules condense into nanoparticles and are collected [59]. This method is fairly versatile, but demands high temperature and vacuum and generally forms solid spherical particles.
- Solution-based synthetic pathways for nanoparticle creation have ranged from simple precipitation reactions to much more complex self-assembly-based routes. In general, simple precipitation leads to formation of agglomerates of nanoparticles, and the size distribution generally varies widely. These problems led to research into synthetic procedures that would result in nanoparticles that are stable and have narrow size distributions. Solution-phase synthesis of semiconductors is often preferred, because it is mild (carried out at ambient temperature and pressures) and can be used to form reasonably good volumes of semiconductor- quantum dots, particles with low polydispersities and novel optical properties [50, 51, 56, 57, 60]. It is even possible to cap the surface of the particles with organic molecules, which controls the size of nanoparticles [53, 55].
- The more conventional route to creating nanostructured materials is of course through top-down lithographic methods [61, 62], electron beam writing [63], focused ion-beam lithography [64], x-ray-lithography [65], scanning probe lithography [66], and microcontact printing [67].

All these techniques can create nanostructures on the scale ranging from tens to hundreds of nanometers, only on very flat substrates, can be quite slow and expensive. Of course, the general problem with self-assembly is that it is not possible to highly control the spatial position of the nanostructure exactly, and thus it is still a long way to go before we create highly functional self-assembled electronic circuits.

12.5.1   MICELLAR ROUTES TO NANOPARTICLE FORMATION

Micelles are self-assembled structures formed from surfactant molecules and at least one of the precursors of the inorganic nanoparticles is in solution. The result is that every micelle in solution work as vast numbers of discrete nanoreactors which individually contain a given concentration of precursor of the inorganic phase. A given number of nanoparticles per micelle may be formed on reaction between precursor and reductant or so. The overall polydispersity is thus influenced by the micelle size. If it is made possible to create a mechanical dispersion of micelles of similar size, then it would be easy to create a colloidal solution containing nanoparticles with a very narrow size distribution. The use of complex macromolecules to form particles of only a specific size can be done by taking cues from biology. A virus particle is a best example of potential nanoreactors to mimick from biology. Nanoparticles with right size distributions if we can load the interior of the virus particles with the precursors and reductants, capping agents, etc.

   Most of the nanoparticle synthesis pathways created solid semiconductor nanoparticles with spherical morphology. However, the synthesis of complex morphologies is exciting and interesting, because even advanced and sophisticated techniques like e-beam lithography produce nanoparticles of the order of 10 nm, which are often considered as too large to lie in desired quantum confinement and other desired properties [63]. Hence, e-beam patterning or other top-down processing routes fail to produce complex morphologies. The possibility of creating complicated morphologies was studied for CdS nanoparticles which formed dendritic structures under Langmuir monolayers [68]. Subsequently, strategies that are based on self-assembly were used for the synthesis of complex morphologies other than spherical for semiconductor nanoparticles. Alivisatos and coworkers [69, 70] demonstrated the formation of nanocrystals of CdSe nanorods with aspect ratios of 30:1, as well as arrow-, teardrop-, tetrapod-, and branched tetrapod- morphologies [69, 70].

12.5.2   SEMICONDUCTOR NANOSTRUCTURES

These composite materials exhibit novel properties significantly higher than either the inorganic or organic phase alone, as has actually been found in a vast range of materials. Composite materials having toughness

[71–73], increased thermal stability [74], sophisticated electronically [75,76], enhanced chemical selectivity [77] have been developed over the time. Even without the organic phase, periodically nanostructured semiconductors have huge promise and potential in the field of solid-state science and technology attributed to their both electronic and catalytic activity. A periodically nanostructured semiconductor might showcase itself as an array of antidots (a material with a periodic array of scattering centers closely spaced than the mean free path of electrons traveling through them) [78,79].

The emphasis earlier was on synthesis of nanoparticles with lower polydispersity index, and not on developing superlattice structures. However, by way of controlled growth and chemical functionality, nanocrystals of many materials, have been obtained in the form of superlattice structures [55]. These structures may exhibit properties over and above simple quantum effects. The individual crystallites in these structures are characterized by segregated thin layers of organic molecules rather than continuous mineral structures, which contain self-assembling molecules used for the cause of regulating the diameter and polydispersity of the nanoparticles. During synthesis, the organic phase self-assembles to form a shell (cap) around the nanoparticles, imparting solubility to the nanoparticles, thereby provide better processing ability in tune with the organic compounds. Because of the controlled orderliness in the size and shape, these nanoparticles (organically coated) assemble into crystalline form with long range periodicity,similar to the behavior of other organic materials. The next level of complexity in nanostructure formation is the development of nanostructures with complex, and requisite morphologies. Here, self-assembly and nanostructure formation (biological concepts) are applicable most. For example, in biology, complex predefined structures at nanometer scale is very common, although the length scale is extremely difficult to control in synthetic materials. However, self-assembly in conjunction with the materials synthesis strategies known so far, hold great potential for the creation of complex composite nanostructures.

12.6   LIQUID-CRYSTAL TEMPLATING FOR INORGANIC NANOSTRUCTURES

This approach is aimed at imparting the periodic structure (organizational order) of liquid crystals to a mineral phase. Liquid crystals offers an ideal matrix for the formation of nanocomposite materials, because in liquid crystals too possess the characteristic 1–10 nm length scales similar to that shown by semiconductor nanostructures. Furthermore, the periodicity in the liquid crystals structure can have very long-range order, and thus subsequently the periodic nanostructure also has huge potential for long-range order, which is of great interest in many of the applications. Creation of long-range nanoperiodic order in materials such as semiconductors by using liquid-crystal templating approach is therefore a goal of many of the research groups across the world. Semiconductor nanocomposite structures with long-range periodicity come in several forms, like an array of embedded second phase material, a thin film with a periodic topography, or a periodically porous material. Highly porous,. Periodically nanostructured semiconductor materials could be quite interesting from the point of view of solution-based chemistry. For example, semiconducting phase with photoconductivity and zeolite-like pore structure together could make them right candidates for photochemical degradation of health hazardous compounds or for conducting the shape-selective chemistry. Thin films may be of great technological importance, due to wide range of their potential uses both as supported and freestanding thin films. Further if we could predefine a nanoperiodic array of features in semiconductor thin films it may open up new vistas of application areas, like electronic devices, sensors, and filter membranes. Three-dimensional semiconductor structures may have unique optical or electronic properties, based on their characteristic length scale.

12.6.1   LYOTROPIC LIQUID-CRYSTAL TEMPLATING

Lyotropic liquid-crystal templating is an approach for nanocomposite formation that makes use of the self-assembled structure of a liquid crystal to control the structural growth of an inorganic material. When thus the liquid crystal provides a 'template' for the inorganic phase then laters structure is a replica the former. The most vital feature of liquid crystal templating of inorganic material is the lyotropic liquid crystal. Lyotropic liquid crystals contain of two covalently bonded components, one of which is usually an amphiphile, which is a molecule with two or more physically distinct components, and the other a solvent. The amphiphile is hydrophobic, and the solvent is hydrophilic, e.g., soaps. The dual properties of an amphiphile lead to the quite interesting self-assembly of these molecules in solution by means of surface segregation, formation of micelles [80,81] and vesicles [82,83], as well as host of LC structures [84,85].

Amphiphiles exhibit very rich, and complex phase behavior with variation in solvent concentration. In the dilute amphiphiles, micelles form, and in the concentrated amphiphiles (even solvent free), some amphiphiles exhibit either liquid crystalline or crystalline phases [86].

The three most common phases observed in mixtures of water and amphiphile are:

- hexagonal,
- lamellar; and
- cubic.

Similar to the structures observed for block copolymers [87], lyotropic liquid crystals can be designed and developed in congruence with the volume fraction of the various components [88, 89].

Nanostructured inorganics formed in many mesoporous oxide systems use coassembly, as the process by which, many biological processes use the order found in a preformed structure. The order present in an organic mesophase has been utilized to directly template the growth of an inorganic mesophase; liquid crystal templating has been the most sought after and powerful technique for the said purpose. Morphologies with oblong or cubic crystallites or microporous reticulated structures have been obtained in the earlier efforts [90–92]. In the recent past, by using liquid-crystal templating, the periodically nanostructured semiconductors have been synthesized which duplicate the symmetry and dimensionality of the precursor liquid crystal [11, 93–96]. Liquid-crystal templating seems to be a general pathway for synthesizing semiconductor nanostructures [103, 104]. When compared the characteristic dimensions of the materials synthesized by liquid-crystal templating with lithographic techniques former have smaller dimensions than the latter, and are often obtainable by using bulk synthesis, unlike lithography.

The order so obtained in the nanostructured systems was found to be influenced by the counterion for the metal [95]. One advantage of the liquid crystal templating is that there are a great number of amphiphilic liquid crystals, with lattice constants (few nm to tens of nm), and possessing lamellar, hexagonal, cubic, and bicontinuous phases [84,105, 106]. Many of these systems can mineralize, generating an array of novel structures and properties, particularlly, II–VI semiconductor nanostructures [11, 93,

95], a lamellar phase liquid crystal formed from oligo (vinyl alcohol) (23) oleyl ester [93]. Other lyotropic phases, such as a variety of bicontinuous and cubic liquid crystals [84, 105, 107], may also yield interesting mineral nanostructures. Thus, when this molecule is hydrated it forms micelles which pack closely, forming a cubic phase [106]. As a specific example, a hexagonal mesophase (50 vol. % aqueous 0.1 M Cd(OAc)$_2$ and 50 vol. % (EO) 10 oleyl template) an inorganic/organic nanocomposite of CdS and amphiphile when exposed to H2S gas [93, 108–109].

For example, the nanostructures of the semiconducting materials like CdS and ZnS synthesized by precipitation method doped with their nitrate salts have hexagonal symmetry with a periodicity and dimensionality in tune with that of the template. The hexagonal nanostructure however is not necessarily evident in TEM, because of randomly oriented nanoparticles in the field of view [95]. When ZnS is synthesized from its acetate salt as a precursor, only porous, spherical polycrystalline particles are formed. The average particle size of the semiconductor material, both CdS and ZnS synthesized from their respective nitrate salts are approximately five times coarser than created from their acetate salts as precursors because of difference in their electron scavenging behavior. This size difference is clearly evident in low magnification electron micrographs. The lamellar morphology can be confirmed with the help of the TEM [94]. Mineral growth taking place in the hexagonal and lamellar phases result into interesting, and regulated nanostructures. [110]. Although the underlying mechanism is yet to unraveled in totality, the result was hollow spheres with in diameter (20–200 nm), which can be seen in both TEM and SEM [95].

Direct templating of an inorganic by an organic liquid crystal phase may be influenced by following factors :

- the thermodynamic stability of the mesophase throughout the mineral growth process
- the stability of the mesophase while addition of mineral precursors, and
- the order of the liquid crystal governed by the the mineral precipitation process.

Material scientists observed that the textures seen under polarized optical microscopy are the same for the pure mesophase and a mesophase that contains the precursor salt shows that the doping doesn't bring about any radical change in the order in the mesophase. Nuclear magnetic resonance (NMR) can also be used to confirm the structure of liquid crystalline mesophases. 2H NMR spectra obtained from both cadmium ion-doped and undoped mesophases [96] to confirm that the characteristic molecular order of the mesophase was not perturbed to any great extent by ion doping. For both mesophases, the same quadrupole splitting was observed. Ionic doping if disturb the structure of the mesophase, the splitting would decrease [111, 112].

12.6.2   LIQUID-CRYSTAL TEMPLATING FOR THIN FILMS

The liquid crystal templating of thin films by self-assembled organic structures find significant applications in both technology and scientific arena. Thin-film templating is structurally close to the bulk templating of inorganic materials, which generally give rise to periodically structured thin films, which have great potential for different applications. Templating with organic structures is especially unclear as the potential to create structural characteristics scaled down than by almost any top-down approach, because it exploits the nanoscale molecular order inherent in self-assembled organic structures which decides the structure of the ultimate thin film.

A few important points to be kept in mind for the successful thin-film templating by liquid crystals are:

- the self assembled matrix must be compatible with the substrate.
- with some process, the inorganic material must be grown on the substrate by chemical and electrochemical pathways.
- other conventional methods of thin-film deposition demand high vacuum, which is not compatible with lyotropic liquid crystals
- the synthetic routes for liquid-crystal templating of thin films are relatively straightforward.

Most studies have used electrochemical techniques to bring about the material deposition as follows:

- First, a precursor containing lyotropic liquid crystal is interfaced with the substrate.
- Under the influence of an applied potential, material is electrochemically grown at the liquid-crystal/substrate interface.

Nanostructured materials that have been formed through this technique covers a variety range of of metals, selenium, and tellurium [97, 99–104, 113]. It may also be possible to electrodeposit other interesting host of materials like semiconductors.

12.6.3 BLOCK-COPOLYMER TEMPLATING

Block copolymers are a widely studied family of materials that form both 2D and 3D structures at marginally longer length scales than that observed for liquid crystals. Similar kind of phase behavior is observed, with systems interconverting between like lamellar, hexagonal and cubic phases with change in the relative volume fraction of the two blocks [87]. Much more complex morphologies can be created with triblock systems. The block copolymer systems are characterized by the periodicity ranging from about 5 nm to hundreds of nanometers and is influenced by the molecular weight of the block copolymer. The increase in molecular weight of the block copolymer, leads to increase in its characteristic length scale too.

Block copolymers are generally solvent-free and can be subjected to higher temperatures and under vacuum without perturbing the self-assembled structure unlike lyotropic liquid crystals; leading to use of high-vacuum material growth and processing techniques. Usually the chemistry of the block copolymer is designed such that one of the two bocks can be taken off by using dry etch with the help of ozone or other reactive compound to create the porous structured material, which will subsequently work as a template for nanostructure generation.

The procedure for block copolymer templating of nanostructures usually is as follows:

- a thin film of some block copolymer is spun-coated in presence of a solvent over a substrate and allowed to self-assemble.
- one of the blocks of the polymer is taken off by use of ozone etching.
- substrate is coated with a thin polymer film containing a periodic nanoscale void structure.
- removal of solid polymer film if any that covers the void structure, the polymer film is then subsequently used as a mask.
- material can be made to evaporate either through the polymer film to the substrate, or can be grown electrochemically from the substrate

up through the polymer film, or the polymer film can be used as an etch mask.

- the ultimate result is material structured to be a exact replica of either the polymer film (when the polymer is used as an etch mask) or the pore structure of the polymer film (when material is deposited in the pores) in all cases.
- at the end, the polymer film is taken off either with solvent or reactive ion etch, leaving behind nanostructured templated features on a substrate [114–121].

12.6.4   COLLOIDAL TEMPLATING

Biologically inspired nanocomposite materials, should include developments in the recent past on the front of colloidal crystal templating of photonic materials. The primary objective of this approach is to use the 3D periodic structure of synthetic opals to guide the structure of a second phase material. This approach is not exactly biologically inspired, but should more appropriately be called as 'naturally inspired', because opals, although natural, are more of geological in origin, than biological,. Further the characteristic length scale of the material generated is 10–20 nm, the characteristic dimension is often relatively high (500 nm). Most of the applications of these materials are optical, which demands the length scale should not be too small than the wavelength of the light that one desires to tune up. However, the templated structure may be embedded with some smaller features (few nm). Colloidal templating of materials is therefore characterized by inspiration from nature and its relationship with many biological processes.

The interest in microperiodic 3D structures has grown tremendously due to the exciting potential of such materials, particularly in the area of photonics [122]. Such 3D structures, often termed photonic crystals, are the extension of the well-known dielectric stack into three dimensions. Although the colors that occur in opals, which stem from diffraction of white light by planes of highly ordered submicrometer silica spheres, are our inspiration; for practical application, synthetic approaches are needed to create materials and structures with the necessary refractive index and periodicity to meet the requirements for most optical applications, which opals simply do not have.

12.6.5   PHOTONIC BANDGAP MATERIALS

A particularly interesting class of optical structures are the so-called photonic bandgap materials. For example, a microperiodic material consisting of low-refractive-index spheres arranged in a face-centered-cubic array in a matrix with a high index of refraction, and having a lattice constant on the order of the wavelength of light (visible or infrared), could be such a photonic band-gap material [123]. Similar to how a dielectric stack has a stop-band for light in a given frequency range, this material would not allow light in a given frequency range to travel through it in any direction. In essence, it would be an omnidirectional, perfectly lossless, mirror.

The synthesis of these structures however is exceedingly difficult. Layer-by-layer fabrication of photonic crystals using state-of-the-art VLSI tools, e.g., deep UV photolithography, chemical vapor deposition (CVD), chemical-mechanical polishing, has been demonstrated [3], but formidable processing difficulties limit the formation of large area and truly 3D structures. When appropriately formed, self-assembled colloidal crystals are natural candidates for the construction of photonic crystals. Good crystal quality is achieved only with colloids that have very low size polydispersity (<5 %), which currently limits the choice of materials to SiO2 or polymers, both of which have a fairly low index of refraction around 1.5, which is much smaller than that required for most optical applications. This has led researchers to take a two-stage templating approach. In a first step the desired microperiodic structure is assembled by using colloids. In a second step this structure is used as a template to build a complementary structure with a material having a higher index of refraction [124].

A range of approaches have been suggested to maximize the index contrast, including sol–gel [125–127], chemical vapor deposition [128–131], imbibing of nanoparticles [132–134], reduction of GeO_2 to Ge [135], electroless [136] and electrochemical deposition [137], and melt imbibing [138].

In addition, polymers have been used to infill colloidal crystals, and in one report, the colloidal particles were less than 100 nm in diameter, which, although perhaps not interesting from an optical standpoint, may have potential for separation membranes and confined chemical reactor spaces [139].

The sol–gel infilling of colloidal crystal templates is intriguing to consider as a route to 3D porous materials [125–127], although it is somewhat limited in application for photonic materials for several reasons.

Another pathway to macroporous materials is to fill the interstitial space of a colloidal crystal with nanoparticles, followed by removal of the colloidal template. This has some advantages over sol–gel infilling, in that the contraction of the structure upon removal of the template from a nanoparticle filled colloidal crystal is significantly less than that seen upon removal of the template from a sol-gel filled system, and a much larger subset of materials can be prepared as nanoparticles, including semiconductors, metals, and ceramics. The first example of semiconductor nanoparticle infilling of colloidal template used II–VI semiconductor nanoparticles [132]; since then, Er-doped TiO_2 nanoparticles, for example, have been filled into a colloidal template, followed by removal of the template to generate a macroporous solid [140].

The use of CVD as a pathway to filling colloidal crystals at first may seem counterintuitive. After all, CVD generally is most efficient at coating planar surfaces, and it would seem almost impossible to fill structures with deep pores, such as the interstitial space of a 3D colloidal crystal. However, significant strides have been made in the past few years, and now virtually complete infilling of colloidal structures with both Si and Ge via CVD has been demonstrated [128–131].

Electrodeposition-based infilling is intriguing for several reasons and has the potential to be general with respect to both characteristic lattice constant and material.

Semiconductors are interesting candidates for photonic crystals, primarily because of their high refractive indices and generally robust nature. For example, CdS has a refractive index of 2.5, and materials such as GaP, Si, and Ge have indices of 3.4, 3.5, and 4.0, respectively. However, routes to creating periodic macroporous structures from such materials are limited because of their very high melting points and low solubility in common solvents. To date, the II–VI semiconductors CdS and CdSe [137, 141], and ZnO [142], have been electrochemically grown through colloidal templates, resulting, after dissolution of the template, in macroporous semiconductor films.

Real progress in optically interesting materials may await the electrochemical deposition of materials such as GaP, Ge, and Si, which, because they have refractive indices >3, may result in materials with 3D photonic band gaps. Routes to the electrodeposition of such materials have been demonstrated [143], but problems, such as hydrogen gas evolution and generally harsh conditions, need to be solved before success in these areas is likely.

Electrodeposition of conducting polymers (electropolymerization) through self-assembled colloidal crystals, followed by removal of the colloidal template, is a promising route to achieving active macroporous materials.

Electrochemical growth of conducting polymers is a fairly well developed field, and many procedures for growing solid films have been published [144]. There are, however, only a few reports on the growth of porous conducting polymer films. Fibers of polypyrrole, poly(3-methyl-thiophene), and polyaniline were formed in the early 1990s by electrodeposition from the appropriate monomer solution through a porous membrane [145]. The first example of electrochemical deposition of a conducting polymer around a colloidal template was in 1992, when polypyrrole was grown around latex particles [146]. Only in the past few years have researchers been exploring the possibility of the templated growth of conducting polymers for photonic applications.

The general procedure of colloidal templating of conducting polymers involves:

- colloidal crystal formation on a conducting substrate,
- electrochemical deposition or growth from solution, and
- dissolution of the colloidal template with an appropriate solvent.

For example, polypyrrole was grown potentiostatically from a solution of pyrrole in acetonitrile through a colloidal crystal composed of SiO_2 spheres with a mean diameter (238 nm) assembled on F-doped SnO_2-coated glass, subsequent removal of the colloidal template with aqueous HF [147]. Macroporous polypyrrole, polyaniline, and polybithiophene films have been polymerized on similar lines through a colloidal crystal assembled from 500 nm and 750 nm polystyrene spheres, on a substrate of gold coated glass. The polystyrene template was then removed with toluene [148]. Polypyrrole and polythiophene macroporous films were deposited through colloidal crystals assembled from 150 nm and 925 nm polystyrene spheres, on glass deposited with indium tin oxide; the polystyrene was removed with tetrahydrofuran [149].

Metallic macroporous ordered replicas of colloidal assemblies have a wide spectrum of applications including filtration, separation, and catalysis. Further, they might possess quite interesting electrical, magnetic, or optical properties. A well-known example of this is the scarlet red color of a nanosized colloidal dispersion of gold nanoparticles. A latest example of amazing behavior is the substantiallly high light transmission through small holes (<200 nm) shown by thin metallic films [150]. Theoretical calculations [151–153] on ordered 3D arrays of metallo-dielectric spheres show that these techniques show lot much of promise for the design of materials with full photonic bandgap in the visible region of the electromagnetic spectrum.

The advantage of metallo-dielectric structures against pure dielectric structures is that it should be easier to achieve a full band-gap in the visible region which is extremely difficult, to create with latter ones having have an index of refraction >3 and very low absorption in the visible region of the electromagnetic spectrum, This has made it possible to develop synthetic pathways to generate metallo-dielectric colloidal core-shell particles with sizes in the sub-micron range [154, 155] and metallic shell thicknesses or cores small enough to show resonance effects. Vos et al. [156] made gold replicas of colloidal crystals made of silica (radius 113 nm) and polystyrene (radius 322 nm).

There have dimensional stability in the dried, sintered colloid and the final replica, although some cracking is noticed during the drying and sintering process, showing that the electrochemically deposited gold is dense and robust structurally. This is a comparative advantage over other methods like infilling macroporous structures with high-dielectric materials, by employing liquid-phase or sol–gel chemistry [126, 127], and infiltration with nanoscale particles [132], in which tremendous shrinkage of the matrix is seen, which amounts to severe crack formation, and warping of the colloidal structure. Other electrodeposited materials like Ni, Pt, and a SnCo alloy [157, 158], Pd, Pt, and Co [159]; electroless deposition have also been tried [136].

The latest work has shown that templating of the interstitial space of highly ordered colloidal holds a lot much of promise for creating macroporous photonic crystals from a range of materials like oxides, semiconductors, metals, polymers, and glasses. The 3D macroperiodic materials so developed have close-packed macropores ranging in diameter from 100 nm to a few micrometers, providing for modulating light ranging from deep UV to the infrared. However, problems with the infilling technique has to be overcome before this approach to design and develop the photonic structures give promising potential for applications.

12.7 CONCLUSION

The confluence of knowledge drawn from branches like nanoscience, biotechnology, and materials chemistry offers a huge promise and potential for the discovery, design, development and fabrication of innovative and novel advanced composite materials. Biological systems have to be studied thoroughly to explore lot much of information which is yet to be unraveled. However now the focus should be on how current body of knowledge on biological systems can help develop highly functional nanocomposites is of paramount importance which would lead to the creation of advanced materials. For example, many natural systems use to advantage the self-assembly to develop a plethora of highly functional and exciting materials, and today we are creating synthetic systems by mimicking the natural systems. However, we must by adopting the design rules expressed by biological systems as biological organisms work with a limited amount of materials and invest years before they create nanocomposite structures, so, the onus should be on creating the materials not only by direct mimicking of biology, but to create them more productive on applying them to synthetic systems. The investigation biologically inspired nanocomposite materials will therefore go a long way in the time to come for the design and development of demand-driven innovative, novel, advanced synthetic materials for a host of application areas if we tap the maximum potential of it.

KEYWORDS

- **biomimetic nanocomposites**
- **nanobiocomposites**
- **synthetically derived nanocomposites**

REFERENCES

1. Corma, A., (1997). From microporous to mesoporous molecular sieve materials and their use in catalysis. *Chem. Rev., 97*, 2373–2419.
2. Brinker, C. J., (1998). Oriented inorganic films. *Curr. Opin. Colloid Interface Sci., 3*, 166–173.
3. Soten, I., & Ozin, G. A., (1999). New directions in self assembly: Materials synthesis over 'all' length scales. *Curr. Opin. Colloid Interface Sci., 4*, 325–337.
4. Antonietti, M., (2001). Surfactants for novel templating applications. *Curr. Opin. Colloid Interface Sci., 6*, 244–248.
5. Sayari, A., & Hamoudi, S., (2001). Periodic mesoporous silica-based organic: Inorganic nanocomposite materials. *Chem. Mater., 13*, 3151–3168.
6. Stroscio, J. A., & Eigler, D. M., (1991). *Science, 254, 1319–1326.*
7. Whitesides, G. M., Mathias, J. P., & Seto, C. T., (1991). Molecular self-assembly and nanochemistry: A chemical strategy for the synthesis of nanostructures. *Science, 254,* 1312–1319.
8. Mann, S., & Ozin, G. A., (1996). Synthesis of inorganic materials with complex form. *Nature, 382,* 313–318.
9. Braun, P. V. & Stupp, S. I. (1996). Nanostructures: Special Issue: Nanostructured Materials, *Chem. Mater., 8*, 1569–1882.
10. Stupp, S. I., LeBonheur, V., Walker, K., Li, L. S., Huggins, K. E., Keser, M., & Amstutz, A., (1997). Supramolecular materials: Self-organized nanostructures. *Science, 276,* 384–389.
11. Stupp, S. I., & Braun, P. V., (1997). Molecular manipulation of microstructures: Biomaterials, ceramics, and semiconductors. *Science, 277*, 1242–1248.
12. Liu, J., Kim, A. Y., Wang, L. Q., Palmer, B. J., Chen, Y. L., Bruinsma, P., Bunker, B. C., Exarhos, G. J., Graff, G. L., Rieke, P. C., et al., (1996). Self-assembly in the synthesis of ceramic materials and composites. *Adv. Colloid Interface Sci., 69*, 131.
13. Shenton, W., Pum, D., Sleytr, U. B., & Mann, S., (1997). Synthesis of cadmium sulfide superlattices using self-assembled bacterial S-layers. *Nature, 389*, 585–587.
14. Neeraj, R. C. N. R., (1998). Metal chalcogenide-organic nanostructured composites from self-assembled organic amine templates. *J. Mater. Chem., 8*, 279–280.
15. Schnur, J. M., (1993). Lipid tubules: A paradigm for molecularly engineered structures. *Science, 262*, 1669–1676.
16. Archibald, D. D., & Mann, S., (1993). Template mineralization of self-assembled anisotropic lipid microstructures. *Nature, 364*, 430.
17. Kresge, C. T., Leonowicz, M. E., Roth, W. J., Vartuli, J. C., & Beck, J. S., (1992). Ordered mesoporpous molecular sieves synthesized by a liquid crystal template mechanism. *Nature, 359*, 710–712.
18. Beck, J. S., Vartuli, J. C., Kennedy, G. J., Kresge, C. T., Roth, W. J., & Schramm, S. E., (1994). *Chem. Mater., 6*, 1816–1821.
19. Monnier, A., Schuth, F., Huo, Q., Kumar, D., Margolese, D., Maxwell, R. S., Stucky, G. D., Krishnamurty, M., Petroff, P., Firouzi, A., et al., (1993). Cooperative formation of inorganic-organic interfaces in the synthesis of silicate mesostructures. *Science, 261*, 1299–1303.

20. Huo, Q., Margolese, D. I., Ciesla, U., Feng, P., Gier, T. E., Sieger, P., Leon, R., Petroff, P. M., Schuth, F., & Stucky, G. D., (1994). Generalized synthesis of periodic surfactant/inorganic composite materials. *Nature, 368*, 317–321.
21. Firouzi, A., Kumar, D., Bull, L. M., Besier, T., Sieger, P., Huo, Q., Walker, S. A., Zasadzinski, J. A., Glinka, C., Nicol, J., et al., (1995). Cooperative organization of inorganic-surfactant and biomimetic assemblies. *Science, 267*, 1138–1143.
22. Attard, G. S., Glyde, J. C., & Goltner, C. R., (1995). *Nature, 378*, 366–368.
23. Beck, J. S., & Vartuli, J. C., (1996). *Curr. Opin. Solid State Mater. Sci., 1*, 76.
24. Hinman, M. B., Jones, J. A., & Lewis, R. V., (2000). *Trends Biotechnol., 18*, 374.
25. Hayashi, C. Y., Shipley, N. H., & Lewis, R. V., (1999). *Int. J. Biol. Macromol., 24*, 271.
26. Gosline, J. M., Guerette, P. A., Ortlepp, C. S., & Savage, K. N., (1999). *J. Exp. Biol., 202*, 3294.
27. Hayashi, C. Y., & Lewis, R. V., (2000). *Science, 387*.
28. Thiel, B. L., Viney, C., & Jelinski, L. W., (1996). b-Sheets and spider silk. *Science, 273*, 1477–1480.
29. Simmons, A. H., Michal, C. A., & Jelinski, L. W., (1996). Molecular orientation and two-component nature of the crystalline fraction of spider dragline silk. *Science, 271*, 84–87.
30. Lazaris, A., Arcidiacono, S., Huang, Y., Zhou, J. F., Duguay, F., Chretien, N., Welsh, E. A., Soares, J. W., & Karatzas, C. N., (2002). Spider silk fibers spun from soluble recombinant silk produced in mammalian cells. *Science, 295*, 472–476.
31. Harrison, C. C., (1996). Evidence for intramineral macromolecules containing protein from plant silicas. *Phytochem., 41*, 37–41.
32. Mann, S., (2002). *Biomineralization: Principles and Concepts in Bioinorganic Materials Chemistry*. Oxford: Oxford University Press.
33. Schultze-Lam, S., Harauz, G., & Beveridge, T. J., (1992). Participation of a cyanobacterial S layer in fine-grain mineral formation. *J. Bacteriol., 174*, 7971–7981.
34. Schultze-Lam, S., Fortin, D., Davis, B. S., & Beveridge, T. J., (1996). Mineralization of bacterial surfaces. *Chem. Geol., 132*, 171–181.
35. Weiner, S., & Addadi, L., (1997). Design strategies in mineralized biological materials. *J. Mater. Chem., 7*, 689–702.
36. Weiner, S., Traub, W., & Wagner, H. D., (1999). Lamellar bone: Structure-function relations. *J. Struct. Biol., 126*, 241–255.
37. Weiner, S., & Wagner, H. D., (1998). The material bone: Structure mechanical function relations. *Annu. Rev. Mater. Sci., 28*, 271–298.
38. Douglas, K., Clark, N. A., & Rothschild, K. J., (1986). Nanometer molecular lithography. *Appl. Phys. Lett., 48*, 676–678.
39. Douglas, K., Clark, N.A., & Rothschild, K. J., (1990). Biomolecular/solid-state nanoheterostructures. *Appl. Phys. Lett., 56*, 692–694.
40. Coffer, J. L., Bigham, S. R., Li, X., Pinizzotto, R. F., Rho, Y. G., Pirtle, R. M., & Pirtle, I. L., (1996). Dictation of the shape of mesoscale semiconductor nanoparticle assemblies by plasmid DNA. *Appl. Phys. Lett., 69*, 3851–3853.
41. Mirkin, C. A., Letsinger, R. L., Mucic, R. C., & Storhoff, J. J., (1996). A DNA-based method for rationally assembling nanoparticles into macroscopic materials. *Nature, 382*, 607–609.

42. Alivisatos, A. P., Johnsson, K. P., Peng, X. G., Wilson, T. E., Loweth, C. J. Jr, Bruchez, M. P., & Schultz, P. G., (1996). Organization of 'nanocrystal molecules' using DNA. *Nature, 382*, 609–611.

43. Alivisatos, A. P., Schultz, P. G., Peng, X. G., Loweth, C. J., & Caldwell, W. B., (1999). DNA-based assembly of gold nanocrystals. *Angew. Chem., Int. Ed. Engl., 38*, 1808–1812.

44. Soto, C. M., Srinivasan, A., & Ratna, B. R., (2002). Controlled assembly of mesoscale structures using DNA as molecular bridges. *J. Am. Chem. Soc., 124*, 8508–8509.

45. Brown, S., (1992). Engineered iron oxide-adhesion mutants of the *Escherichia coli* phage lambda receptor. *Proc. Natl. Acad. Sci. U.S.A., 89,* 8651–8655.

46. Brown, S., (1997). Metal recognition by repeating polypeptides. *Nat. Biotechnol., 15*, 269–272.

47. Whaley, S. R., English, D. S., Hu, E. L., Barbara, P. F., & Belcher, A. M., (2000). Selection of peptides with semiconductor binding specificity for directed nanocrystal assembly. *Nature, 405*, 665–668.

48. Lee, S. W., Mao, C. B., Flynn, C. E., & Belcher, A. M., (2002). Ordering of quantum dots using genetically engineered viruses. *Science, 296*, 892–895.

49. Addadi, L., & Weiner, S., (1992). Control and design principles in biological mineralization. *Angew. Chem., Int. Ed. Engl., 31*, 153–169.

50. Weller, H., (1993). Colloidal semiconductor Q-particles: Chemistry in the transition region between solid state and molecules. *Angew. Chem., Int. Ed. Engl., 32*, 41–53.

51. Weller, H., (1993). Quantized semiconductor particles: A novel state of matter for materials science. *Adv. Mater., 5*, 88–95.

52. Weller, H., (1996). Optical properties of quantized semiconductor particles. *Philos. Trans. R. Soc. London, Ser. A, 354*, 757–766.

53. Murray, C. B., Norris, D. J., & Bawendi, M. G., (1993). *J. Am. Chem. Soc., 115*, 8706.

54. Dabbousi, B. O., Murray, C. B., Rubner, M. F., & Bawendi, M. G., (1994). Langmuir-Blodgett manipulation of size-selected cdse nanocrystallites. *Chem. Mater., 6*, 216–219.

55. Murray, C. B., Kagan, C. R., & Bawendi, M. G., (1995). Selforganization of CdSe nanocrystallites into three-dimensional quantum dot superlattices. *Science, 270*, 1335–1338.

56. Alivisatos, A. P., (1995). Semiconductor nanocrystals. *MRS Bull., 20*, 23–32.

57. Peng, X., Wilson, T. E., Alivisatos, A. P., & Schultz, P. G., (1997). Synthesis and isolation of a homodimer of cadmium selenide nanocrystals. *Angew. Chem., Int. Ed. Engl., 36*, 145–147.

58. Brus, L. E., (1994). Electron-electron and electron-hole interactions in small semiconductor crystallites: The size dependence of the lowest excited electronic state. *J. Chem. Phys., 80*, 4403–4409.

59. Siegel, R. W., (1996). Creating nanophase materials. *Sci. Am., 275*, 74–79.

60. Fendler, J. H., & Meldrum, F. C., (1995). The colloid chemical approach to nano-structured materials. *Adv. Mater., 7,* 607–632.

61. Geppert, L., (1996). Semiconductor lithography for the next millennium. *IEEE Spectrum, 33*, 33–38.

62. Levenson, M. D., (1995). *Solid State Technol.,* 81.

63. Chang, T. H. P., Thomson, M. G. R., Yu, M. L., Kratschmer, E., Kim, H. S., Lee, K. Y., Rishton, S. A., & Zolgharnain, S., (1996). *Microelectron. Eng., 32*, 113.

64. Matsui, S., & Ochiai, Y., (1996). *Nanotechnology, 7*, 247.

65. Smith, H. I., Schattenburg, M. L., Hector, S. D., Ferrera, J., Moon, E. E., Yang, I. Y., & Bukhardt, M., (1996). *Microelectron. Eng., 32*, 143.

66. Marrian, C. R. K., & Snow, E. S., (1996). *Microelectron. Eng., 32*, 173.

67. Zhao, X. M., Xia, Y., & Whitesides, G. M., (1997). *J. Mater. Chem., 7*, 1069.

68. Fendler, J. H., (1994). *Membrane-Mimetic Approach to Advanced Materials*. Berlin: Springer-Verlag.

69. Peng, X. G., Manna, L., Yang, W. D., Wickham, J., Scher, E., Kadavanich, A., & Alivisatos, A. P., (2000). Shape control of CdSe nanocrystals. *Nature, 404*, 59–61.

70. Manna, L., Scher, E. C., & Alivisatos, A. P., (2000). Synthesis of soluble and processable rod-, arrow-, teardrop-, and tetrapod-shaped CdSe nanocrystals. *J. Am. Chem. Soc., 122,* 12700–12706.

71. Berman, A., Addadi, L., & Weiner, S., (1988). *Nature, 331*, 546–548.

72. Berman, A., Addadi, L., Kvick, A., Leiserowitz, L., Nelson, M., & Weiner, S., (1990). *Science, 250*, 664–667.

73. Berman, A., Hanson, J., Leiserowitz, L., Koetzle, T. F., Weiner, S., & Addadi, L., (1993). *Science, 59*, 776–779.

74. Messersmith, P. B., & Stupp, S. I., (1995). High-temperature chemical and microstructural transformations of a nanocomposite organoceramic. *Chem. Mater., 7*, 454–460.

75. Mitzi, D. B., Feild, C. A., Harrison, W. T. A., & Guloy, A. M., (1994). Conducting tin halides with a layered organic-based perovskite structure. *Nature, 369*, 467–469.

76. Mitzi, D. B., Wang, S., Feild, C. A., Chess, C. A., & Guloy, A. M., (1995). Conducting layered organic-inorganic halides containing <110>- oriented perovskite sheets. *Science, 267*, 1473–1476.

77. Feng, X., Fryxell, G. E., Wang, Q. L., Kim, A. Y., Liu, J., & Kemner, K. M., (1997). Functionalized monolayers on ordered mesoporous supports. *Science, 276*, 923–926.

78. Weiss, D., Roukes, M. L., Mensching, A., Grambow, P., Klitzing, K., & Weimann, G., (1991). Electron pinball and commensurate orbits in a periodic array of scatters. *Phys. Rev. Lett., 66*, 2790–2793.

79. Hansen, W., Kotthaus, J. P., & Merkt, U., (1992). In: Hansen, W., Kotthaus, J. P., & Merkt, U., (eds.), *Electrons in Laterally Periodic Nanostructures* (Vol. 35, pp. 279–380). San Diego: Academic Press.

80. Schechter, R. S., & Bourrel, M., (1988). *Microemulsions and Related Systems: Formation, Solvency, and Physical Properties*. New York: Marcel Dekker.

81. Tanford, C., (1974). *J. Phys. Chem., 78*, 2469.

82. Rosoff, M., (1996). *Vesicles*. New York: Marcel Dekker.

83. Ringsdorf, H., Schlarb, B., & Venzmer, J., (1988). *Angew. Chem., Int. Ed. Engl., 27*, 114–158.

84. Laughlin, R. G., (1994). *The Aqueous Phase Behavior of Surfactants*. San Diego: Academic Press.

85. Degiorgio, V., & Corti, M., (1985). *Physics of Amphiphiles: Micelles, Vesicles and Microemulsions*. Amsterdam: Elsevier Science Pub. Co.

86. Israelachvili, J., (1985). Thermodynamic and geometrical aspects of amphiphile aggregation into micelles, vesicles, and bilayers, and the interactions between them.

In: Degiorgio, V., & Corti, M., (eds.), *Physics of Amphiphiles: Micelles, Vesicles and Microemulsions* (p. 24).

87. Bates, F. S., (1991). Polymer-polymer phase behavior. *Science, 251*, 898–905.

88. Wennerstrom, H., (1979). *J. Colloid Interface Sci., 68*, 589–590.

89. Tiddy, G., (1980). *Phys. Rep., 57*, 1.

90. Fribreg, S. E., & Wang, J., (1991). *J. Dispersion Sci. Technol., 12*, 387–402.

91. Walsh, D., Hopwood, J. D., & Mann, S., (1994). Crystal tectonics: Construction of reticulated calcium phosphate frameworks in bicontinuous reverse microemulsions. *Science, 264*, 1576–1578.

92. Yang, J. P., Qadri, S. B., & Ratna, B. R., (1996). Structural and morphological characterization of pbs nanocrystallites synthesized in the bicontinuous cubic phase of a lipid. *J. Phys. Chem., 100*, 17255–17259.

93. Braun, P. V., Osenar, P., & Stupp, S. I., (1996). Semiconducting superlattices templated by molecular assemblies. *Nature, 380*, 325–328.

94. Osenar, P., Braun, P. V., & Stupp, S. I., (1996). *Adv. Mater., 8*, 1022.

95. Tohver, V., Braun, P. V., Pralle, M. U., & Stupp, S. I., (1997). Counter ion effects in liquid crystal templating of nanostructured CdS. *Chem. Mater., 9*, 1495–1499.

96. Braun, P. V., Osenar, P., Tohver, V., Kennedy, S. B., & Stupp, S. I., (1999). Nanostructure templating in inorganic solids with organic lyotropic liquid crystals. *J. Am. Chem. Soc., 121*, 7302–7309.

97. Attard, G. S., Bartlett, P. N., Coleman, N. R. B., Elliott, J. M., Owen, J. R., & Wang, J. H., (1997). Mesoporous platinum films from lyotropic liquid crystalline phases. *Science, 278*, 838–840.

98. Attard, G. S., Edgar, M., & Goltner, C. G., (1998). Inorganic nanostructures from lyotropic liquid crystal phases. *Acta Materialia, 46*, 751–758.

99. Elliott, J. M., Birkin, P. R., Bartlett, P. N., & Attard, G. S., (1999). Platinum microelectrodes with unique high surface areas. *Langmuir, 15*, 7411–7415.

100. Attard, G. S., Leclerc, S. A. A., Maniguet, S., Russell, A. E., Nandhakumar, I., & Bartlett, P. N., (2001). Mesoporous Pt/Ru alloy from the hexagonal lyotropic liquid crystalline phase of a nonionic surfactant. *Chem. Mater., 13*, 1444.

101. Attard, G. S., Leclerc, S. A. A., Maniguet, S., Russell, A. E., Nandhakumar, I., Gollas, B. R., & Bartlett, P. N., (2001). Liquid crystal phase template mesoporous platinum alloy. *Microporous Mesoporous Mater., 44*, 159–163.

102. Nelson, P. A., Elliott, J. M., Attard, G. S., & Owen, J. R., (2002). Mesoporous nickel/nickel oxide: A nanoarchitectured electrode. *Chem. Mater., 14*, 524–529.

103. Nandhakumar, I., Elliott, J. M., & Attard, G. S., (2001). Electrodeposition of nano-structured mesoporous selenium films (H-I-eSe). *Chem. Mater., 13*, 3840.

104. Gabriel, T., Nandhakumar, I. S., & Attard, G. S., (2002). Electrochemical synthesis of nanostructured tellurium films. *Electrochem. Commun., 4*, 610–612.

105. Schick, M. J., (1987). *Nonionic Surfactants, Physical Chemistry*. New York: Marcel Dekker.

106. Wanka, G., Hoffmann, H., & Ulbricht, W., (1994). Phase diagrams and aggregation behavior of poly(oxyethylene)-poly(oxypropylene)-poly(oxyethylene) triblock copolymers in aqueous solutions. *Macromolecules, 27*, 4145–4159.

107. Fontell, K., (1990). Cubic phases in surfactant and surfactant-like lipid systems. *Colloid Polym. Sci., 268*, 264–285.

108. Lo, I., Florence, A. T., Treguier, J. P., Seiller, M., & Puisieux, F., (1977). The influence of surfactant HLB and the nature of the oil phase on the phase diagrams of nonionic surfactant-oil water systems. *J. Colloid Interface Sci., 59*, 319–327.

109. Treguier, J. P., Seiller, M., Puisieux, F., Orecchioni, A. M., & Florence, A. T., (1977). Effect of a hydrophilic surfactant and temperature on water-surfactant-oil diagrams. *In First Expo. Cong. Int. Technol. Pharm.: Assoc. Pharm.*, 75–87.

110. Braun, P. V., & Stupp, S. I., (1999). CdS mineralization of hexagonal, lamellar, and cubic lyotropic liquid crystals. *Mater. Res. Bull., 34*, 463–469.

111. Blackburn, J. C., & Kilpatrick, P. K., (1992). Using deuterium NMR line shapes to analyze lyotropic liquid crystalline phase transitions. *Langmuir, 8*, 1679–1687.

112. Schnepp, W., Disch, S., & Schmidt, C., (1993). 2H NMR study on the lyomesophases of the system hexaethylene glycol dodecyl methyl ether/water: Temperature dependence of quadrupole splitting. *Liq. Cryst., 14*, 843–852.

113. Attard, G. S., Goltner, C. G., Corker, J. M., Henke, S., & Templer, R. H., (1997). Liquid-crystal templates for nanostructured metals. *Angew. Chem., Int. Ed. Engl., 36*, 1315–1317.

114. Park, M., Harrison, C., Chaikin, P. M., Register, R. A., & Adamson, D. H., (1997). Block copolymer lithography: Periodic arrays of_1011 holes in one square centimeter. *Science, 276*, 1401–1404.

115. Park, M., Chaikin, P. M., Register, R. A., & Adamson, D. H., (2001). Large area dense nanoscale patterning of arbitrary surfaces. *Appl. Phys. Lett., 79*, 257–259.

116. Li, R. R., Dapkus, P. D., Thompson, M. E., Jeong, W. G., Harrison, C., Chaikin, P. M., Register, R. A., & Adamson, D. H., (2000). Dense arrays of ordered GaAs nanostructures by selective area growth on substrates patterned by block copolymer lithography. *Appl. Phys. Lett., 76*, 1689–1691.

117. Thurn-Albrecht, T., Schotter, J., Kastle, C. A., Emley, N., Shibauchi, T., Krusin-Elbaum, L., Guarini, K., Black, C. T., Tuominen, M. T., & Russell, T. P., (2000). Ultrahigh-density nanowire arrays grown in self-assembled diblock copolymer templates. *Science, 290*, 2126–2129.

118. Kim, H. C., Jia, X. Q., Stafford, C. M., Kim, D. H., McCarthy, T. J., Tuominen, M., Hawker, C. J., & Russell, T. P., (2001). A route to nanoscopic SiO2 posts via block copolymer templates. *Adv. Mater., 13*, 795.

119. Lin, Z. Q., Kim, D. H., Wu, X. D., Boosahda, L., Stone, D., LaRose, L., & Russell, T. P., (2002). A rapid route to arrays of nanostructures in thin films. *Adv. Mater., 14*, 1373–1376.

120. Bal, M., Ursache, A., Touminen, M. T., Goldbach, J. T., & Russell, T. P., (2002). Nanofabrication of integrated magnetoelectronic devices using patterned self-assembled copolymer templates. *Appl. Phys. Lett., 81*, 3479–3481.

121. Shin, K., Leach, K. A., Goldbach, J. T., Kim, D. H., Jho, J. Y., Tuominen, M., Hawker, C. J., & Russell, T. P., (2002). A simple route to metal nanodots and nanoporous metal films. *Nano Lett., 2*, 933–936.

122. Joannopoulos, J. D., Meade, R. D., & Winn, J. N., (1995). *Photonic Crystals: Molding the Flow of Light*. Princeton: Princeton University Press.

123. Busch, K., & John, S., (1998). Photonic band gap formation in certain self-organizing systems. *Phys. Rev. E, 58*, 3896–3908.

124. Velev, O. D., & Kaler, E. W., (2000). Structured porous materials via colloidal crystal templating: From inorganic oxides to metals. *Adv. Mater., 12*, 531–534.
125. Velev, O. D., Jede, T. A., Lobo, R. F., & Lenhoff, A. M., (1997). Porous silica via colloidal crystallization. *Nature, 389*, 447–448.
126. Holland, B. T., Blanford, C. F., & Stein, A., (1998). Synthesis of macroporous minerals with highly ordered three-dimensional arrays of spherical voids. *Science, 281*, 538–540.
127. Wijnhoven, J. E. G. J., & Vos, W. L., (1998). Preparation of photonic crystals made of air spheres in titania. *Science, 281*, 802–804.
128. Zakhidov, A. A., Baughman, R. H., Iqbal, Z., Cui, C. X., Khayrullin, I., Dantas, S. O., Marti, I., & Ralchenko, V. G., (1998). Carbon structures with three-dimensional periodicity at optical wavelengths. *Science, 282*, 897–901.
129. Míguez, H., Blanco, A., Meseguer, F., López, C., Yates, H. M., Pemble, M. E., Fornés, V., & Mifsud, A., (1999). Brag diffraction from indium phosphide infilled fcc silica colloidal crystals. *Phys. Rev. B, 59*, 1563–1566.
130. Blanco, A., Chomski, E., Grabtchak, S., Ibisate, M., John, S., Leonard, S. W., Lopez, C., Meseguer, F., Miguez, H., Mondia, J. P., et al., (2000). Largescale synthesis of a silicon photonic crystal with a complete three-dimensional bandgap near 1.5 micrometers. *Nature, 405*, 437–440.
131. Vlasov, Y. A., Bo, X. Z., Sturm, J. C., & Norris, D. J., (2001). On-chip natural assembly of silicon photonic bandgap crystals. *Nature, 414*, 289–293.
132. Vlasov, Y. A., Yao, N., & Norris, D. J., (1999). Synthesis of photonic crystals for optical wavelengths from semiconductor quantum dots. *Adv. Mater., 11*, 165–169.
133. Subramania, G., Constant, K., Biswas, R., Sigalas, M. M., & Ho, K. M., (1999). Optical photonic crystals fabricated from colloidal systems. *Appl. Phys. Lett, 74*, 3933–3935.
134. Subramanian, G., Manoharan, V. N., Thorne, J. D., & Pine, D. J., (1999). Ordered macroporous materials by colloidal assembly: A possible route to photonic bandgap materials. *Adv. Mater., 11*, 1261–1265.
135. Míguez, H., Meseguer, F., Lopez, C., Holgado, M., Andreasen, G., Mifsud, A., & Fornes, V., (2000). Germanium FCC structure from a colloidal crystal template. *Langmuir, 16*, 4405–4408.
136. Jiang, P., Cizeron, J., Bertone, J. F., & Colvin, V. L., (1999). Preparation of macroporous metal films from colloidal crystals. *J. Am. Chem. Soc., 121*, 7957–7958.
137. Braun, P. V., & Wiltzius, P., (1999). Electrochemically grown photonic crystals. *Nature, 402*, 603–604.
138. Braun, P. V., Zehner, R. W., White, C. A., Weldon, M. K., Kloc, C., Patel, S. S., & Wiltzius, P., (2001). Epitaxial growth of high dielectric contrast three dimensional photonic crystals. *Adv. Mater., 13*, 721–724.
139. Johnson, S. A., Ollivier, P. J., & Mallouk, T. E., (1999). Ordered mesoporous polymers of tunable pore size from colloidal silica templates. *Science, 283*, 963–965.
140. Jeon, S., & Braun, P. V., (2003). Hydrothermal synthesis of Er-doped luminescent TiO2 nanoparticles. *Chem. Mater., 15*, 1256–1263.
141. Braun, P. V., & Wiltzius, P., (2001). Electrochemical fabrication of 3-D microperiodic porous materials. *Adv. Mater., 13*, 482–485.
142. Sumida, T., Wada, Y., Kitamura, T., & Yanagida, S., (2001). Macroporous ZnO films electrochemically prepared by templating of opal films. *Chem. Lett., 1*, 38–39.

143. Pandey, R. K., Sahu, S. N., & Chandra, S., (1996). *Handbook of Semiconductor Electrodeposition*. New York: Marcel Dekker.

144. Gurunathan, K., Vadivel, M. A., Marimuthu, R., Mulik, U. P., & Amalnerkar, D. P., (1999). Electrochemically synthesized conducting polymeric materials for applications towards technology in electronics, optoelectronics and energy storage devices. *Mater. Chem. Phys., 61*, 173–191.

145. Martin, C. R., (1994). Nanomaterials: A membrane based synthetic approach. *Science, 266*, 1961–1966.

146. Koopal, C. G. J., Feiters, M. C., Nolte, R. J. M., Deruiter, B., & Schasfoort, R. B. M., (1992). Third generation amperometric biosensor for glucose-polypyrrole deposited within a matrix of uniform latex particles as mediator. *Bioelectrochem. Bioenerg., 29*, 159–175.

147. Sumida, T., Wada, Y., Kitamura, T., & Yanagida, S., (2000). Electrochemical preparation of macroporous polypyrrole films with regular arrays of interconnected spherical voids. *Chem. Commun.,* 1613–1614.

148. Bartlett, P. N., Birkin, P. R., Ghanem, M. A., & Toh, C. S., (2001). Electrochemical syntheses of highly ordered macroporous conducting polymers grown around self-assembled colloidal templates., *J. Mater. Chem., 11*, 849–853.

149. Cassagneau, T., & Caruso, F., (2002). Semiconducting polymer inverse opals prepared by electropolymerization. *Adv. Mater., 14*, 34–38.

150. Ebbesen, T. W., Lezec, H. J., Ghaemi, H. F., Thio, T., & Wolff, P. A., (1999). Extraordinary optical transmission through sub-wavelength hole arrays. *Nature, 391*, 667–669.

151. Moroz, A., (1999). Three-dimensional complete photonic-band-gap structures in the visible. *Phys. Rev. Lett., 83*, 5274–5277.

152. Moroz, A., (2000). Photonic crystals of coated metallic spheres. *Europhys. Lett., 50*, 466–472.

153. Zhang, W. Y., Lei, X. Y., Wang, Z. L., Zheng, D. G., Tam, W. Y., Chan, C. T., & Sheng, P., (2000). Robust photonic band gap from tunable scatterers. *Phys. Rev. Lett., 84*, 2853–2856.

154. Oldenburg, S. J., Averitt, R. D., Westcott, S. L., & Halas, N. J., (1998). Nanoengineering of optical resonances. *Chem. Phys. Lett., 288*, 243–247.

155. Graf, C., & Van Blaaderen, A., (2002). Metallodielectric colloidal core-shell particles for photonic applications. *Langmuir, 18*, 524–534.

156. Wijnhoven, J., Zevenhuizen, S. J. M., Hendriks, M. A., Vanmaekelbergh, D., Kelly, J. J., & Vos, W. L., (2000). Electrochemical assembly of ordered macropores in gold. *Adv. Mater., 12*, 888–890.

157. Xu, L., Zhou, W. L., Frommen, C., Baughman, R. H., Zakhidov, A. A., Malkinski, L., Wang, J. Q., & Wiley, J. B., (2000). Electrodeposited nickel and gold nanoscale meshes with potentially interesting photonic properties. *Chem. Commun.,* 997–998.

158. Luo, Q., Liu, Z., Li, L., Xie, S., Kong, J., & Zhao, D., (2001). Creating highly ordered metal, alloy, and semiconductor macrostructures by electrodeposition, ion spraying, and laser spraying. *Adv. Mater., 13*, 286–289.

159. Bartlett, P. N., Birkin, P. R., & Ghanem, M. A., (2000). Electrochemical deposition of macroporous platinum, palladium and cobalt films using polystyrene latex sphere templates. *Chem. Commun.,* 1671–1672.

160. Kokorina, V. F., (1996). *Glasses for Infrared Optics*. Boca Raton, FL: CRC Press.

161. Dunin-Borkowski, R. E., McCartney, M. R., Frankel, R. B., Bazylinski, D. A., Posfai, M., & Buseck, P. R., (1998). Magnetic microstructure of magnetotactic bacteria by electron holography. *Science, 282*, 1868–1870.

162. Zaremba, C. M., Morse, D. E., Mann, S., Hansma, P. K., & Stucky, G. D., (1998). Aragonite-hydroxyapatite conversion in gastropod (abalone) nacre. *Chem. Mater., 10*, 3813–3824.

163. Ziv, V., Sabanay, I., Arad, T., Traub, W., & Weiner, S., (1996). Transitional structures in lamellar bone. *Microsc. Res. Technique, 33*, 203–213.

164. Wong, K. K. W., Douglas, T., Gider, S., Awschalom, D. D., & Mann, S., (1998). Biomimetic synthesis and characterization of magnetic proteins (magnetoferritin). *Chem. Mater., 10*, 279–285.

165. Yang, J., Meldrum, F. C., & Fendler, J. H., (1995). Epitaxial growth of size-quantized cadmium sulfide crystals under arachidic acid monolayers. *J. Phys. Chem., 99*, 5500–5504.

166. Rosevear, F. B., (1968). Liquid crystals: The mesomorphic phases of surfactant compositions. *J. Soc. Cosmetic Chemists, 19*, 581–594.

INDEX

A